Addiction and Self-Control

Perspectives from Philosophy, Psychology, and Neuroscience

EDITED BY NEIL LEVY

OXFORD
UNIVERSITY PRESS

OXFORD
UNIVERSITY PRESS

Oxford University Press is a department of the University of Oxford.
It furthers the University's objective of excellence in research, scholarship,
and education by publishing worldwide.

Oxford   New York
Auckland   Cape Town   Dar es Salaam   Hong Kong   Karachi
Kuala Lumpur   Madrid   Melbourne   Mexico City   Nairobi
New Delhi   Shanghai   Taipei   Toronto

With offices in
Argentina   Austria   Brazil   Chile   Czech Republic   France   Greece
Guatemala   Hungary   Italy   Japan   Poland   Portugal   Singapore
South Korea   Switzerland   Thailand   Turkey   Ukraine   Vietnam

Oxford is a registered trademark of Oxford University Press
in the UK and certain other countries.

Published in the United States of America by
Oxford University Press
198 Madison Avenue, New York, NY 10016

Library of Congress Cataloging-in-Publication Data
Addiction and self-control : perspectives from philosophy, psychology, and neuroscience / edited by
Neil Levy.
   pages cm. — (Oxford series in neuroscience, law, and philosophy)
ISBN 978–0–19–986258–0 (alk. paper) — ISBN 978–0–19–931468–3 (updf)   1. Substance abuse—
Treatment.   2. Addicts.   3. Self-control.   I. Levy, Neil, 1967– editor of compilation.
RC564.A558 2013
362.29—dc23
2012049466

9 8 7 6 5 4 3 2 1
Printed in the United States of America
on acid-free paper

CONTENTS

CONTRIBUTORS

George Ainslie studies impulsiveness and self-control as intertemporal conflict within individuals (picoeconomics). He is the author of *Picoeconomics: The Strategic Interaction of Successive Motivational States within the Person* and *Breakdown of Will*, and he has published widely in psychological, economic, philosophical, and legal literature. He is a research psychiatrist at the Department of Veterans Affairs Medical Center, Coatesville, PA, and professor in the School of Economics, University of Cape Town, South Africa.

Nomy Arpaly is an Associate Professor of Philosophy at Brown University. She is the author of *Unprincipled Virtue, Merit, Meaning and Human Bondage* and various articles.

Kent Berridge is the James Olds Collegiate Professor of Psychology and Neuroscience at the University of Michigan (Ann Arbor, USA).

Owen Flanagan is James B. Duke Professor of Philosophy and Professor of Psychology and Neuroscience at Duke University, Durham, NC. He is the author of *Varieties of Moral Personality: Ethics and Psychological Realism* and *Consciousness Reconsidered* and other books.

Natalie Gold is a Senior Research Fellow at King's College London, where she leads the European Research Council–funded project "Self-Control and the Person: An Inter-Disciplinary Account."

Richard Holton is Professor of Philosophy at MIT. He currently works mainly in action theory and moral psychology, and is the author of *Willing, Wanting, Waiting*.

Jeanette Kennett is Professor of Moral Psychology in the Department of Philosophy at Macquarie University, Sydney, Australia. She is lead investigator on an Australian Research Council–funded project on Addiction and Moral

Identity, which has supported work on her contribution to this volume. She has published widely on moral agency and its impairments.

Neil Levy is an Australian Research Council Future Fellow at the Florey Institute of Neuroscience and Mental Health, Australia. He has published widely on the topics of free will and moral responsibility, addiction, philosophical psychology, applied ethics, and many other topics.

Nicholas A. Nasrallah completed his J.D. at Yale Law School and his doctorate in psychology at the University of Washington. His research generally focuses on the intersection between law and decision theory.

Steve Pearce is a consultant psychiatrist in Oxford, UK, where he runs the Complex Needs Service, a specialist NHS service for people with personality disorders and related conditions. He is the editor of the *International Journal of Therapeutic Communities* and president of the British and Irish Group for the Study of Personality Disorder.

Hanna Pickard is a therapist at the Complex Needs Service, a specialist NHS service for people with personality disorders and related conditions, and a philosopher of mind and psychiatry. She holds a Wellcome Trust Biomedical Ethics Clinical Research Fellowship at the Oxford Centre for Neuroethics and is a Fellow of All Souls College. Her research explores philosophical issues that arise out of clinical practice and related science. Current projects include the nature of responsibility and blame within the clinic and its potential use within the criminal justice system and prisons, addiction, self-harm, violence, emotions, and psychosis.

Don Ross is Professor of Economics and Dean of Commerce at the University of Cape Town, and Program Director, Methodology, at the Center for Economic Analysis of Risk at Georgia State University. His main current areas of research are in economic methodology, the experimental estimation of utility function distributions in heterogeneous populations, the picoeconomics and neuroeconomics of impulsive choice, game-theoretic models of human sociality, and the unification of the sciences by reference to the statistical and stochastic character of reality at all scales of modeling. He is the author or editor of 12 books and numerous articles.

Timothy Schroeder is an Associate Professor of Philosophy at Ohio State University. His *Three Faces of Desire* (Oxford University Press, 2004) presents a theory of desire that lies at the intersection of moral psychology and the philosophy of mind; he has also written on norms, concepts, consciousness, and deliberation.

Walter Sinnott-Armstrong is Chauncey Stillman Professor of Practical Ethics in the Philosophy Department and the Kenan Institute for Ethics at Duke University. He publishes widely in normative moral theory, meta-ethics, applied ethics, moral psychology and neuroscience, philosophy of law, epistemology, informal logic, and philosophy of religion.

Mark E. Walton is a Wellcome Trust Research Fellow and University Research Lecturer at the University of Oxford. His laboratory focuses on how different aspects of value are learned and represented by particular brain circuits and how these are used to guide decision making.

Gideon Yaffe is Professor of Law and Professor of Philosophy at Yale Law School. He has published books and articles about agency and criminal responsibility, including *Attempts* (Oxford University Press, 2010) and "Lowering the Bar for Addicts" (in *Addiction and Responsibility*, Poland and Graham, eds., 2011).

1

Addiction and Self-Control

Perspectives from Philosophy, Psychology, and Neuroscience

NEIL LEVY

One of the defining features of addiction is an impairment of self-control: addicts are people who (to all appearance) find it especially difficult to bring their behavior into line with their best judgments. Addicts often *report* a loss of control, and theorists have often used the language of loss of control to describe addiction. Indeed, loss of control over behavior has often been seen as definitive of addiction; the *Diagnostic and Statistical Manual of Mental Disorders*, fourth edition (DSM-IV) makes unsuccessful efforts to control substance use and use for longer periods than intended two of the seven criteria for a diagnosis of substance dependence (any three of the seven must be present for a positive diagnosis).

Addiction, especially addiction to nicotine and alcohol, is a serious public health problem, leading to an enormous number of early deaths. But loss of control manifests itself and causes harms in many arenas other than substance addictions. Process addictions like pathological gambling also produce great harms. Loss of control is also an enormous and growing problem in spheres beyond addiction: consider the inexorable increase in obesity, which is now a major contributor to the global burden of disease. Obesity typically (though not always) arises from thousands of quotidian and banal losses of control. An agent eats slightly more, or slightly more often, than he or she intends on thousands of occasions; from these small incidents may arise severe health problems, including heart disease, cancer, and diabetes. Losses of control also manifest themselves in impulsive spending, failures to save for retirement, and dozens of other behaviors that cause social and individual problems.

Despite the ubiquity of losses of control, the phenomenon remains ill-understood. How does it come about—*does* it come about—that rational agents act contrary to their own best judgments? How, and why, would an agent who judges she ought to refrain from consuming (cake, sex, drugs) and who retains voluntary control over her bodily movements nevertheless consume the object of her desire? It has frequently been supposed that addictive behavior is *compelled*: the addict is caused, perhaps by the strength of her cravings, to consume her drug of choice regardless of what she judges. But there is strong evidence to reject the compulsion thesis, at least insofar as compulsion is taken literally. First, addicts often do refrain from consuming their drug, for longer or shorter periods, and they do so in response to normal kinds of incentives. Second, consuming a drug requires an elaborate series of actions to procure the drug; it is implausible to think that this whole series of actions is compelled.

The failure of the compulsion thesis has motivated some thinkers to argue that addictive behavior does not involve an impairment of self-control at all. Gene Heyman, most recently and forcefully, has argued that addiction is a disorder of choice: addicts choose to consume their drugs utilizing the same mechanisms of assessment and volition as nonaddicts use to choose other rewarding goods (Heyman 2009). Heyman's argument is powerful, but he pays little attention to a wealth of evidence emerging (especially) from cognitive neuroscience about the ways in which the mechanisms involved in addiction seem to be different from those engaged in ordinary choice. Moreover, Heyman's view leaves it somewhat mysterious why addiction is a chronic relapsing disease: his perspective seems to predict that once the incentives to remain drug free are in place, addicts should have less trouble abstaining than they actually do.

This volume is motivated by the belief that understanding addiction, and loss of self-control more generally, requires a scientifically informed and philosophically sophisticated perspective on human agency. Human psychology is sometimes stranger than we might imagine from the armchair: the scientific perspective may reveal insights that are at odds with our folk psychological preconceptions, but which illuminate our behavior. Philosophy can help us to better understand these scientific insights and to integrate them with our experiences and self-conception as agents. In other words, understanding addiction requires the synthesis or coordination of work on the subpersonal mechanisms involved in behavior with the personal level at which we understand ourselves. Progress on these difficult issues will come, therefore, from the interchange between researchers in diverse fields—neuroscientists, psychologists, and philosophers—who are prepared to listen respectfully and learn from one another.

The Oxford Centre for Neuroethics assembled just a group of researchers in Oxford in May 2010. Our conference, *Addiction and Self-Control*, explored the loss of self-control apparently seen in addiction from a variety of perspectives.

Participants included leading neuroscientists, psychologists, and philosophers. Following this very successful event, most of the participants agreed to contribute papers to a volume that would expand on and develop the themes explored in the conference. The papers collected here are very different from the papers presented in Oxford (for one thing, several of the contributors to the volume couldn't make it to Oxford). Rather, they build on the papers presented and the interchange that followed. We believe that this unique interdisciplinary forum represents the cutting edge of work on addiction and on pathologies of human agency.

THE PAPERS

George Ainslie's work on hyperbolic discounting is an indispensable reference point in the landscape of the literature concerning loss of self-control (Ainslie 2001). Human beings—and other animals—prefer immediate rewards to delayed rewards: we discount rewards for delay. Ainslie demonstrated that our discount function is hyperbolic: that is, the discount function is itself sensitive to delay. As a consequence, our discount curves can cross: though when competing rewards (health and junk food; fidelity and sex; and so on) are distant, we might prefer the first to the second, as the opportunities for the second become imminent, our delay curves become steeper and our preferences might reverse. Hyperbolic discounting predicts that we will have a very hard time exercising self-control. Of course, though we do have a hard time exercising self-control, we do often succeed in resisting temptations (or else we would never be able to save for retirement, or write books). Part of the explanation for our (limited) success at self-control is due to our ability to manipulate the available rewards, by self-binding or by bundling rewards with punishments (for instance, by putting our money in a long-term savings account with heavy penalties for early withdrawal). But we sometimes seem to exercise self-control by exerting *willpower*. How do we do it?

Ainslie suggests that bundling our choices is a big part of the answer. If we choose bundles of rewards at once—a whole series of smaller/sooner versus larger/later rewards at the same time—we are more likely to choose the larger/later rewards. Of course, we do not often actually choose series of rewards at the same time, but Ainslie argues that we can simulate this kind of bundled choice by seeing our choices as test cases. When I choose between a smaller/sooner and a larger/later reward, I can and should see my choice as predicting how I will behave on later occasions. If I choose the smaller/sooner reward now, I cannot trust myself on future occasions to choose the larger/later reward; conversely, if I make a commitment now to the larger/later reward, I provide evidence that I can be trusted on future occasions. Ainslie suggests we model these choices as a prisoner's dilemma in which successive selves face the option of defecting or cooperating with one another. Seeing one's choice as predictive of future choices is seeing it as iterated; and of course cooperation is the dominant strategy in an iterated prisoner's dilemma.

Not content with the significant contributions he has already made to our thinking, Ainslie continues to innovate. His paper in this volume is an exciting extension of his work on hyperbolic discounting to the process addictions (if "addictions" they be). His exemplar is problem gambling. As he points out, problem gambling is on the surface paradoxical. Gamblers ostensibly pursue a reward in the form of money, yet they choose a means that—as they know— has an expected payoff lower than zero. If gamblers pursue money, they have chosen a spectacularly inefficient means of pursuing it. Problem gambling therefore seems to require some kind of explanation. One explanation cites neuroadaptations: problem gamblers do not exercise normal control over their behavior because they are addicted. Ainslie pursues a very different, and very provocative, approach (while recognizing that the neuroadaptation approach may explain some gambling, or play some role together with other explanations in most problem gambling). He suggests that for gamblers, money is what Alfred Hitchcock called a MacGuffin: it is the ostensible target of pursuit, but its real role is to structure the pursuit.

The key to understanding problem gambling, Ainslie suggests, is to recognize that we habituate to reward. This is most especially a problem for people in the overdeveloped world, in which so many of our basic rewards are freely available. Reward for these abundant goods is dependent on our appetites, but their easy availability leads to the diminishing of appetite. We may therefore do better, hedonically, by limiting our access to goods, even when these goods do not compete with larger/later rewards. Thus, for instance, we may impose a rule on ourselves of not eating until dinner time, so as to enjoy the feeling of satisfying hunger, rather than simply consuming an equivalent amount of calories throughout the day. Gambling—and not just problem gambling—is rewarding because it makes the payoff uncertain. The player may derive a greater hedonic value from winning n than from retaining it, because she has ceded control over the money to external forces. The potential loss stimulates her appetite for the money and reverses the effects of habituation (perhaps she needs actual loss to stimulate appetite; thus, she may derive hedonic reward from winning n even when her expenditure in pursuit of money is $> \$n$).

Refreshing appetites requires that we arrange obstacles to our satisfaction. However, we cannot do this too self-consciously: the game is worth the candle when we see the obstacles as necessary. We must engage in a kind of self-deception when we deliberately place obstacles in the way of our own satisfactions. We become skilled at misdirection, in the service of an inefficient pursuit of reward. Gambling is ripe for exploitation as misdirection, because we can easily see it as instrumental: we gamble (we tell ourselves) because of the chance of a big payday. But the real rewards come from the unexpected payoffs, even if the payoffs are smaller than the expenditure.

Ainslie notes that the cognitive distortions that seem characteristic of problem gamblers—the so-called gambler's fallacy, for instance—persist even in the face of correction. He suggests that we ought to see their retention as the product of misdirection: the gambler refuses to steadfastly examine her own beliefs, because they serve a function for her. To some extent, he suggests, we ought to see problem gamblers as *successfully* pursuing a larger/later reward, but the reward is directly hedonic, not monetary.

Ainslie actually proposes two somewhat independent explanations of process addictions. Whereas one turns on refreshing appetites for real rewards, the other turns on the structuring of endogenous rewards: rewards (like those of imagination) that are under our control. Since endogenous rewards are available *ad lib*, we need to find convincing strategies for delaying them, or else habituation soon undermines their value. Misdirection may indeed play a role in the explanation of endogenous reward. It is worth noting that Ainslie's larger project of explaining self-control and its loss requires an explanation of endogenous rewards, since self-control requires that agents forgo material satisfactions in favor of delayed rewards that are enjoyed by later person-stages. If misdirection is required to explain endogenous reward, a disconcerting consequence seems to follow: that self-control—which many philosophers have seen as an exemplar of rational behavior—depends on some degree of cognitive opacity or self-deception. Perhaps, however, misdirection is not required to explain *all* endogenous reward. Pascal Boyer (2008) has suggested that mental time travel may have evolved to allow earlier person-stages to vicariously enjoy delayed rewards, by delivering a simulacrum of these rewards to the earlier person-stage. Whether a view like Boyer's, turning on the present delivery of future reward via imaginative identification, can be developed into a rival explanation of gambling remains to be explored.

Don Ross's paper is a response to Ainslie's. He suggests that the perspective Ainslie offers, while powerful, fails to distinguish between genuine addicts and other people who suffer problems with loss of control. The intraperson bargaining mechanisms may become ineffective in each of us were we to accumulate evidence that we can't be trusted to exercise self-control. Nothing more than a self-fulfilling prophecy is needed to explain ordinary loss of control. This mechanism may, Ross concedes, be at work in addicts, too. But genuine addicts differ from those of us who (merely) suffer deficits with regard to self-control in ways that Ainslie does not acknowledge, and which his picoeconomic apparatus is blind to. First, properties of gambling—in particular, its unpredictable payoff structure—explain why it is more likely to result in extensive self-control problems than other activities, but these properties do their explanatory work only in conjunction with facts about the neural reward system (in particular, the way that dopamine spikes signaling reward respond to unexpected reward, rather than just to reward *simpliciter*; other properties of classic drugs of abuse explain how they directly hijack dopaminergic systems). Thus, ignoring neurochemistry leaves us unable to explain why certain activities are more likely to lead to self-control problems than others. Second, by explaining the nature of loss of control, in terms of the production of cravings and intrusive thoughts, on the one hand, and the weakening of synaptic inhibitory mechanisms, on the other, neuroscience explains why the loss of control caused by pathological gambling, alcohol, and addictive drugs is likely to be far more difficult to overcome than the loss of control caused by regular consumption of, say, food.

Ross does not claim that the neuroadaptations characteristic of addiction directly cause the loss of control. Rather, he understands control as top-down modulation of automatic processes, and the neuroadaptations as both causing more powerful priming of the motor systems and weakening the resources needed for effortful control. To that extent, though he suggests that addiction may be a genuine taxon and addicts categorically different from those of us who tend to lose self-control in more quotidian ways, the mechanisms involved in the reassertion of control are likely to be the same in addicts and nonaddicts. Neuroscience explains why the task facing the addict is harder than the task facing us, and why their resources for addressing the task are more meagre, but the task is of the same kind.

Natalie Gold takes an approach to self-control (abstracting away from the extra complications introduced by addiction) that is in some ways broadly similar to Ainslie's. Like Ainslie, she believes that self-control problems can be modeled as iterated prisoner's dilemmas where the players are transient selves. Self-control requires the current transient self to forgo a reward so that a greater benefit can accrue to later selves or (as Gold prefers to think of it) to the extended series as a whole.

Gold uses a neglected resource to model this intertemporal and intrapersonal problem: literature on team agency. Team reasoning often has the same structure: individuals may benefit themselves by pursuing selfish ends or benefit the team instead by cooperating. Gold argues that in the team agency context, cooperation can be increased by having members "frame" the choices appropriately. If the agent sees her options through the frame of team reasoning, defection will be less salient. If the "team" frame has a motivational grip on her, she is likely to act to benefit the team. In the intrapersonal case, the probability that the agent will exercise self-control rises if she frames her choices as a problem for herself over time. If this perspective captures an important element in self-control, loss of control may arise from a lack of identification with the self over time.

This perspective generates predictions and also suggests practical remedies. It predicts that lack of self-control will be associated with relative lack of self-identification. Gold notes that there is evidence that this is true with regard to sufferers from borderline personality disorder (psychopaths also seem to present with a combination of low self-identification and impulsivity; see Levy, forthcoming). The practical remedies it suggests will increase the salience of the self as a temporally extended entity and increase identification with the self. Again, Gold points to existing evidence that such techniques may improve self-control.

It is likely, as Gold notes, that ordinary people implicitly conceive of themselves as selves extending over time. That raises the question of why self-control problems are ubiquitous. Perhaps as a result of experience we acquire an implicit commitment to a near-term self-concept (there is evidence that as people mature their discount curves become less hyperbolic). But for many self-control problems the costs of defection are never salient enough for us to achieve a genuine, visceral commitment to avoiding them that is not mediated by top-down, effortful processing. Think of the costs of smoking or small indulgences: the costs may be borne many years later. Different self-control problems may make different demands on us, depending on when and how the costs of defection will be experienced, and may therefore demand different frames.

Owen Flanagan writes about Alcoholics Anonymous (AA) with the authority that comes from being a renowned naturalistic philosopher and a long-time participant in AA meetings. He argues that the second perspective, that of the participant, should not be regarded as epistemically privileged because AA functions as what Foucault called an *episteme*. It is designed to provide an epistemological framework into which members fit their experience of alcoholism, and it places members under great pressure to describe, or redescribe, their phenomenology to fit the AA mould. For this reason, Flanagan suggests, first-person reports from within AA are shaped (more than most first-person reports: though Flanagan is silent on the question, I suspect he would accept that the biases he identifies are absolutely pervasive) by the confirmation bias and self-fulfilling prophecy. Key tenets of AA are false, or apply only to some subset of alcoholics, or at best are only partially true. It is not true, for instance, that alcoholism involves the loss of control, in any very strong sense of that phrase, though it certainly involves great difficulties in exercising self-control.

Yet, Flanagan argues, despite the fact that AA misdescribes alcoholism, it works: it works at least as well as, perhaps better than, any other program. Why does it work? Flanagan suggests that AA should be seen as a repository of practical wisdom about self-control and recovery. Further, it offers a form of cognitive-behavioral therapy for members, therapy strengthened and made effective by the fact that it also offers very concrete distractions (for instance, mentors who one can call upon) and alternative social activities to provide competition for drinking. In his recent book, Gene Heyman (2009) makes the crowding out of competing activities central to the explanation of substance abuse. This focus on the way in which AA works (in part) by buttressing the attractiveness of such competing activities seems to fit nicely with his model. It may also be that the rhetoric of "loss of control" utilized by AA encourages the use of Ainslie-style self-prediction mechanisms, causing the alcoholic to see her abstention as a sign of regaining control and therefore as predictive of future abstention.

Walton and Nasrallah suggest that understanding the loss of control seen in addiction requires understanding normal value and rule-guided decision making. They argue that decision making is produced by multiple mechanisms that may compete for control over behavior. These mechanisms respond to different incentives—hedonic value, costs, social rules, and so on—and may pull in different directions. They argue that the heterogeneity of mechanisms involved in decision making is incompatible with any picture of choice as involving a simple competition between "reason" and "affect." The value of a response or a behavior to an organism is not a unitary property; instead, it is multidimensional and components of value may dissociate in unintuitive ways. Even within the frontal lobe, different regions encode different dimensions of value, implying that the association of cognitive control with frontal mechanisms is oversimplistic. The perspective offered here also suggests that identical failures of control may have quite different causes. An addict may give in to temptation due to aberrant encoding of the value of alternatives, or due to failure to inhibit impulses, for instance.

Understanding which components of decision making mechanisms are dysfunctional may play an important role in guiding judicial and social responses to addiction, Walton and Nasrallah argue. For many addicts, failures of self-control may result from impairments in mechanisms sensitive to longer term consequences of actions, so that behavior is driven by mechanisms that respond to benefits alone. This entails that deterrence will be relatively ineffective with regard to these addicts: penalties for drug use simply won't register sufficiently well to modulate behavior. As an aside, it is worth mentioning that I have argued elsewhere, on the basis mainly of behavioral data, that addicts are generally more responsive to rewards than punishments, and have suggested that this might entail that carrots ought to play a proportionally larger role in our response to addicts and sticks a proportionally smaller one (Levy, 2013). Walton and Nasrallah's arguments seem to support this claim.

Walter Sinnott-Armstrong's broad-ranging paper also focuses on the relationship between responsiveness to incentives and control. He argues that the question he poses in the title of his paper—"are addicts responsible?"—is misleading. According to the account of control defended by Sinnott-Armstrong, addiction undermines reasons-responsiveness to different degrees in different individuals in different circumstances. Addiction covers a broad spectrum of cases; accordingly, different addicts possess the wherewithal for moral responsibility to different degrees. Further, the same addict may be responsible to different degrees for the same behavior, depending on the circumstances.

Like Walton and Nasrallah, Sinnott-Armstrong notes that control fractionates, in ways that are counterintuitive. In the face of this evidence, Sinnott-Armstrong suggests, courts need to make a decision on where to draw the line regarding culpability. This decision is not entirely arbitrary, since the legal system is normatively constrained in various ways; nevertheless, it must be made on ultimately pragmatic grounds. However, if control does not merely fractionate, but fractionates in the systematic way that Walton and Nasrallah suggest, the legal system might be able to draw the lines of culpability to better match the neuroscience without sacrificing its pragmatic aims. Indeed, there may be a case for saying that the law *ought* to adjust its criteria for culpability to match the contours of human capacities.

Walton and Nasrallah explicitly assume throughout their paper that addiction is a brain disease. In one sense, I suggest, this is misleading: though their paper constitutes powerful evidence that we cannot understand, or tailor social policies to, addiction without understanding brain mechanisms, the concrete suggestions they offer resituate the addict in an environment. It is by altering incentives and changing cues that they suggest that we respond to addiction. Jeanette Kennett's paper broadens the focus even further, away from the neuroscience of addiction—indeed, away from any explanation that focuses on psychological features of the addict alone—and toward the social setting of the addict. She takes aim, in particular, at my own work. In "Resisting 'Weakness of the Will'" (Levy 2011) I argued that weakness of the will did not constitute a discrete psychological phenomenon, but was instead a manifestation of a broader phenomenon: the driving of behavior by system 1 processes. Strength of will, in contrast, results from effortful overcoming of impulses stemming from system 1. Kennett argues (plausibly) that this framework fails to capture the forces driving the behavior of many addicts. Some addicts may be something akin to wantons: they do not even attempt to resist the impulse to consume drugs, because they may (sometimes rightly) believe that no larger/later reward is available to them. It is not that these addicts—Kennett calls them resigned addicts—lack a conception of a life worth leading, as do true wantons; instead, they believe (again, quite possibly rightly) that deferring gratification will not allow them to have a chance at a better life. Their choice may be being homeless and stoned or homeless and sober enough to reflect on what they have lost (or never had) and how little chance they have of regaining it. These addicts believe (often correctly) that they have no realistic prospect of jobs, relationships, and homes, and they have no incentive to exercise effortful self-control. These addicts do not need more self-control, and the dual-process model is of little relevance to understanding their predicament.

Even in many of these cases, though, I suspect that effortful self-control may play some important role. Achieving the goods constitutive of a life worth living is, as Heyman reminds us, sometimes a hill-climbing exercise. That is, it may be true that for me to achieve the goods I really value, I may have to worsen my situation right now and for some time into the future. Addicts like those that Kennett describes may often be in this position. The homeless addict may know that if he abstains tonight, he faces a truly miserable night on the streets (much worse than a stoned night on the streets, bad as that is). He may also know that if he abstains, he raises the probability that in the medium term— once he has acquired some training and some help—he may get off the street. In that case, he faces a self-control problem. Because the rewards are distant, and very uncertain, they are unlikely to exert a very powerfully motivating effect on him; nevertheless, part of the explanation of why he does not seek to abstain tonight might cite failures of system 2 processes.

Pickard and Pearce's paper is perhaps the most committed to the folk psychological explanation of addiction. For them, addictive behavior is explained by reference to the same kinds of concepts—willpower, habit, motivation, and so on—we utilize to explain ordinary behavior, because addictive behavior just *is* ordinary behavior, though perhaps an extreme instance of it. Pickard and Pearce draw on their experience treating patients with personality disorders; they argue that the consumption of drugs by addicts is not compelled. Rather, like many of the other problematic behaviors in which patients engage, it is a means of coping with psychological distress. Accordingly, successful treatment programs aim at providing patients with alternatives means of coping, thereby expanding the scope of their agency. However, central to the aim of enabling patients to free themselves of their addictions is recognizing, and bringing the patients to recognize, that they already possess a significant degree of control over their behavior.

Pickard and Pearce cite a mass of evidence, including their own clinical observations, in support of the claim that addicts do not suffer from a compulsion to use. They cite, for instance, the fact that addicts who enter their therapeutic program are required as a condition of entry to abstain from drug taking. The fact that their patients succeed in meeting this requirement shows that for them drug use was not compulsive. They responded to a perfectly ordinary incentive (the support of a therapeutic community) and thereby demonstrated that they possessed a general capacity to respond to ordinary incentives.

But the claim that the capacity to respond to one ordinary incentive is evidence of the existence of a capacity to respond to any ordinary incentive is exactly the claim that Walton and Nasrallah dispute. If you doubt the inference from the first capacity to the second, evidence for the existence of the first capacity should not allay your doubt. What is needed, to put the doubt to rest, is evidence that addicts—in the circumstances in which they find themselves, and without special help—have a truly domain-general capacity to respond to incentives. The real difficulty here is that the same problems that arise with regard to the identification of incentives—which ones count as ordinary, and responses to which are evidence for capacities that generalize to different cases—also arise with regard to circumstances (capacities are manifested across a range of circumstances) and with regard to special help (what counts as too special?). Pickard and Pearce note, for instance, that addicts often believe that they can't control their behavior. On their view, addicts are simply wrong. But perhaps self-fulfilling beliefs are the kind of thing we ought to hold fixed in assessing capacities? It seems to me, at least, that the debate here is still in its infancy; neither side is in a position to be very confident in its claims. It is worth noting, however, that Pickard and Pearce's demanding conception of compulsion entails that it is not merely addicts who are not in the grip of compulsions—neither are sufferers from disorders on the obsessive-compulsive spectrum. This conclusion will be too counterintuitive for many people to accept.

The next three papers, like Don Ross's, center on the correct interpretation of the role of dopamine in the development of addiction. The dopamine system is widely held to be a learning system. Dopamine release is a signal that the world contains more rewards than was predicted. Natural rewards (say, food) result in the release of dopamine. Once an organism has learned that a cue predicts a natural reward, the cue (and not the reward itself) results in the release of dopamine: it is the cue that is unexpected, since the reward itself is expected, given the cue. Drugs of addiction all hijack the dopamine system, in one way or another: unlike natural rewards (that is, the rewards to which the dopamine system is designed, by evolution, to be sensitive to), these drugs cause the release (or increase the availability) of dopamine directly. The upshot is this: while cues predictive of the availability of the drug result in the release of dopamine, release of dopamine also occurs when the drug is consumed. Whereas the dopamine system adapts to natural rewards, so that consumption of the expected reward is treated by the system as the normal course of events, it cannot adapt to drugs of addiction, and their consumption is treated as showing that the world is better than expected. Yaffe's paper and Schroeder and Arpaly's paper attempt to assign a content to the signal. For Yaffe, the dopamine signal is associated with, or partially constitutes, the person's *valuing* of the cause of the signal. For Schroeder and Arpaly, the signal is associated with, or partially constitutes, the person's *desire* for the cause. For Holton and Berridge, in contrast, the signal has no content: rather, it causes the person to form the disposition to experience a desire in response to cues predictive of the cause of the spike.

Yaffe's view seems the least revisionary of the three; he argues that the best interpretation of the neurobiology of addiction will understand it as underpinning folk psychological states. Yaffe thinks that this is important, because it entails that addicts act in accordance with their values when they consume drugs; this matters, in turn, because the degree to which an action is expressive of an agent's values is directly relevant to how much blame attaches to the agent.

One possible objection to Yaffe is that the notion of "value" he defines is not in fact the one that features in folk psychology. Yaffe defines value in a way that is designed to entail that an agent's values may be fleeting, but some philosophers think that values cannot be fleeting: an agent values a state of affairs only insofar as she is disposed to take it as reason giving across a sufficiently long stretch of time. Yaffe's notion is explicitly stipulative: he recognizes that his notion of valuing may not match up with the notion in much ordinary discourse. But he maintains that the criminal law is particularly concerned with the values agents have (however fleetingly) at the time of action. That, he contends, is the justification for the law's exclusion of evidence about the agent at other times (e.g., past convictions). So the notion of value he defines is at least important for judgments of criminal blameworthiness. Whether Yaffe is right about this claim, and—if so—whether the law is justified in associating blameworthiness with fleeting facts, is a question worth pursuing.

Yaffe identifies the dopamine signal as a *part* of the valuing system. He claims that the signal can only play its action-guiding role, motivating the organism to pursue expected value, if the organism represents the cause of the signal as worth pursuing, hence, as reason giving. But even if he is right, there seems to be a gap between a signal constituting part of the valuing system and the organism valuing the state of affairs that is the object or cause of the signal. If the valuing system has other components, and these components may dissociate from the dopamine signal, then it may be that the organism fails to value the cause of the signal. If that were so, we could explain concurrent exercises of self-control by appealing to other elements of the valuing system, which underwrite the organism's genuine values. As it stands, Yaffe seems committed to holding that concurrent exercises of self-control (say, when an addict succeeds in resisting a drug) are akratic, which seems counterintuitive.

One of Yaffe's targets in his paper is Timothy Schroeder's (2010) interpretation of the dopamine signal. His paper is followed by a restatement of this view. Schroeder and Nomy Arpaly (a major theorist of moral responsibility, with whom Schroeder has collaborated in the past) argue that the dopamine signal causes cravings for addictive drugs. On the theory of moral responsibility that Schroeder and Arpaly have developed, together and separately (Arpaly and Schroeder 1999; Arpaly 2002, 2006), agents are morally blameworthy only for actions that express their ill will or moral indifference, where to have ill will is to have an intrinsic desire for something that is wrong or bad, and to be morally indifferent is to fail to have an intrinsic desire for that which is right or good. Since blameworthiness turns for them on agents' desires, the important question is whether cravings are desires.

Their answer is yes, but only partially. The craving is caused by a dysfunction of the dopaminergic system, caused by drugs of addiction driving up the signal directly. As a consequence, the dopamine signal *misrepresents* the true reward value of the drug. The addict desires drugs, but the motivational force of the craving is greater than the desire. Insofar as the addict desires drugs, and this desire is a partial cause of a wrongful act, she is blameworthy, but insofar as the action is caused by motivational forces exceeding her desire, her blame is mitigated.

It is only if the motivational force of the cravings cannot be reduced to the motivational force of a desire that addicts' blame can be mitigated, on Schroeder and Arpaly's view. In addition to desire, they argue, there are two motivational forces at work: habit and expectations. The expectations generate negative feelings, which they argue cannot be identified with desires. The dopamine release is generated by a combination of intrinsic desires and expectations, which combine with habits to generate behavior. The degree of blameworthiness is a function of the degree to which the action is driven by desire; since the action is also driven by unconscious expectations and habits, the agent is not fully blameworthy for the action.

It is worth noting that the view developed here has consequences that will be seen by many to be harsh. Consider the case with which they open their paper. Driven by cravings, David Carr left his two infant daughters for hours in the car on a freezing night in order to get cocaine. Schroeder and Araply argue that Carr's terrible (but thankfully harmless) action deserves our condemnation, because it was driven (or at any rate partially explained) by an imperfect intrinsic desire for the good. A moral paragon would not have acted as he did. However, it seems harsh to blame someone for an action that *only* a moral paragon would have avoided. Schroeder and Arpaly mitigate Carr's blame because he did not express "monstrous moral indifference" in his behavior, but it is hard to see how his behavior is evidence of moral indifference *at all*.

Richard Holton, an influential moral philosopher, and Kent Berridge, a neuroscientist whose work on addiction is widely discussed, contribute the third of the three papers focusing on the dopamine signal. They reject the view that the

dopamine signal causes valuing or desires. Rather, it plays a role in the generation of a disposition to experience cravings, where a craving is a state midway
between a desire and an intention. A craving is not an instrumental desire—a
desire for pleasure, or relief, or what have you. Rather, it generates an intrinsic motivation and issues in an impulse that, unless checked by an exercise of
self-control, leads to action. Holton and Berridge argue that work by Wyvell
and Berridge (2000) demonstrates that dopamine generates cue-conditioned
cravings rather than an expectation of reward. Wyvell used amphetamines to
sensitize rats to a sugar reward. Sensitized rats who learned to associate a tone
with the availability of sugar pressed the lever to deliver sugar frantically, but
sensitized rats who simply had the lever made available to them did not press
it any more frequently than control rats. Since there is no reason to think that
rats in either condition had different expectations about how rewarding sugar
would be, the tone seems to be a direct cause of motivation, independent from
beliefs or expectations. Since cravings can cause behavior that is at variance
with agents' beliefs, Holton and Berridge reach a conclusion that is directly in
conflict with Yaffe's: (some) addicts act akratically.

Holton and Berridge note that their theory might be expanded to encompass
process (and substance) addictions that do not centrally involve a dysfunction
of the dopamine system: there may be other causal routes to cue-driven cravings that are insulated from beliefs and which can be inhibited only by an exercise of self-control. It may be that the neuroscience of addiction will force such
an expansion in any case. Following George Koob (Koob and Le Moal 1997,
2008), and others, some neuroscientists believe that dopaminergic dysfunction is a relatively small and perhaps inessential part of the neuroadaptations
associated with addiction. These neuroscientists emphasize long-term depression of reward circuitry and increased activity in antireward circuitry, the result
of opponent processes adapting to the chronic presence of addictive drugs.
Whether the incentive salience story can be adapted to recognize the role of
allostatic change remains to be explored.

The field of addiction research—or rather, the many overlapping fields of
addiction research, encompassing the natural and social sciences, as well as
the humanities and law—is enormous and growing. Important discoveries are
being made day by day, and we are gradually coming to better understand the
mechanisms involved in addiction, relapse, and recovery, as well as how addiction differs from other failures of self-control. It would be foolish to pretend
that this collection constitutes the last word; as the field evolves, some views
may be superseded entirely, while others will require amendment or supple-
mentation. For anyone who wants to grasp the state of the art in self-control
research, however—and that ought to include anyone who wants to understand human agency and its failures and strengths—the papers collected here

are indispensable. They represent some of the world's best thinking on how we achieve our goals and why we often fail.

REFERENCES

Ainslie, G. 2001. *Breakdown of Will.* Cambridge: Cambridge University Press.

Arpaly, N. 2002. *Unprincipled Virtue: An Inquiry Into Moral Agency.* Oxford: Oxford University Press.

Arpaly, N. 2006. *Merit, Meaning and Human Bondage: An Essay on Free Will.* Princeton, NJ: Princeton University Press.

Arpaly, N., and Schroeder, T. 1999. Praise, Blame and the Whole Self. *Philosophical Studies* 93: 161–188.

Boyer, P. 2008. Evolutionary Economics of Mental Time-Travel? *Trends in Cognitive Sciences* 12: 219–223.

Heyman, G. 2009. *Addiction: A Disorder of Choice.* Cambridge, MA: Harvard University Press.

Koob, G.F., and Le Moal, M. 1997. Drug Abuse: Hedonic Homeostatic Dysregulation. *Science* 278: 52–58.

Koob, G.F., and Le Moal, M. 2008. Addiction and the Brain Antireward System. *Annual Review of Psychology* 59: 29–53.

Levy, N. 2011. Resisting Weakness of the Will. *Philosophy and Phenomenological Research* 82: 134–155.

Levy, N. 2013. Punishing the Addict: Reflections on Gene Heyman. In Thomas Nadelhoffer (ed.), *The Future of Punishment.* Oxford: Oxford University Press, 233–246.

Levy, N. forthcoming. Psychopaths and Blame: The Argument from Content. *Philosophical Psychology.*

Schroeder, T. 2010. Irrational Action and Addiction. In D. Ross, H. Kincaid, D. Spurrett, and P. Collins (eds.), *What Is Addiction?* Cambridge, MA: MIT Press, 391–407.

Wyvell, C.L., and Berridge, K.C. 2000. Intra-Accumbens Amphetamine Increases the Conditioned Incentive Salience of Sucrose Reward: Enhancement of Reward "Wanting" Without Enhanced "Liking" or Response Reinforcement. *Journal of Neuroscience* 20: 8122–8130.

2

Money as MacGuffin

A Factor in Gambling and Other Process Addictions

GEORGE AINSLIE

Alfred Hitchcock's genius was in his timing. The experience he sold, which for years he produced better than any competitor, was suspense. His characters were always chasing something, but for Hitchcock this something was arbitrary—what he called a MacGuffin. The uranium being stashed away in *Notorious* could just as well have been diamonds or hidden evidence or a toxic virus, and the emotional arc of the movie would have been the same. The MacGuffin was a necessary but nonspecific component of the suspense. The management of this suspense was what required timing, the crescendo of threats and reprieves as the protagonists approached their goal, culminating in an exhilarating climax. At that point the MacGuffin had become unnecessary. Other directors have often thrown it away at the end—the treasure of the Sierra Madre, the diamond-studded necklace in *Titanic*—like a female impersonator tossing off his wig. The crucial question for us, though, is why it was valuable to begin with.

This conference is about addiction, a problem that is perhaps the greatest challenge to our confidence in human rationality. The problem of addiction is not confined to a few seductive molecules. Addictive preferences are woven deeply into the fabric of civilized life, including those for normal substances (food, chocolate), structured activities that do not require a substance (gambling, day trading), emotional patterns (thrill seeking, destructive personal relationships), and the most elementary and pervasive form of regretted choice, procrastination (Andreou & White, 2010). There have been many attempts to formulate a technical definition of addiction, but the results never coincide exactly with ordinary usage. For instance, the emergence of physiological signs of withdrawal has been a favorite of authors who want to restrict "addiction" to the realm of substance use, but discontinuing even heavy use of cocaine does not lead to physiological withdrawal, whereas stopping intense gambling activity sometimes does (Blaszczynski et al., 2008). We do not have to settle on the proper definition. The challenge to rationality is the same whether someone has an addiction or just a bad habit, as long as the person herself perceives the habit to be both bad and hard to break.

In rational choice theory (RCT) an individual maximizes expected future utility according to an exponential discount curve,

$$\text{Present value} = \text{Value}_0 \times \delta^{\text{Delay}} \quad \text{Formula 1}$$

where Value_0 = value if immediate and $\delta = (1 - \text{discount rate})$.

The obvious question that addiction poses RCT is, what motivates someone to repeatedly choose what she herself often sees as a poorer option, even if she is trying to stop choosing it? Furthermore, when someone is seduced by a fudge sundae or cocaine high, she chooses immediate consumption in one modality despite larger, later losses in others—health, wealth, safety. The problem gambler seeks wealth despite the likelihood of actually losing this same wealth. Thus, the present discussion must address a second question as well: What is there in this internally inconsistent proposition that seduces the gambler?

A night at the casino has something of the structure of a suspense film. You make repeated small plays, winning a little or losing a little, but building up a sum for the evening that will be either a win or a loss. There is as much lore in the gambling industry as there is in the film industry on how to pace the bets and structure the risks. Certainly the optimal patterns differ. Unlike the invariant win in a Hitchcock movie, the odds favor an overall loss at the casino. But our second question arises in both fields: How does the threat of loss generate value, in such a way that the prospective combination of loss and restoration is worth more than the prospect of staying secure? The question has relevance beyond the confines of fiction and gambling, but they provide simplified examples, stripped of noncontributory properties.

Suspense fiction is a modality of reward that does not depend on money or the things that money can buy. A similar modality, thrill born of suspense, is well recognized as what adds the value needed to make gambling a winning hedonic activity. But this phenomenon raises a third, more unsettling question: When our physical senses are not involved, where does our reward come from? That is, when we do not need to obtain a specific turnkey to unlock our reward process, what do we need? The conventional answer is that we are rewarded by the prospect of getting physical rewards at some time in the future—that when we seek money or power or reputation, they are just tokens backed by the promise of physical rewards. It is obvious that such tokens come to function on their own, just as token currencies can function without being convertible to gold; but the properties of this independent rewarding power have not been explored.[1] Just as token currencies have specific requirements, such as a widespread expectation of being accepted, and specific vulnerabilities, such as a proneness to inflation, nonphysical reward must also have its own requirements and constraints. In recent years the discovery of mirroring centers in the brain has suggested a neural substrate for one such highly valued process, vicarious experience, but not how vicarious experience translates into reward (see Preston & de Waal, 2002, and Ainslie & Monterosso's commentary, 2002). Vicarious experience is only one kind of imagination, and even that has not been explored in cases where its object is not present to at least one of the senses.

The possibility of nonphysical addictions (or addiction components) brings this ignorance into sharp focus and provides an extreme example that any theory of nonphysical reward must accommodate. I will describe how an alternative to the exponential delay discount curves of RCT permits answers to the three questions I have listed as raised by problem gambling: (1) What leads a person to temporarily prefer poorer alternatives? (2) What leads her to prefer the prospect of less to more of the same good? (3) What leads her to value goods that lack the physical capacity to induce reward? Hyperbolic discounting itself is a well-established empirical finding, and I will give only a brief summary here. The value of risk per se is best explored in light of how nonphysical rewards function, a difficult process to study experimentally but one for which hyperbolic discounting can at least clarify the components (see related discussion in Ainslie, 2001, pp. 161–197, and 2003).[2]

A REVIEW OF HYPERBOLIC DISCOUNTING

This approach originated in controlled experiments suggesting that rewards exert attraction in inverse proportion to their delays. Richard Herrnstein initially reported that nonhuman animals tend to sample two concurrent streams of reward in proportion to the mean rates, amounts, and immediacies of those

1. The internal reward process is thought of as a way of predicting the "real" rewards that have obvious adaptive usefulness. But although rewardingness evolved as a proxy for adaptiveness, within an organism the rewardingness itself is sovereign. Just as organisms can be seen as mere vehicles for passing on genes, functionally rewards are just means to stimulate the internal reward process. Occasions that excite this process without leading to adaptive goods are not false, just unattached, but therefore vulnerable to the deterioration I will be describing.

2. Texts of many Ainslie references are available at www.picoeconomics.org.

rewards (the "matching law"; 1961), a pattern he later found in humans as well (1997). Application of the matching law to single (discrete, i.e., not streamed) choices between smaller sooner (SS) and larger later (LL) rewards by the current author yielded four specific predictions (Ainslie, 1975, 1992):

1. The decline in rewarding effect with delay is described better by a value function that is inversely proportional to delay (hyperbolic discount curve) than by a function that declines by a constant proportion of remaining value for each unit of delay (exponential discount curve; Figure 2.1). That is, data on the evident value of a single prospective reward at varying delays will be described better by a hyperbolic than by an exponential function of those delays. The most commonly used form of the hyperbolic curve has been

$$\text{Present value} = \text{Value}_0 \, / \, [1 + (k \times \text{Delay})] \qquad \text{Formula 2}$$

   where Value_0 = value if immediate and k is degree of impatience (Mazur, 1987).

2. Preferences between some pairs of an SS reward and an LL alternative at varying delays but with a constant lag between SS and LL rewards will favor LL rewards when both are distant, but shift to SS alternatives when they become closer.

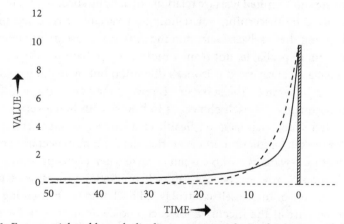

Figure 2.1 Exponential and hyperbolic discount curves drawn from a reward that would be worth 10 units if immediate, with slopes adjusted so that each is worth 1 unit of reward at 10 units of delay (hyperbolic k = 0.9; exponential δ = 0.794). The value of the reward at any given delay is represented by the height of the curve at that point. The hyperbolic curve (solid line) is steeper at short delays, but has a higher tail.

3. During the period when an LL reward is preferred, subjects will sometimes choose behaviors whose only function is to prevent their own subsequent choice of the SS alternative.
4. Subjects choosing between a whole series of SS/LL pairs at once will have a greater tendency to choose the LL rewards than will subjects choosing between the same pairs one at a time. A subsidiary prediction is that human subjects who perceive current choices between SS and LL rewards as test cases—examples that predict their own future preferences between similar pairs of rewards—will prefer LL rewards more than they do when they see the pair of alternatives as an isolated choice. That is, people may create *bundles* of interdependent expectations by predicting their future choices *recursively* on the basis of each current choice.

Subsequent work by both economists and psychologists has largely confirmed these predictions, both in nonhuman animals and in human subjects[3] under conditions that do not invite calculation (Ainslie, 2007; Ainslie & Monterosso, 2003; Green & Myerson, 2004; Hofmeyr et al., 2010; Kirby, 1997; Kirby & Guastello, 2001). The first three findings suggest that our successive motivational states regularly conflict in a way that prevents durable resolution, and that we must find ways to avoid or forestall our own foreseeable temporary preferences if we want to make sure that our current preference will be followed. The fourth finding suggests a way of managing temporary preferences, which fits intuitive descriptions of both willpower and freedom of will. The gist is that a combination of imperfect self-prediction and a tendency to temporarily prefer SS rewards sets up a limited warfare relationship among successive selves, which can be resolved by discerning—or defining—a variant of repeated prisoner's dilemma among these selves: Defection in the present case makes defection in future cases more probable, not from a motive of retaliation (which would be present in a classical repeated prisoner's dilemma) but by making cooperation seem likely to be wasted. The stake of LL reward may be aggregated from the evident consequences of each choice, as in binges with hangovers, or may be an anticipated state, such as good health or adequate savings. The necessary element for the self-prediction process is that the person's expectation of getting a category of LL reward as a whole is put at stake when each opportunity within a definable set of SS rewards occurs. This self-prediction process is recursive, in that each estimate of future self-control is fed back into the estimating process, thus forming part of the incentive for each choice. Our criteria for deciding which choices constitute lapses are often called *personal rules*.

---

3. Most experiments now award human subjects one of their actual choices, selected randomly, but the results have been reported not to differ from studies in which subjects chose between hypothetical rewards (Madden et al., 2003).

I have developed this model of will elsewhere (Ainslie, 2001, 2005, 2011, 2012). Its importance for the present discussion is that efficient intertemporal bargaining entails making choices in predictable ways, that is, not surprising yourself when you can avoid it. Ironically, the mechanism that rewards this regularity is also the one that arguably makes the will free.

SELF-CONTROL IS ONLY HALF OF RATIONALITY

The phenomenon of hyperbolic discounting might seem to imply that rationality consists of foreseeing your temporary preferences and forestalling them either by judicious use of Ulysses-like commitments or by making resolutions that can function as self-enforcing contracts—willpower. However, rationality as willpower leaves something out, and may create a problem in its own right—not just the "rule worshipping" of Mintoff and others (2004), but your systemization of your own choices, which become less hedonically satisfying as they become more regular. Hyperbolic discount functions predict this limitation as well. I will not discuss most of will's side effects here (see Ainslie, 2001, pp. 143–160), but to understand substance-free addictions, we will need to find an aspect of rationality that does not entail will as it is usually understood, and may even be spoiled by it.

In older models of motivation deprivation states had a negative valence. Circumstances imposed needs on you, and you got pleasure from reducing them. Your appetites were like steam boilers, in which pressure was aversive and your motivation was to get rid of it. You would avoid deprivation states if you could and seek to remain in a Nirvana-like calm. A little thought revealed this model to be absurd. It would mean that people should eat to avoid hunger, and that the loss of sexual libido caused by certain medicines would be a benefit rather than an unfortunate side effect. We now regard deprivation states as making appetites possible;[4] appetites are what make possible reward in general and satisfaction in particular.[5]

---

4. Appetite is the capacity to be rewarded in a given modality. Modalities are defined by the processes that satiate one while leaving another fresh (such as hunger versus thirst), which are modestly known in the case of physical rewards (Herrnstein, 1977) and almost unknown for endogenous rewards (see below, and Ainslie, 1992, pp. 243–256).

5. I use "satisfaction" as a special case of "reward," the most general term for the mechanism that makes processes that have just happened more likely to recur. Satisfaction is reward that is subjectively desirable, which means reward that does not bring on reward-inhibiting components to form vivid but aversive experiences such as pains and negative emotions. In this usage, pain is an appetite that at the very least makes attention to it rewarding, and arguably draws us into the emotional engagement that creates aversion ("protopathic" pain; Melzack et al., 1963). Urges that are avoided when foreseen in advance could thus be thought of as *negative appetites*—itches, for instance, or the urge to panic.

Historically, the dysphoria of unsatisfied appetites has been the main driving force of human behavior, but modern societies are expert at solving that problem. We are used to eating when we want, having analgesics available for pain, and being neither too hot nor too cold. Control of conception and treatment of venereal disease have greatly reduced barriers to sexual satisfaction *ad lib.* Beyond such concrete rewards there are limitless activities and relationships that now provide most of our satisfaction, and perhaps always have. We know a great deal about how to satisfy appetites. Only rarely has the converse problem come into focus: What do we do when appetites become too slight? If our appetites are not like boilers but like waves on the ocean, which we ride up to have the pleasure of coasting down, what do we do if we find ourselves becalmed?

Reward by an abundant good is largely determined by appetite. The problem for modern societies is that however robust our sources of satisfaction, our appetites are perishable. At the most elementary level, repeated stimulation of any sense organ leads to fatigue, a temporary decline in function. But familiar scenarios lose their power to excite even after periods of rest; this is not fatigue, but habituation, a learned anticipation that forestalls curiosity or suspense. From the standpoint of evolution, it is undoubtedly adaptive for intense satisfactions to fade away into habit as we get efficient at obtaining them. This process keeps us motivated to explore our environment, both when we are young and inept and when we have become master problem solvers. If our reward mechanisms operated in strict proportionality to how much of some external stimulus we could get, then a reward rate that was sufficient to shape our behavior when we were beginners would lead us to rest on our laurels once we had become adept at getting it. But instead, as we learn an activity, the reward it generates increases only at first, and then decreases again because our appetite does not build as much before it is satisfied.

> The paradox is that it is just those achievements which are most solid, which work best, and which continue to work that excite and reward us least. The price of skill is the loss of the experience of value—and of the zest for living (Tomkins, 1978, p. 212).

While habituation makes our skills at getting goods more effective, it makes our attempts to enjoy these goods less effective. Here we begin to see the divergence of two kinds of effectiveness, presaging a split in rationality itself, which will figure increasingly in our discussion.

Because hyperbolic discount curves give disproportionate weight to imminent prospects, we cannot just blend appetite and satisfaction in optimal mixtures, like breathing out and breathing in. Small satisfactions that can be had immediately will outweigh delayed satisfactions that, compared from a distance, would seem worth the delay. As soon as a wave rises a little from the surface of the sea, we get an urge to coast down it. The properties of appetites are often such that rapid consumption brings an earlier peak of reward but reduces the total amount of reward that the appetite makes possible. Where we have free access to an activity that rewards more intensely the greater our appetite for it, we tend to consume it faster than we should if we were going to get the most reward over time from that appetite. Hyperbolic discounting predicts that in a conflict of satisfaction patterns between the long but delayed versus the brief but soon, an organism that discounts the future hyperbolically is primed to choose brief but soon. Similarly, if an increase in intensity can be had at the cost of duration, that increase, too, is apt to be chosen. This problem makes no sense in a world of exponential discounting. In an exponential world, an adept consumer should simply gauge what the most productive way to exploit an appetite would be, and pace her consumption accordingly. We would entertain ourselves optimally by waiting for just enough appetite and then satisfying it. By contrast, common experience teaches that a reward that we indulge in *ad lib* becomes unsatisfactory for that reason itself. To get the most out of any kind of reward, we have to have—or develop—limited access to it.

The effect of limiting access to a reward that is otherwise freely available can be modeled with a diagram. Assume for simplicity that appetite grows linearly and is exhausted linearly with consumption. The value of consumption is the summed, hyperbolically discounted value of each of its instants. If there is a factor that delays consumption from the instant at which the consumption could, if immediate, compete with available alternatives—the instant it reaches what could be called the market level of reward—that factor may substantially increase the product of [value × duration] before the appetite satiates (Figures 2.2a and 2.2b).

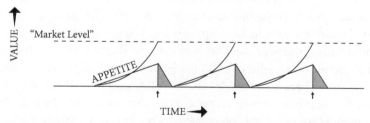

Figure 2.2a A simple model of appetite that grows in a straight line until the reward it makes possible (stippled area) is worth harvesting, then grows again. The choice to harvest it occurs when a hyperbolic discount curve from the estimated sum of the moments in the stippled area reaches a competitive market level. Without a delay factor, the reward is harvested as soon as the choice is made (at arrows).

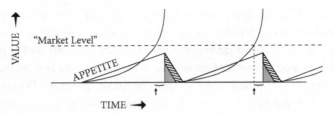

Figure 2.2b Increased reward (stripes) resulting from increased appetite when there is an obligatory delay (brackets) in consumption of the reward between the instant of choice, when its discounted value rises to market level (arrows), and when the reward can be consumed. The obligatory delay allows the discounted value of the reward to rise well above market level before consumption occurs.

These relationships are obvious with concrete satisfactions. For instance, spending our day with snacks at hand can lead to the pattern of eating called grazing, which may be an efficient way to get some other task done but undermines the potential pleasure of dining. The solution is to commit ourselves to deprivations, such as a personal rule against eating between meals. A basic example of creating hedonic gain from net neutrality is the sauna—you make yourself hot for the pleasure of making yourself cold, instead of staying at room temperature and looking for satisfaction in some other activity. Examples with more punch include the threatening experiences that we expect to create exhilaration: climbing dangerous mountains (see Loewenstein, 1999), sponsoring a social event that is at risk for failing, or signing up for a grueling training rotation such as surgery in a medical internship. The privation entailed in such activities is often such that we have to commit ourselves in advance—at least in resolution—because we would otherwise not choose them on the morning when we had to set out. It may be that there is no limit to this logic, that enormous deprivations can lead to enormous gains—some religions suggest giving away all our possessions and becoming mendicants—but as the deprivation required increases, fulcrums that provide the motivational leverage necessary to accept it become increasingly hard to find. The !Kung people of the Kalahari Desert are said to have appeared unusually happy when they lived in cultural isolation under conditions of extreme deprivation, but they nevertheless chose to live squalid lives on the bottom rungs of modern civilization when that option became available (Glantz & Pearce, 1989). However, as long as consumption requires physical action, commitment is at least possible. Physical commitment is apt to be unavailable when a rewarding activity is mental.

Among imaginative organisms most reward is endogenous. When we are free of, or have satiated, our physical deprivation states, most of the reward we seek comes from expectations we construct of the future, our rehearsal of the past, and occasions for emotion that we have in the present, which are often but not necessarily connected to physical rewards. We conjure up so much that is not in our current sensory fields that we live as if in a video game, cultivating some scenarios and trying to avoid others, able even to prevent the intrusion of physical reality in many cases, but unable to prevent the intrusion of remembered or imagined horror in other cases. Much (I would say most) satisfaction that modern people experience from goods of various kinds is actually available *ad lib*, within our psyches, and what we buy from the world is only some kind of sheet music that lets us pace it.[6] We get the most satisfaction from emotion, even turning fear and grief into positive experiences (as in horror films and tear-jerkers, respectively). Sensual pleasure is a poor second, although we do use imagination to heighten it by cultivating appetites for various patterns of sight, sound, taste, and touch. As Wallace Stevens said, "We live in the mind." There has been no good term for the reward that does not require an association with physical events; it could be called mental reward, self-reward, or process reward, but these terms all have extraneous connotations. Elsewhere I have used "emotional" reward (Ainslie, 2001), since emotions are its best examples, even though "emotion" connotes an intensity that many examples do not have. "Imaginary" would suit, except that it connotes a falsehood or delusion. "Self-generated" reward is literally what I mean, but its connotation of deliberateness is also misleading. Here I will try out "endogenous" to refer to those rewards not governed strictly by sensory experience.

The neural mechanics of choice is becoming known. We try out scenes before entering them. This cannot yet be measured with the necessary specificity in people, but many studies have shown a rhesus monkey entertaining choices in its intraparietal cortex until an action threshold is reached (Glimcher, 2009). Even a rat in a maze has been found to model the maze in its hippocampus, and can be seen lighting up one arm of this mental maze and then the other over fractions of a second as it hesitates at a choice point (Johnson & Redish, 2007). This is the process that psychologist Edward Tolman described seventy years ago as vicarious trial and error (VTE; Tolman, 1939), but the concept fell into disuse. Nonhuman subjects are mostly weighing these possible scenes for how much concrete reward they will deliver and how soon, but humans' larger brains can create scenes that are worth staying in for their own sake.[7]

6. Some of this reward is "conditioned," of course; but since it mostly lacks a believable unconditioned stimulus, the relationship to laboratory conditioning is a limited analogy. For the many problems of conditioned reward models, see Ainslie, 2001, pp. 19–22, and 2010a.

7. Brain imaging has begun to supply some information about the construction of scenarios. Significantly, the same few parts of the brain, largely in prefrontal and medial temporoparietal lobes, seem to be active in all the major kinds of imagination—our memories of the past, the future we construct from those memories, the experience we attribute vicariously to others, and even, to some extent, the locations where these scenes might occur (Spreng et al., 2009).

We bring up a memory so as to relive a scene, or a plan so as to anticipate one, or another person's experience so as to model one, and may stay engaged with any of them for a considerable time without necessarily being moved to any actual behavior. Still, we cannot arbitrarily designate which of our imaginings will repay us for the time they take. We are constrained by whatever principle governs reward by imagination, and we are obliged to find this reward by VTE. There is no reason to think that a situation with endogenous rewards is different from that with physical rewards in cases where those rewards are freely available. We mentally try out whether we are ready for another cup of coffee, just as a rat that can self-administer unlimited cocaine can be seen emitting small striatal neuronal bursts to try out whether its appetite for cocaine has returned (Phillips et al., 2003, p. 616). In the same way we try out our imaginings for how they feel. In a marketplace based on prospective reward, a scenario[8] competes for our engagement against alternatives such as preparing coffee, taking a nap, or imagining something else. The question that must be answered is, how can scenarios without prospective external rewards, or with prospective external rewards that are extensively subject to interpretation, compete against alternatives with rewards that are nearby and certain? In other words, what makes a scenario worth spending time in?

Certainly its effect on external events is part of the answer: Is a given train of imagination instrumentally useful? That is, is it a plan or hypothesis about environmental contingencies, or some other mental process that is not rewarding in its own right but that will help bring about a situation that is? Conventionally we place a value on the rewarding effect a scenario would have if it predicted external events, then correct this value for the probability and delay of those events, and choose according to the resulting belief. But a great amount of imagination is not used to bring about or avoid events. People often seek out pleasant memories or are drawn into reliving horrid ones.[9] We buy large amounts of fiction—novels, cinema, video games—sometimes to the extent of impairing our real lives. Even our goal-directed plans are based on beliefs that are notoriously malleable, not only in the direction of wishful thinking but also toward hypochondria, obsessional doubt, paranoid jealousy, and the exaggerated worry that some cognitive therapists have called "catastrophizing" (Ellis & Grieger, 1977; subtler examples in Elster, 2010).

---

8. By "scenario" I mean any imagined or mooted sequence of experience—a concept as general as the constructionists' "text," but implying an element of choice according to which one text is selected over another on the basis of reward. Adding a basis for selection corrects the constructionists' disregard of incentive (see Ainslie, 1993).

9. Here is an illustration of the distinction between rewards and satisfactions (see note 6). Horrid memories compete on the basis of a rewarding component, but they are not satisfactions.

These distortions of planning are not simply mistakes. Some thinkers might argue that people's notorious overvaluation of highly improbable events—the phenomenon that sells both high-jackpot lotteries and dismemberment insurance—is purely cognitive, an artifact of bad heuristics; but publishing the odds in lotteries does not seem to reduce enthusiasm for them. Likewise, objective reassurance has little effect on hypochondria. Superstitions resist scientific correction, and science itself has repeatedly been revealed to be cherishing false assumptions because of their reassuring tractability. People sometimes say they behave so as to go to heaven, the VTE of which has certainly not been shaped by experience; this is also true of young workers' expectations for retirement or anyone's plan for a remote period in her life. Ostensibly these plans are instrumental, but people's persistent ignoring of realistic information about them suggests that they serve another purpose to a greater or lesser extent. Future scenarios may or may not come true, but to be entertained at all they have to deliver reward in the present, whether in the form of satisfaction or of giving in to an unwelcome appetite. The planned/fantasied retirement, vacation, or social victory must have a current savoring value, and the feared/fantasied disease, loss, or humiliation must urge itself on present attention in the form of current dread. To the extent that present reward is governed by something other than stochastic prediction, it represents another selective factor for scenarios—beyond their instrumental role—that could be called *hedonic*. But what are the constraints on hedonic selection?

Endogenous reward comes to be governed by occasions. As I argued above, hyperbolic impatience makes the imagining of even desirable scenarios *ad lib* relatively unrewarding because it condenses the appetizing phase, as in grazing. When one occasion for reward is as good as another, they will replace each other as soon as each is slightly fresher or temporarily more desirable, and the imagining will have the quality of a daydream. Conversely, if there is a unique or relatively rare—*singular*—occasion that stands out from the others, it will make the corresponding imagination more robust. The creation of singular occasions is elementary in a game such as solitaire: We bind ourselves with a personal rule that defines steps toward a scarce outcome. Such a rule has to be strict, but it will be self-enforcing, since if we cheat we undermine the suspense that is the sole purpose of the game.[10] Solitaire pays off poorly if we just imagine winning, or cheat. It pays off most when we win with optimal infrequency; only that scenario induces enough appetite to make the game more rewarding than not playing at all. Solitaire has, after all, no instrumental use. Setting up a challenge—making it important, "betting on it"—is the basic process for exploiting

10. "Solitaire is the one game that requires absolute honesty." Madame Armfeldt in *A Little Night Music*.

endogenous reward, most apparent in games and puzzles without instrumental purpose, but discernible in a great deal of human endeavor. In pursuing any long task we have to define what benchmarks will count as accomplishments, and hence as occasions for self-congratulation; here, too, wishful thinking will erode their rewarding effect. In another noninstrumental example, we can turn to fiction to provide a string of occasions for endogenous reward, which are undermined if we read ahead, surf television channels, or disengage emotionally from the scary parts of a film. In the rare cases where an author offers a choice of contradictory outcomes—for instance, in the alternate endings of John Fowles' novel, *The French Lieutenant's Woman*—the same dysphoric feeling arises as with the temptation to cheat at solitaire.[11] The power of occasions to deliver endogenous reward depends on the person's discipline of accepting one particular source of them, and on the singularity of the occasions it offers.

There are many degrees of this singularity. Solitaire is only one game among many, and you can always put down one novel and read another—although five hundred pages into *War and Peace* the sunk cost is bound to have some committing effect. With more commitment a particular source of occasions gains power, even, hypothetically, a daydream. A believable example is depicted in Robert Coover's novel, *The Universal Baseball Association Inc., J. Henry Waugh, Proprietor* (1968). Here the protagonist experiences emotions so entirely according to a dice-driven baseball fantasy that it becomes more important to him than the real events of his life. When a rare throw requires him to kill his favorite character, he faces what could be called a crisis of belief, pitting the anguish of grief against his devaluation of the game if he cheats on the outcome. His rules for testing reality within his game had become as confining as someone else's for testing objective reality. To a lesser extent fictional works may achieve a degree of uniqueness by becoming cultural icons—as Schelling describes (1986) for the grief occasioned by the death of Lassie, a fictional collie on an American TV show.

To some extent the singularity principle also governs the power of realistic expectations to occasion endogenous reward. Authentic facts about the world are supposed to be valued for their instrumental usefulness, but at the same time they are a unique pattern of potential occasions. Realistic plans are those that maximize our prospects for external rewards. But milestones in such plans will also be excellent occasions for anticipation (or self-congratulation), a kind of endogenous reward—but only to the extent that we have appetite for that

---

11. To expand this example, I personally did not feel the same disturbance in the film because it depicted parallel plots, in the story and in a company filming the story, assigning one of the two endings to each. I attribute my different reaction to what was a very similar choice of vicarious experiences to the fact that the film did not threaten the convention by which I accept a unique string of occasions for my feelings.

reward. If our plans have worked so well that they no longer excite us, conventional wisdom tells us to take this as an accomplishment and move on to new projects; however, if realistic obstacles arise, creating suspense, the accomplishment will be less but the hedonic outcome may be greater. The hedonic problem, of course, is that we have been relying on the instrumental importance of our plan to make its occasions for reward singular, that is, more than just the results of a game or fantasy. If we catch ourselves introducing obstacles to make the task more exciting, increasing hedonic but reducing instrumental productivity, we belie that importance. To maximize the plan's effectiveness in pacing our reward, we have to believe both in its importance and in the necessity of its obstacles.

Tom Sawyer was brazen about arranging obstacles. In *Huckleberry Finn* he points out the need to Huck:

> Blame it, this whole thing is just as easy and awkward as it can be. And so it makes it so rotten difficult to get up a difficult plan. There ain't no watch-man to be drugged—now there OUGHT to be a watch-man. There ain't even a dog to give a sleeping-mixture to. And there's Jim chained by one leg, with a ten-foot chain, to the leg of his bed: why, all you got to do is to lift up the bedstead.... There won't be nobody nor nothing to interfere with us, and so after all our hard work and trouble this escape'll go off perfectly flat; won't amount to nothing—won't be nothing TO it.

In real life the hedonic maximizer must find ways to keep her instrumental skills from confronting this kind of thinking. Foremost among instrumental skills is her vigilance against distraction from her goals, enforced by the intertemporal bargaining process described above—willpower. Successful bargaining leads to dependable progress toward the rewards that are at stake; but it may also spoil the excitement.

The best occasions are surprises. With mental satisfactions, the only way to stop our minds from rushing ahead to a predictable outcome is to avoid approaches that can be too well learned. Thus, the most valuable occasions will be those that are either (1) uncertain to occur or (2) mysterious—too complex or subtle to be fully anticipated, arguably the rationale of art. To get the most out of endogenous reward, we have to either gamble on uncertainty or find routes that, although certain, will not become too efficient. In short, our occasions have to stay surprising. Intertemporal bargaining results in predictability and in turn depends on it, thus serving to reduce the surprise that refreshes emotional appetites. To avoid confrontation with this effort, the hedonic maximizer must maintain her appetite through *indirection,* that is, through finding activities whose obstacles seem necessary (Ainslie, 2001, pp. 187–197). Since we can sense the emotional consequences of a line of thought before actually pursuing it (Shiffrin & Schneider, 1977), such concealment of purpose probably develops with experience, in the ordinary course of VTE. The important point is that although this process must be considered a form of denial, it not only produces reward in the short term like the denial that abets an impulse, but it also serves to keep two long-term reward strategies—to increase accomplishment and to increase appetite—from interfering with each other. If this motivated reasoning (Kunda, 1990) can avoid obvious violation of our personal rules for testing reality, it may permit a hedonically motivated task to avoid losing its apparent singularity. Thus, the satisfaction that depends on indirection belongs in Jon Elster's insightful category of "states that are essentially by-products" (1981).

The most elementary way to create a significant surprise is to gamble literally—to stake money on a race or a throw of dice. Sophisticated games invite people to risk their reputations, their safety, or their self-esteem in complex social interactions, even when their ostensible expected value is negative. However, such games are vulnerable to close examination that might reveal them to break major personal rules for getting and defending satisfactions. It is true that, in an activity we classify as hedonic to begin with, we recognize the rationality of an intermittent appetizing process—the extreme is the opiate addict's deliberate withdrawal to cheapen her habit—but this is not true of activities we see as instrumental. We would not allow ourselves to throw money away to heighten the satisfaction of earning more, or deliberately reveal an embarrassing secret so we could rebuild our reputations. And yet if we could let the risk of doing so persist alongside our straightforward plans to build our various kinds of wealth, such peril might lead to more net satisfaction than "rational" diligence—even when the objective cost was greater than the instrumental value.

In summary, both instrumental and hedonically motivated activities may serve long-range interests—the former in getting goods that satisfy appetites, the latter in maintaining and refreshing those appetites. They are often the same activity, and not just by coincidence: Instrumental effectiveness is one of the most reliable bases for singularity, so an activity that is hedonically productive, but that can also be authenticated as instrumental, will have a great competitive advantage in the marketplace of choice. If the activity demands significant risk but can still masquerade as instrumental, it may produce more satisfaction than either the most efficient instruments or the cleverest of games by themselves.

GAMBLING MAY BE MORE THAN IMPULSIVE

We can finally address the question of why gambling is such a robust activity in some people—more than an impulse but a life companion, a love affair with

Lady Luck that can take its place among other ostensibly foolish love affairs with partners ranging from rejecting lovers to murderous mountains (e.g., Leamer, 1999). The key in all these activities is the value of risk in refreshing appetite. A perception of risk is almost impossible to achieve without intermittent loss (some physical stimuli such as roller coasters excepted). Since the value of appetite usually cannot be weighed directly against instrumental value, for reasons described above, the question of whether the hedonic gain from the risky activity is worth the instrumental losses is apt to be hard to answer, particularly because hyperbolic discounting will make any answer different from short- and long-range perspectives.

Utility theory expends a great deal of effort in figuring out whether people behave rationally toward the events they value. If we take the gambler at her word that she values money, then her repeated seeking of an activity that can be expected to lose money is a puzzle to utility theory. Proposed explanations tend to focus on cognitive errors—a failure to compute odds correctly, a belief that an improbable string of events will lead to a reversal (the gambler's fallacy) or that an improbable string of events will tend to continue (the hot hand illusion). The gambler's failure to learn from experience is attributed to innumeracy, impulsiveness, or, in an outmoded theory that may have been groping after an important idea, an unconscious wish to lose.[12] The gambler herself believes that the value of gambling comes from the chance to win money, and researchers have taken her word for that. Thus, a recent self-report study found that problem gamblers experienced enough excitement to cause visceral symptoms equivalent to alcohol withdrawal when it stopped—including in a subsample who had both alcohol and gambling problems—but that subjects overwhelmingly "reported that increases in bet size were motivated by increasing chances of bigger wins or for hopes of changing luck rather than for excitement" (Blaszczynski et al., 2008, p. 187). "The majority reported motivations that were more consistent with a cognitive rather than an addiction interpretation of gambling…that the erroneous perceptions pertaining to the gambler's fallacy and luck accounted for their reason to increase bet sizes, not the desire to generate desired levels of arousal or excitement" (*Ibid.*, pp. 188–189). However, this conclusion ignores the necessary presence of a motivational factor that keeps problem gamblers from re-examining their instrumental beliefs.

---

12. "The gambler is a neurotic with an unconscious wish to lose. His logically senseless conviction that he will win is an expression of the fiction of omnipotence in the child who escaped destruction in a real experience. Gambling also activates the latent rebellion against logic, morals and renunciation, a rebellion which is based on the inwardly unrelinquished pleasure principle. Heavy inner retaliation and an unconscious tendency toward self-punishment follow his unconscious aggression. He cannot win in the long run because losing is necessary for his psychic equilibrium" (Berliner, 1945, p. 138).

Someone whose primary goal actually is wealth should eventually do some simple arithmetic, or be driven by experience into taking the word of experts who have calculated the odds.

Gamblers' self-reported rationales are apt to be as unreliable as those of smokers, who regularly fail to report what has been demonstrated to be the essential feature of cigarettes, the nicotine effect (Spielberger,1986). However, smokers confabulate reasons to smoke because the effect of nicotine is not directly sensible (Goldfarb et al., 1970), not because they have a long-range interest in smoking. Gamblers, by contrast, would undermine the instrumental validity of their activity if they failed to view getting money as its key objective. As long as this belief survives, gambling can be a source not just of short-term satisfaction, but of at least relatively long-term satisfaction as well. Gamblers thus have durable incentives to manipulate their instrumental beliefs, although they must also avoid detecting this manipulation. Stimulus-seeking personalities, in whom habituation occurs especially quickly, may consistently prefer a life of "wasting" resources on gambling to one of quiet desperation, even when they say they acknowledge the waste and seem to be making efforts to end it. They face an ongoing struggle between acknowledging the primacy of their hedonic return from gambling and maintaining the belief in its instrumental effectiveness, which is what keeps it from deteriorating into fantasy.

To the extent that the gambler chooses patterns with negative expected value, we have reason to believe that the money has become a MacGuffin— the object of a hedonic game that is justified by its instrumental believability but which is actually shaped by its production of satisfaction in its own right. We may make mistakes about this attribution, of course. The gambler may sometimes make unmotivated cognitive miscalculations, just as conventional theory says. Conversely, in pursuing patterns' MacGuffin value she may happen to choose those that actually have a positive instrumental value. This might be true if she were gambling on stocks, for instance, instead of dice. The giveaway is her reliance on the activity to produce ongoing emotional reward without the kinds of delays that are normal in instrumental investing. In stock market investing she would be led to day trading, which is apt to have negative expected value because of her hedonic need to get frequent payoffs. Even in mainstream investors current hedonic value can be seen competing against instrumental efficiency in such phenomena as the sunk cost fallacy (Arkes & Blumer, 1985). The same distinction is visible within gambling, where a successful race track punter bets on a minority of races, and a poker player who consistently makes money restricts her bets to a small minority of hands (McCormack & Griffiths, 2011). The distinction is evident in many professions that have a high hedonic potential, for instance, in dealers in collectibles, who are distinguished from the amateurs who support them by not showing the instrumentally irrational but hedonically potent phenomenon of loss aversion (Haigh & List, 2005). A MacGuffin is especially insidious when the value it adds to a purely instrumental activity is hard to weigh. With enough talent and discipline, skill-based gambling, day trading, and dealing in collectables are instrumentally productive, and there is no bright line marking how much talent or discipline is enough.

MacGuffin-based addictions are a special class, distinguishable from simple dissipations like drug taking or sexual excess in that they have parasitized the person's instrumental endeavors. Nor is such parasitism necessarily short-sighted. The element of risk may be a durable support for appetite and thus may increase the person's long-term satisfaction over what purely instrumental activities could do. Seen from a hedonic perspective, a gambler's losses are investments in the emotional impact of her eventual wins, and are undesirable only to the extent that they interfere with richer long-term emotional activities or, of course, cause her to go broke. Even without the appetite factor, defining a string of wins and losses by its first win and discounting that win hyperbolically will yield a positive expected value for a string with no net undiscounted cash return (Rachlin, 1990). But this is true only in the period just before this win. Counting the appetite-renewing effect of suspense, the string might seem to be an improvement over predictable wealth maintenance even when viewed from a distance. Authenticated as part of a project for gaining wealth, such strings may have more long-term preferability than a steady income.

Even counting its long-term hedonic value, gambling can be an addiction as ordinarily understood: an activity that is strongly motivated in the short run but which the person is motivated to control or avoid from the perspective of distance. Its appetizing effect pays off especially in the immediate future, and alternative activities are apt to become less possible to the extent that a person becomes preoccupied with it—as is the case with other addictions. Neurophysiological observations in problem gamblers include a sensitization to gambling-related cues and an absence of habituation that are similar to the findings in cocaine addiction (summarized in Ross et al., 2008), suggesting incidentally that drugs may not supply anything that cannot be had from highly effective pacing patterns of endogenous reward. However, pacing intense reward by gamblers requires their outcomes to be of singular importance. The effect cannot be achieved at church casino nights, nor can the rich avoid staking significant portions of their riches. To appease the enmity, as it were, of the person's instrumental interests, gambling to this degree must seem to have instrumental validity.

The determinant of when gambling will become addictive may lie less in its payoffs and costs than in what satisfaction the person sees as alternative to it.

The sequences of intense craving and glorious satisfaction that gambling entails seem to appeal especially to people who feel beset by their failure to solve problems in their ordinary lives, and who therefore need gambling's intensity to keep their attention from being drawn back to this failure. When problem gamblers are interviewed in depth about their motives, they acknowledge some form of mood manipulation just as substance addicts do—blocking out their problems, "buzz," filling a void—in the service of escaping life problems (Wood & Griffiths, 2007), which, of course, come to form part of their appetites for gambling. To be a net source of satisfaction, gambling requires the same moderation as other potentially addictive activities, and lacks benchmarks for where that moderation stops. Furthermore, for most people the long-term hedonic value of risk is better exploited in economic and social activities that have a wider range of choices and outcomes than are available in the stereotyped bets of conventional gambling games.

The value of money has a significant MacGuffin component in many of a wealthy society's activities—when we pursue it as a token of accomplishment or victory rather than for the sake of what we plan to buy with it (see also Lea & Webley, 2006). However, we nowhere see it separated from its instrumental purpose as much as we do in addictive gambling. Just as the example of procrastination offers a chance to study the hyperbolic discounting of reward without having to deal with an arousal factor (Ainslie, 2010b), the study of gambling may let us observe the arousal of appetite without the participation of a physical object, and particularly to observe the coexistence of this arousal with a rationality that does not recognize its value. Ross and his collaborators were right to call addictive gambling "the template of 'basic' addiction, the form on which all other addictions are complications" (2008, p. 163).

An understanding of gambling and other non-substance addictions requires exploration of the vast human topic of endogenous rewards—those rewards that are always at hand in our mental repertoires, without needing to be unlocked by innately programmed stimuli. I have hypothesized that such rewards can exist without leading to self-reward-at-will because the hyperbolic function with which we discount delayed rewards leads to rapid habituation of any endogenous rewards that we do not bind to adequately singular and surprising occasions. I propose that the pursuit of risky instrumental tasks—exemplified by gambling to make money—often generates such occasions, but only if getting the endogenous reward is perceived as subordinate to the task's instrumental purpose. This contingency sets up an incentive to be inefficient at evaluating the instrumental value of the risky tasks, an irrationality that may nevertheless produce both short- and long-term increases in reward because it supports the refreshment of appetite.

ACKNOWLEDGMENT

This material is the result of work supported with resources and the use of facilities at the Department of Veterans Affairs Medical Center, Coatesville, PA, USA. The opinions expressed are not those of the Department of Veterans Affairs or of the US Government. I thank Jenna Haley for background research, and an anonymous referee for incisive criticisms.

REFERENCES

Ainslie, G. (1975) Specious reward: A behavioral theory of impulsiveness and impulse control. *Psychological Bulletin* 82, 463–496.

Ainslie, G. (1992) *Picoeconomics: The Strategic Interaction of Successive Motivational States within the Person*. Cambridge University Press.

Ainslie, G. (1993) A picoeconomic rationale for social constructionism. *Behavior and Philosophy* 21, 63–75.

Ainslie, G. (2001) *Breakdown of Will*. Cambridge University Press.

Ainslie, G. (2003) Uncertainty as wealth. *Behavioural Processes* 64, 369–385.

Ainslie, G. (2005) Précis of *Breakdown of Will*. *Behavioral and Brain Sciences* 28(5), 635–673.

Ainslie, G. (2007) Can thought experiments prove anything about the will? In D. Spurrett, D. Ross, H. Kincaid, & L. Stephens (eds.), *Distributed Cognition and the Will: Individual Volition and Social Context*. MIT Press, pp. 169–196.

Ainslie, G, (2010a) Hyperbolic discounting versus conditioning and framing as the core process in addictions and other impulses. In D. Ross, H. Kincaid, D. Spurrett, & P. Collins (eds.), *What Is Addiction?* MIT Press, pp. 211–245.

Ainslie, G. (2010b) Procrastination, the basic impulse. In C. Andreou & M. White (eds.), *The Thief of Time: Philosophical Essays on Procrastination*. New York: Oxford University Press, pp. 11–27.

Ainslie, G. (2011) Free will as recursive self-prediction: Does a deterministic mechanism reduce responsibility? In Jeffrey Poland & George Graham (eds.), *Addiction and Responsibility*. MIT Press, pp. 55–87.

Ainslie, G. (2012) Pure hyperbolic discount curves predict "eyes open" self-control. *Theory and Decision* 73, 3–34. doi:10.1007/s11238-011-9272-5

Ainslie, G., & Monterosso, J. (2002) Hyperbolic discounting lets empathy be a motivated process. *Behavioral and Brain Sciences* 25, 20–21.

Ainslie, G., and Monterosso, J. (2003) Building blocks of self-control: Increased tolerance for delay with bundled rewards. *Journal of the Experimental Analysis of Behavior* 79, 83–94.

Andreou, C., & White, M. (2010) *The Thief of Time: Philosophical Essays on Procrastination*. New York: Oxford University Press.

Arkes, H.R., & Blumer, C. (1985) The psychology of sunk cost. *Organizational Behavior and Human Decision Processes* 35, 124–140.

Berliner, B. (1945) Abstract of *The Gambler: A Misunderstood Neurotic*: E. Bergler, that appeared in *Journal of Criminal Psychopathology*, IV, 1943, pp. 379–393. *Psychoanalytic Quarterly* 14, 138–139.

Blaszczynski, A., Walker, M., Sharpe, L., & Nower, L. (2008) Withdrawal and tolerance phenomenon in problem gambling. *International Gambling Studies* 8, 179–192.

Coover, R. (1968) *The Universal Baseball Association, Inc., J. Henry Waugh, Prop.* Random House.

Ellis, A., & Grieger, R. (1977) *R.E.T.: Handbook of Rational-Emotive Therapy.* Springer.

Elster, J. (1981) States that are essentially by-products. *Social Science Information* 20, 431–473. Reprinted in Elster, J. (1983) *Sour Grapes: Studies in the Subversion of Rationality.* Cambridge University Press, pp. 43–108.

Elster, J. (2010) Self-poisoning of the mind. *Transactions of the Royal Society B* 365, 221–226.

Glantz, K., & Pearce, J. (1989) *Exiles from Eden: Psychotherapy from an Evolutionary Perspective.* New York: Norton.

Glimcher, P.W. (2009) Choice: Towards a standard back-pocket model. In P. W. Glimcher, C. Camerer, R. A. Poldrack, & E. Fehr (eds.), *Neuroeconomics: Decision Making and the Brain.* Elsevier, pp. 503–521.

Goldfarb, T.L., Jarvik, M.E., & Glick, S.D. (1970) Cigarette nicotine content as a determinant of human smoking behavior. *Psychopharmacologia Berlin* 17, 89–93.

Green, L., & Myerson, J. (2004) A discounting framework for choice with delayed and probabilistic rewards. *Psychological Bulletin* 130, 769–792.

Haigh, M., & List, J.A. (2005) Do professional traders exhibit myopic loss aversion? An experimental analysis. *Journal of Finance* 60 (1): 523–534.

Herrnstein, R. (1961) Relative and absolute strengths of response as a function of frequency of reinforcement. *Journal of the Experimental Analysis of Behavior* 4, 267–272.

Herrnstein, R.J. (1977) The evolution of behaviorism. *American Psychologist* 32, 593–603.

Herrnstein, R.J. (1997) *The Matching Law: Papers in Psychology and Economics.* H. Rachlin & D. Laibson (eds.). Sage.

Hofmeyr, A., Ainslie, G., Charlton, R., & Ross, D. (2010) The relationship between addiction and reward: An experiment comparing smokers and non-smokers. *Addiction* 106, 402–409.

Johnson, A., & Redish, D.A. (2007) Neural ensembles in CA3 transiently encode paths forward of the animal at a decision point. *Journal of Neuroscience* 12, 483–488.

Kirby, K.N. (1997) Bidding on the future: Evidence against normative discounting of delayed rewards. *Journal of Experimental Psychology: General* 126, 54–70.

Kirby, K.N., & Guastello, B. (2001) Making choices in anticipation of similar future choices can increase self-control. *Journal of Experimental Psychology: Applied* 7, 154–164.

Kunda, Z. (1990) The case for motivated reasoning. *Psychological Bulletin* 108, 480–498.

Lea, S.E.G., & Webley, P. (2006) Money as tool, money as drug: The biological psychology of a strong incentive. *Behavioral and Brain Sciences* 29, 161–209.

Leamer, L. (1999) *Ascent: The Spiritual and Physical Quest of Legendary Mountaineer Willi Unsoeld.* Quill.

Loewenstein, G. (1999). Because it is there: The challenge of mountaineering...for utility theory. *Kyklos* 52, 315–344.

Madden, G.J., Begotka, A.M., Raiff, B.R., & Kasten, L.L. (2003) Delay discounting of real and hypothetical rewards. *Journal of Experimental & Clinical Psychopharmacology* 11, 139–145.

Mazur, J.E. (1987) An adjusting procedure for studying delayed reinforcement. In M.L. Commons, J.E. Mazur, J.A. Nevin, & H. Rachlin (eds.), *Quantitative Analyses of Behavior V: The Effect of Delay and of Intervening Events on Reinforcement Value*. Erlbaum, 55–73.

McCormack, A., & Griffiths, M.D. (2011) What differentiates professional poker players from recreational poker players? A qualitative interview study. *International Journal of Mental Health and Addiction* XX, 1–15. doi:10.1007/s11469-011-9312-y

Melzack, R., Weisz, A.Z., & Sprague, L.T. (1963) Stratagems for controlling pain: Contributions of auditory stimulation and suggestion. *Experimental Neurology* 8, 239–247.

Mintoff, J. (2004) Rule worship and the stability of intention. *Philosophia* 31, 401–426.

Phillips, P.E.M., Stuber, G.D., Helen, M.L.A.V., Wightman, M.R., & Carelli, R.M. (2003) Subsecond dopamine release promotes cocaine seeking. *Nature* 422, 614–618.

Preston, S.B., & de Waal, F.B.M. (2002) Empathy: Its ultimate and proximate basis. *Behavioral and Brain Sciences* 25, 1–20.

Rachlin, H. (1990) Why do people gamble and keep gambling despite heavy losses? *Psychological Science* 1, 294–297.

Ross, D., Sharp, C., Vuchinich, R., & Spurrett, D. (2008) *Midbrain Mutiny: The Picoeconomics and Neuroeconomics of Disordered Gambling*. MIT Press.

Schelling, T.C. (1986) The mind as a consuming organ. In J. Elster (ed.), *The Multiple Self*. Cambridge University Press, 177–195.

Shiffrin, R.M., & Schneider, W. (1977) Controlled and automatic human information processing: II. Perceptual learning, automatic attending, and a general theory. *Psychological Review* 84, 127–190.

Spielberger, C.D. (1986) Psychological determinants of smoking behavior. In R.D. Tollison (ed.), *Smoking and Society: Toward a More Balanced Assessment*. Lexington Books, 89–134.

Spreng, R.N., Mar, R.A., & Kim, A.S.N. (2009) A common neural basis of autobiographical memory, prospection, navigation, theory of mind, and the default mode: A quantitative meta-analysis. *Journal of Cognitive Neuroscience* 21 (3), 489–510.

Tolman, E.C. (1939) Prediction of vicarious trial and error by means of the schematic sowbug. *Psychological Review* 46, 318–336.

Tomkins, S.S. (1978) Script theory: Differential magnification of affects. *Nebraska Symposium on Motivation* 26, 201–236.

Wood, R.T.A., & Griffiths, M.D. (2007) A qualitative investigation of problem gambling as an escape-based coping strategy. *Psychology and Psychotherapy: Theory, Research and Practice* 80, 107–125.

3

The Picoeconomics of Gambling Addiction and Supporting Neural Mechanisms

DON ROSS

George Ainslie's picoeconomic account of the widespread attractiveness of gambling, and more specifically of addiction to gambling (this volume, Chapter 2), may cause puzzlement in readers who are accustomed to thinking of addiction as a brain disorder. The picoeconomic model, after all, involves dynamics that ascribe considerable cognitive sophistication to subcognitive processes. For the addicted and nonaddicted gambler alike, the money at stake is, according to Ainslie, a MacGuffin—the apparent reward that justifies the activity, but which is in fact not the actual object of pursuit. "Gamblers," Ainslie tells us, "may...have durable incentives to manipulate their instrumental beliefs, although they must also avoid detecting this manipulation.... They face an ongoing struggle between acknowledging the primacy of their hedonic return from gambling and maintaining the belief in its instrumental effectiveness that keeps it from deteriorating into fantasy." Even the reader who finds the story beguiling in its characterization of the subtlety of addictive self-deception—as manifest in all of the great literary depictions of addiction, such as de Quincy (1821) and Dostoyevsky (1867)—may struggle to see how it could be thought to be the consequence of a brain disorder. Why, if Ainslie is right, can we not successfully treat gambling addicts simply by convincing them that gambling is *not* instrumentally effective, thereby dismantling their delicately maintained house of cards? Is Ainslie's account not a throwback to the kind of clever Freudian constructions of subconscious mental complexity that clinical neuroscience consigns to a prescientific era in psychiatry?

In this comment, I will provide grounds for thinking that this kind of worry rests on a false dichotomy. Ainslie's picoeconomics of gambling provides the basis for a case study of the way in which mentalistic and neuroscientific models of behavioral phenomena can be used to complement one another. The complementarity in question is not well pursued in the way that philosophers often attempt, by constructing more or less elaborate stories about metaphysical relationships between "mental states" (or events) and "physical states" (or events) (e.g., as in Kim 1998 and elsewhere). The bargaining subselves of Ainslie's account should not be regarded as proposed processing modules in the brain. They are instead competing narratives the addict could tell to rationalize her emotions, and their mutual incompatibility supports the ambivalence—strenuous efforts to stop addictive consumption, punctuated by relapses and binges— that frustrate both the economic modeler's and the exasperated helper's efforts to locate underlying rationality. As narratives, the picoeconomic subselves are virtual entities, in the sense of Dennett (1991)—recurrent patterns that triangulate among observed behavior, confabulated self-reconstructions, and social probes that call for normative rationalization. However, notwithstanding the fact that picoeconomics does not *reduce*[1] to any neuroscientific description, it is properties of the brain that explain why the patterns Ainslie characterizes constitute a common human syndrome. Such facts are indeed crucial to a more complete explanation of gambling addiction, because they provide a clearer basis for the distinction between the addict and the nonaddict than Ainslie is able to suggest using picoeconomic ideas alone, and to explain why addicts cannot generally be simply hectored into adopting less destructive behavior.

Let us first reinforce the cogency of Ainslie's account of what attracts people to gambling by means of a simple thought experiment. Suppose that a group of devoted gamblers encounter a casino operated by an altruistic patron who wants to transfer wealth to them in the way that, according to his observations, they seem to most enjoy. In this wonderful casino all bets always win: the fruit icons on the slot machines always resolve in agreement, the roulette wheel always stops on the sign for the square that holds the most chips, and so on. Imagine further that individual payoffs are small enough, and with sufficiently low variance, to prevent the gamblers from either becoming so rich that they devote all their time to scholarship, sex, or drugs instead, or from obsessively pursuing rare jackpots. I take it as obvious that although the gamblers would initially be delighted, in short order their attitudes toward the casino would change. Soon they would no longer look forward with pleasurable anticipation to their sessions on the gaming floor. They would no doubt continue to put in long such sessions. But they would treat getting up and going to the casino as an

1. Or quasi-reduce; see Ross & Spurrett (2004).

obligation, and sitting at the slot machine or the blackjack table as *work*. From time to time they would invent occasions for taking some time off to relax and have fun. This pattern would characterize addicts[2] and nonaddicts alike.

This thought experiment should almost be enough, in itself, to convince us that for gamblers money is a MacGuffin, just as Ainslie argues. What motivates people to gamble is the reward of the suspenseful activity; minus the suspense, the same activity would be a dull routine. But the suspense is not *intrinsic* to the activity abstracted from its social and economic context. Most gamblers cannot sustain interest in playing for matchsticks or worthless chips; something of real value must be at stake. In consequence, longer-range rewards that could be purchased if the stakes were not gambled away compete against the immediate value of the entertaining excitement, and the gambler is in the situation of ambivalent choice that Ainslie has devoted his career as a scholar to elaborating through the model of hyperbolic discounting.

Ainslie thus provides a highly persuasive account of what people want from gambling, even if we regard it as incomplete insofar as it is not grounded in neuroscience. However, I also suggest that Ainslie's account of the difference between nonaddicted and addicted gamblers is incomplete in a more specific and dissatisfying way. Addicted gamblers, Ainslie avers, are those who become "preoccupied" with gambling and use the stimulation it provides as a substitute for rewards they cannot enjoy from other aspects of their lives, either because the rewards in question are put out of reach by circumstances and limited ability or because they are achievable but arouse insufficient appetite. This indeed corresponds with the self-reports of many diagnosed pathological gamblers. However, clinical data are ambiguous with regard to cause and effect here. *Perhaps* gambling addicts begin as bored people who finally find, in the casino or the betting track, an environment that arouses their emotions. However, the evidence is at least as consistent with the hypothesis that increasing attention to gambling causes some people—those who become addicts—to lose the interest they formerly took in their family and social lives, their careers, and their previous hobbies (Lesieur 1979). Thus, although picoeconomics convincingly relates the source of gambling's attractiveness to the nature of the addict's internal motivational conflict, it does not offer a fully satisfactory account of what distinguishes the addicted from the nonaddicted gambler. Here is where neuroscience can be called on to add crucial explanatory leverage.

The basic currency of proximate reward for the relevant system in the brain is dopamine—more specifically, spikes of phasic dopamine uptake across receptors in the ventral striatum (VS). These spikes occur not in response to anything

---

2. Ross et al. (2008) argue that the imagined circumstance would be a (sadly unrealistic) *cure* for gambling addiction.

that constitutes a reward for the person in light of her cognitive goals, but to stimuli that the striatal circuit becomes conditioned to associate with unpredictable personal-scale payoffs—such as gambling outcomes. This constitutes the neural realization of the phenomenon Ainslie describes in this volume, whereby people become habituated to rewards they have learned how to reliably harvest, and are motivated to devote energy to learning new relationships between environmental contingencies and means of exploiting them for gain. Unpredicted gains produce rewarding dopamine spikes, whereas fully expected ones do not, because the dopamine system evolved to motivate mobile animals to speculate and explore. This mechanism is the basis for everyday learning in humans and other mobile animals.

In this context, the gambling environment has special characteristics. Precisely because outcomes are set up so as to be systematically unpredictable, the system never exhausts opportunities for learning, and its expectations are subject to continuous nonstabilizing readjustment through dopamine spikes, in response to cues the gambler generates for herself by rolling dice or putting coins in slots. It may be objected here that in games of pure chance the learning opportunity is an illusion: there is only one simple pattern relating cues to outcomes, namely, the limiting relative frequency of wins and losses. The answer to this objection lies in the mechanism's impenetrability to frontal cognitive processes. The striatal dopamine circuit is a gadget driven by a simple conditioning rule—likely a temporal difference algorithm (Sutton & Bartow 1998; McClure, Berns, & Montague 2003)—that evolved long in advance of the frontal cortex. One of the things it cannot learn—though of course the person as a whole can—is that in the fixed rule spaces of commercial gambling, once frequencies are successfully estimated there is nothing more to learn.[3]

The fact that the person can appreciate a limit to practical learning that the dopamine circuit cannot is plausibly the condition that makes sense of the fact that the typical nonaddicted gambler can appreciate the futility of strategizing in games of chance while continuing to derive pleasant excitement from playing them. She exercises her willpower—to borrow Ainslie's conceptual language—not by suppressing striatal dopamine spikes that are occasioned by gambles, but by controlling the dopamine system's influence over motor responses. She decides when to play, and then lets her "stupid" dopamine mechanism provide her with the resulting excitement. Thus, she retains her power to *stop* playing

---

3. Empirical evidence for the inability of the dopamine circuit to learn higher-order statistical patterns is reported on the basis of a single-cell neural recording experiment conducted by Lee et al. (2005). Monkey neurons that encode learned best responses in games where randomization among strategies is the optimal response stabilize short of the ideal, oscillating around the equilibrium mix by continually overadjusting and underadjusting to the most recent rounds of play.

once she has exhausted her chosen stake or the time she had budgeted for this form of entertainment.

It is worth emphasizing that this mechanism for willpower involves *interference* with relatively automatic processes. The natural default for dopamine system interaction with other brain circuits is that striatal spikes automatically trigger motor system preparation. This makes good evolutionary sense: having noticed a cue that predicts the appearance of a reward that may be fleeting or trying to escape, an animal should be poised to harvest it through chasing, grabbing, or pouncing. However, evidence suggests that such motor preparation is inhibited by GABA neurons synapsing on cells in the ventromedial prefrontal cortex (VMPFC) that are also synaptic sites for dopamine (Yang et al. 1999; Gulledge & Jaffe 2001). Thus, we might hypothesize that when an ambivalent gambler impulsively throws the dice another time, she allows the dopamine circuit to exercise its customary influence on behavior, whereas when concern for longer-range influences wins out, this is expressed in release of ventromedial GABA.

So far we have merely described neural mechanisms that might implement the psychodynamics as Ainslie describes them for the nonaddicted gambler, including the gambler who is ambivalent and sometimes impulsive. This should not be regarded as furnishing genuine explanatory completion for Ainslie's model, but simply as indicating its possible neural correlates. We noted, however, that Ainslie does not offer a satisfactory hypothesis as to what is distinctively wrong with the gambling *addict*. It is here that neuroscience provides a complementary hypothesis that strengthens the picoeconomic model by closing what would otherwise be an explanatory gap.

The most salient behavioral distinction between gambling or drug addicts and regularly indulgent but nonaddicted counterparts is that the former but not the latter find it difficult to carry out normal activities, or to enjoy normal social relationships, because they are continuously preoccupied with thoughts of consuming their learned addictive rewards. Furthermore, these thoughts are experienced as visceral discomfort,[4] commonly referred to as "cravings." Most

---

4. Philosophers of mind might get anxious about this formulation. Some would say that a thought could be experienced *as* a discomfort, as opposed to *causing* discomfort, only if it was uncomfortable due to its content, for example, someone entertaining a sexual fantasy she found shameful. That is *not* the kind of discomfort associated with cravings. Thus, some philosophers would insist that the addict experiences *two* states that are correlated, and perhaps causally related, in their occurrence. I resist this insistence, preferring my slightly ambiguous formulation to a more precise one that would be unsupported, for now, by any scientific evidence. I reject suggestions that neuroscientifically informed psychology should labor under an obligation to traffic in anything isomorphic to philosophers' intuitively derived discrete experiential "states."

addicts report the highly stressful anhedonia associated with very persistent cravings to be a major motivating factor in their tendency to relapse. The most convincing evidence for the hypothesis that some pathological gamblers are true addicts is the repeated clinical observation of this syndrome among them.

Picoeconomics is not entirely without resources, in its own terms, for understanding preoccupation and craving. One could suggest that the addict is someone whose internal bargaining interests can never stably close a deal on choice of a larger later reward. However, this seems to be a—perfectly reasonable—redescription rather than a step along the road of explanatory progress. *Why*, we are bound to wonder, can some people's subpersonal bargaining dynamics usually reach equilibria that avoid disaster while addicts repeatedly fail to do so? Some neuroscientific evidence helps us to see *why* the suggested picoeconomic description is apt. The brains of addicts show signs of various neuroadaptations, that is, changes in strength of synaptic connections that are correlated with the distribution of neurotransmitter types at the synapses (Steketee 2002). Some of these long-term potentiations (LTPs) vary with specific addictive drugs, and some seem to be common to those drugs that are implicated in addiction. Cocaine addicts, whose neurochemistry most resembles that of people with very high scores on pathological gambling screens, typically show negative LTP in ventromedial GABA synapses correlated with hyperactivity of dopamine 3 (D3) receptors in the nucleus accumbens (NAcc)[5] (Everitt et al. 2001). D3 cells are the dopamine receptors that have for some years been most directly linked to motor response control: animals given agents that block D3 uptake develop Parkinson's symptoms (Baik et al. 1995). D3 activity competes with D1 and D2 activity in the NAcc. This may be important because, in some neurochemical contexts, D1 and D2 activity excites GABA responses in the VMPFC (Steketee 2002).

The GABA-D3 connection does not exhaust the apparent neuroadaptations associated with addiction. For example, serotonin (5-HT) release inhibits excitatory effects of dopamine on subcortical areas, and indeed low tonic serotonin is correlated with both addictive behavior and, independently, with probability of relapse (Chambers et al. 2003). However, the LTP relating reduced GABA and heightened D3 is particularly interesting where cravings are concerned. In the standard theory of the reward circuit, dopaminergic learning integrates expected reward magnitude with both cue salience and motor system preparation (McClure, Daw, & Montague 2003). Cravings are plausibly the phenomenal experience of the body being primed to consume its addictive target, which

---

5. This is a part of the ventral striatum that much evidence suggests to be the core site where the violations in expected reward magnitudes that constitute the basis for temporal difference learning are registered.

persists when the consumption in question does not occur. On this hypothesis, the question of whether thoughts of addictive consumption cause cravings or the other way around may be moot: D3 activity that suppresses GABA response and stimulates motor preparation may be the common mechanism for both preoccupation and craving.

Ainslie (2011) argues that "[t]he unusually great rewardingness for a particular person of a particular modality—drinking, gambling, buying—might reasonably be called a disease, but the resourcelessness that follows her repeated defections in intertemporal bargaining is more like a budgetary crisis. When the addict cannot find enough credibility to stake against her temptations to consume, we might say that she is no longer responsible for her choices—but because of a kind of bankruptcy, not sickness." In light of our reflections here on the neuroscience of addiction, there is solid insight in this comment. The addict is indeed someone who has lost an important resource—strong inhibitory synaptic influences—for damping impulsive choice. But, as Ainslie says, choice it remains: a great deal of data shows that addicts are strongly influenced, in the standard direction, by changes in prices and other rational incentives (Heyman 2009).

Ainslie's comment might be interpreted by some readers as suggesting agreement with the "willpower stock" informal model of self-control and addiction that has been promoted by Baumeister and colleagues (Baumeister & Vohs 2003; Baumeister et al. 2006). According to this conception, willpower is like a muscle that can be strengthened by successful use and weakened by lack of exercise; moreover, what it produces when it is strong enough is a renewable but finite resource. However, Ainslie (2012) criticizes this model, arguing that it is a gratuitously hydraulic interpretation of a mental accounting phenomenon: after periods of being "good" people typically think they are entitled to holidays. As Ainslie objects, Baumeister's account presents addictive targets as exogenous temptations, ignoring the dynamics by which addicts *learn* to make them salient through manipulation of the internal marketplace of reward.

Unfortunately, Ainslie (2011) follows his helpful introduction of his bankruptcy metaphor with an expression of exaggerated skepticism about the prospects for neurochemically based diagnoses of addiction. "There is," he says, "no natural test for whether such bankruptcy 'exists' or not, nor even a test for when we should recognize it." This dismisses a thriving experimental literature aimed at detecting telltale indicators of addictive neuroadaptations[6] and implies an unhappily armchair-based dismissal of the prospects for effective neuropharmacological intervention against addiction. Addicts and nonaddicts may indeed sort along a continuum without sharp boundaries so far as their

6. Madras et al. (2006) is one of several handbook-level surveys.

self-narratives are concerned. However, if neuroeconomic models of addiction (see Ross 2010) are approximately correct in positing equilibrium dynamics for addictive learning, then addicts may *also* form a distinctive taxon with respect to potentially reversible but long-range physiological changes that have been induced in their brains. Some part of the apparently strong genetic influence on risk for addiction (MacKillop et al. 2010) may reside in inherited rates at which such neuroadaptation onsets in response to consumption of addictive agents or indulgence in addictive behaviors. It needlessly undermines the picoeconomic model to suggest that it must *compete* with the search for "natural tests" of the presence of addiction.

This brings us to what I regard as the principal—and important—philosophical lesson of the present comment. Ainslie argues that the addict comes to feel (relatively) powerless in the face of gambling or a drug because, in light of her own history, she can no longer believe in the promises of internal interests that urge patience for the sake of a greater reward; the greater reward, she believes, will never be delivered because the promise will not be kept. Thus, there is no point in her suffering deprivation in the immediate moment. Now, many readers will think that this account would be shown to be a redundant, inexact— even if insightful—high-level *story* if, in fact, what is wrong with the addict is attenuated strength of GABA synapses in the VMPFC and/or low tonic 5-HT. This conviction might contribute to the idea that mentalistic and physiological accounts of addiction are competitors. But this reductionistic attitude is unwarranted. The addict's lack of confidence will indeed tend to exert *causal influence* on her behavior. As the dominant narrative about herself that she will tell, it will influence her level of investment in alternative possible life courses, and infect the confidence of those who might try to help her. This causal influence will affect her brain: the more she chooses to addictively consume, the worse will be her preoccupation and cravings when she is not addictively consuming.

This second, neurodynamic, part of the story is crucial for descriptive and explanatory completeness, because it implies a qualitative difference between the addict and the nonaddict that picoeconomics alone does not: addicts are people who have undergone a specific kind of neuroadaptational change. This implies that although Ainslie's description of the chooser who has lost confidence in her willpower will indeed apply to most addicts—and will *also* be an important predictor of aspects of their behavior—it will also apply to some *non*addicts. This is mainly because not every possible object of an impulsive choice is potentially addictive. For example, Ross et al. (2008) argue that the relationships between cues associated with interpersonal sex and actual interpersonal sexual experiences are too variable in kind, too irregular in pacing, and too extended in time to have the sort of structure that the relatively simple dopamine learning system can encode in an automated D3 spiking response.

Thus, the existence of addiction to interpersonal sex is doubtful.[7] Nevertheless, popular cultural anecdote and clinical experience are replete with instances of people who suffer from guilt and marital distress because they indulge in more sexual opportunities than they think would be best; and Ainslie's description of the "bankrupt will" very plausibly applies to such people. The relationship between willpower and addiction is complex.

The conclusion, then, is against *any* simple philosophical account of the relationship between picoeconomic and neuroscientific models of addiction. They are not alternative descriptions of exactly the same thing. Picoeconomics should not be expected to reduce to a neuroscientific model. Neurochemical models are not distinguished from picoeconomic models by being "causal" or "mechanistic": picoeconomics is a causal, mechanistic hypothesis in good standing, even if the causal patterns in which it traffics are nonlinear and block deterministic prediction in individual cases.[8] Addiction is characteristic of the gamut of psychological patterns, which are best understood on multiple, mutually enlightening scales of integration with complex environments and complex nervous systems.

ACKNOWLEDGMENT

Thanks to George Ainslie for critical comments on an earlier draft.

REFERENCES

Ainslie, G. (2011). Free will as recursive self-prediction. In G. Graham & J. Poland, eds., *Addiction and Responsibility*, pp. 54–87. Cambridge, MA: MIT Press.

Ainslie, G. (2012). Pure hyperbolic discount curves predict 'eyes-open' self-control. *Theory and Decision* 73: 3–34.

Baik, J., Picetti, R., Saiardi, A., Thirlet, G., Dierich, A., Depaulis, A., Le Meur, M., & Borrelli, E. (1995). Parkinson-like locomotor impairment in mice lacking dopamine D2 receptors. *Nature* 377: 424–428.

Baumeister, R., Gailliot, M., DeWall, C., & Oaten, M. (2006). Self-regulation and personality: How interventions increase regulatory success, and how depletion moderates the effects of traits on behavior. *Journal of Personality* 74: 1773–1801.

Baumeister, R., & Vohs, K. (2003). Willpower, choice and self-control. In G. Loewenstein, D. Read, & R. Baumeister, eds., *Time and Decision*, pp. 201–216. New York: Russell Sage Foundation.

7. This point would not apply to consumption of pornography; there may well be pornography addicts. To further complicate the picture, some pornography addicts might use interpersonal sex as medication for their frustrating preoccupation, leading them to seek more sex than they otherwise would.

8. See Ainslie (2011).

Chambers, R.A., Taylor, J., & Potenza, M. (2003). Developmental neurocircuitry of motivation in adolescence: A critical period of addiction vulnerability. *American Journal of Psychiatry* 160: 1041–1052.

Dennett, D. (1991). *Consciousness Explained*. Boston: Little Brown.

De Quincy, T. (1821/1971). *Confessions of an English Opium Eater*. Harmondsworth: Penguin.

Dostoyevsky, F. (1867/2010). *The Gambler*. R. Meyer, trans. Harmondsworth: Penguin.

Everitt, B., Dickinson, A., & Robbins, T. (2001). The neuropsychological basis of addictive behavior. *Brain Research Reviews* 36: 129–138.

Gulledge, A., & Jaffe, D. (2001). Multiple effects of dopamine on layer V pyramidal cell excitability in rat prefrontal cortex. *Journal of Neurophysiology* 86: 586–595.

Heyman, G. (2009). *Addiction: A Disorder of Choice*. Cambridge, MA: Harvard University Press.

Kim, J. (1998). *Mind in a Physical World*. Cambridge, MA: MIT Press.

Lee, D., Conroy, M., McGreevy, B., & Barraclough, D. (2005). Learning and decision making in monkeys during a rock-paper-scissors game. *Cognition and Brain Research* 25: 416–430.

Lesieur, H. (1979). The compulsive gambler's spiral of options and involvement. *Psychiatry* 42: 79–87.

MacKillop, J., McGeary, J., & Ray, L. (2010). Genetic influences on addiction: Alcoholism as an exemplar. In D. Ross, H. Kincaid, D. Spurrett, & P. Collins, eds., *What Is Addiction?*, pp. 53–98. Cambridge, MA: MIT Press.

Madras, B., Colvis, C., Pollock, J., Rutter, J., Shurtleff, D., & von Zastrow, M. (2006). *Cell Biology of Addiction*. Cold Spring Harbor, NY: Cold Spring Harbor Laboratory Press.

McClure, S., Berns, G., & Montague, P.R. (2003). Temporal prediction errors in a passive learning task activate human striatum. *Neuron* 38: 339–346.

McClure, S., Daw, N., & Montague, P.R. (2003). A computational substrate for incentive salience. *Trends in Neuroscience* 26: 423–428.

Ross, D. (2010). Economic models of addiction. In D. Ross, H. Kincaid, D. Spurrett, & P. Collins, eds., *What Is Addiction?*, pp. 131–158. Cambridge, MA: MIT Press.

Ross, D., Sharp, C., Vuchinich, R., & Spurrett, D. (2008). *Midbrain Mutiny: The Picoeconomics and Neuroeconomics of Disordered Gambling*. Cambridge, MA: MIT Press.

Ross, D., & Spurrett, D. (2004). What to say to a skeptical metaphysician: A defense manual for cognitive and behavioral scientists. *Behavioral and Brain Sciences* 27: 603–627.

Steketee, J. (2002). Neurotransmitter systems of the medial prefrontal cortex: Potential role in sensitization to psychostimulants. *Brain Research Reviews* 42: 203–228.

Sutton, R., & Bartow, A. (1998). *Reinforcement Learning: An Introduction*. Cambridge, MA: MIT Press.

Yang, C., Seamans, J., & Gorelova, N. (1999). Developing a neuronal model for the pathophysiology of schizophrenia based on the nature of electrophysiological actions of dopamine in the prefrontal cortex. *Neuropsychopharmacology* 21: 161–194.

4

Team Reasoning, Framing, and Self-Control

An Aristotelian Account

NATALIE GOLD

In the *Nicomachean Ethics,* Aristotle discusses the problem of how someone can intentionally act against his best judgment. The Ancient Greeks called this *akrasia,* or lack of control, and its opposite is self-control. Aristotle's example of akrasia involves someone who is tempted, against his better judgment, to eat something sweet. When the person eats, he is still "under the influence (in a sense) of reason" (1147b1-2).[1] Hence, *self-control* involves the exercise of control over temptations. This usage of the term, which is fairly standard in philosophical discourse, contrasts with a modern colloquial usage, whereby the opposite of having self-control involves losing the ability to intentionally control one's actions.[2] In this paper I will adopt the philosophical usage of "self-control" to refer to overcoming temptations while remembering that, as J. L. Austin said, we can help ourselves to two portions of dessert without ravening and that "We often succumb to temptation with calm and even with finesse" (Austin, 1956–1957, p. 24 n.13).

---

1. All quotations from the *Nicomachean Ethics* refer to the translation by Ross in Barnes (1984) and the standard Bekker page reference is given.

2. The modern usage is at some points implied in Aristotle, for instance, when he says that the akrates "acts with passion and not choice" (1111b13). In determining Aristotle's position, much turns on the interpretation of "choice." But my aim is not to provide an accurate reconstruction of Aristotle; rather, it is to explore an interesting idea that can be divined in his work. (For an interesting reconstruction that is broadly sympathetic to the ideas in this paper, see Moss, 2009.) Interpretive issues, including interpretations that are at odds with those that I use, will be confined to the footnotes.

Aristotle gives a causal account of akrasia, as located in the reasoning process of the akrates. For Aristotle, reasoning is characterized as a syllogism, involving a major and a minor premise. The major premise is a universal principle and the minor premise is a particular one about the situation at hand. In book VI, Aristotle has declared that the second, minor premise is the "starting point" of reasoning (1143b4-6) and that the universals are reached from these particulars, of which we have perception.

Aristotle illustrates the reasoning of the akrates as follows:

Particular premise:	This thing is sweet
Universal premise:	Everything sweet ought to be tasted

———————————————————————————

Conclusion:	This thing ought to be tasted[3]

Opposed to this is a second syllogism, whose conclusion is that the akrates should not taste the thing. But, according to Aristotle, the akrates uses only the universal and not the particular premise of the second syllogism. Although the akrates "has" knowledge of the particular premise s/he does not "use" it (1146b31ff), where "using" should be understood as thinking of the premise or having it before one's mind (Bostock, 2000 pp. 125–126).[4] Hence, Aristotle says that the akrates is ignorant of particular facts that are "within the sphere of perception" (1147a26).

However, Aristotle does not specify the content of the second syllogism, the particular facts that the akrates does not perceive, or the premise that s/he does not use. The Ancients were more concerned with the puzzle of how akratic action could exist than with how people exercise self-control.

This contrasts with decision theory, whose framework suggests that people will always give into temptations and where the puzzle is to explain how people exert self-control. In decision theory, problems of overcoming temptation are naturally modeled within the framework of "dynamic choice," where one person makes a sequence of decisions over time. It is conventional to analyze problems of dynamic choice as if, at each time t at which the person has to make a decision, that decision is made by a distinct *transient agent*, "the person at time t." Each transient agent is treated as an independent rational decision maker. In this framework, self-control is a problem of *diachronic consistency*,

3. It is generally thought that Aristotle intended that the conclusion is also an action. For a minority dissenting view that the conclusion of the syllogism is not identical with the action, see Charles (1984), and for an argument that the conclusion of the syllogism cannot also be an action if akrasia is to exist, see Wiggins (1980).

4. Some commentators favor an interpretation where the proposition that is known but not used is the conclusion of the second syllogism (e.g., Charles, 1984; Urmson, 1988).

where the profile of choices that seems best from the point of view of an early transient agent relies on a choice by a later agent that will not seem best from the later agent's point of view. The early transient agent would like to implement a plan that she cannot rely on her later self to carry through. Standard examples of the problem are going on diets, giving up smoking, and studying for an exam.

One objection to the decision theoretic account is that it provides a neat model of temptation at the expense of an impoverished notion of agency. Agency is entirely vested in the transient agents; there is no notion of a self that extends over time. It is as if every transient agent asks, "What should *I*-now do?" The instruments for achieving self-control are limited to *precommitments*, actions that constrain the choices or alter the incentives that will be available to future selves; making a resolution in the hope that it will affect future behavior is "naive" (Strotz, 1955–1956). There is no sense of an extended agency over time, whereby earlier selves make plans for the person over time that influence later selves because of their status as plans.

In this paper, I place the decision theoretic account of temptation within a framework that allows multiple levels of agency and use this to show how the rational agents of decision theory can achieve self-control. The idea of multiple levels of agency has been articulated at the interpersonal level, where theories of team reasoning allow agents to ask, "What should *we* do?" and identify distinctive modes of reasoning used by people in teams (Bacharach, 2006; Sugden, 1993). I apply team reasoning at the intrapersonal level, modeling the self as a team of transient agents over time. The resulting account of self-control is Aristotelian in flavor, in that it involves reasoning schemas and perception, and it is compatible with some of the psychological findings about self-control.

In order to motivate the application of team reasoning to the problem of self-control, I begin by showing how the problem of self-control can be seen as a prisoner's dilemma. The prisoner's dilemma set-up is not essential to the idea of the person as a team over time, but it is an important aspect of the decision theoretic puzzle of self-control. The prisoner's dilemma is also one of the puzzles of game theory that motivated the development of team reasoning, so analyzing the problem of self-control as a prisoner's dilemma makes very clear the analogy between team reasoning in the interpersonal and the intrapersonal cases.

SELF-CONTROL AS AN INTRAPERSONAL PRISONER'S DILEMMA

In the prisoner's dilemma, individual agents must choose between two strategies, commonly called *defect* and *cooperate*. It is in each individual's interest to defect, but if everyone defects that leads to a worse outcome than if all had cooperated. For instance, pollution is an example of a prisoner's dilemma, with *defect* being to pollute and *cooperate* refraining from polluting.

The reason that the problem of pollution has the form of a dilemma is that there is an *externality*, where each person's action has effects on other players that are not captured in the player's own payoff. To illustrate with an example: the prisoner's dilemma is actualized experimentally in "public goods games" with the cooperative action being investing in a group account (Ledyard, 1995). Money in the group account is multiplied up and shared out among all the players, with the contributor receiving less back than she put in, but the group as a whole receiving more. If there are n players, and f is the factor by which the money is multiplied, $1 < f < n$. So contributing to the group kitty has benefits for the other players, as they receive more money as a result of the agent's investing. But the agent who invests a pound bears a cost of £1 and only gets back $£f/n$, which is less than £1.

We can see that the problem of pollution has the same basic structure. Each individual might prefer the outcome where the air is clean (all *cooperate*) to the outcome where the air is polluted (all *defect*). However, the cost of not polluting (or benefits that the nonpolluter forgoes) is borne entirely by the individual whereas the gains of cleaner air are shared between the whole community.[5]

Problems of self-control can have an analogous structure. Take an individual who is a smoker.[6] Each transient agent might think that it is better for herself, over her lifetime, to be a nonsmoker rather than a smoker, as that reduces the risk of cancer. In order to implement this plan, the transient agent must bear a cost, namely, forgoing the enjoyment of smoking a cigarette. However, the benefit of being a nonsmoker is not all captured by the transient agent. We might think that it is shared across transient agents or even that it accrues entirely to the transient agents at the end of the individual's life. The benefit of not smoking in any period is an *externality*; it is not completely captured by the agent that period.

The plan that the agent would most prefer to implement is to smoke a cigarette today and give up from tomorrow onward (which is analogous to the

---

5. With a very large number of individuals and small incremental benefits, which are hence spread very thin, this can result in the benefits from any one person's action being imperceptible. For discussion of imperceptible benefits see McCarthy and Arntzenius (1997). But it is the dilemma structure that is key to the incentive structure of pollution, regardless of whether or not the benefits are imperceptible.

6. Nicotine is an addictive substance. Arguably, addiction is simply a species of self-control problem (Heyman, 2009), but any reader who thinks that addiction adds extra complications to problems of self-control should either assume our smoker is not an addict or transpose the example to a case that clearly does not involve addiction, such as studying for an exam.

case of pollution, where the most preferred outcome is to pollute while everyone else refrains), but that plan is not realizable because the transient agent of
tomorrow will face the same preference structure and, hence, will not play her
part. So we have a prisoner's dilemma with smoking equivalent to *defect* and
refraining to *cooperate*.

The analogy between the interpersonal and the intrapersonal cases is not
exact. In the intrapersonal case the players do not move simultaneously, and it
is an *asynchronous prisoner's dilemma*. For this to change the analysis, it is not
sufficient that the agents move in sequence. It is also necessary that the second
player knows what the first player did. If the transient agents have perfect recall
of past moves, then, in some respects, a better analogy for the intrapersonal
case is found in Hume's two farmers, who play an asynchronous prisoner's
dilemma:[7]

> Your corn is ripe to-day; mine will be so to-morrow. 'Tis profitable for
> us both, that I shou'd labour with you to-day, and that you shou'd aid me
> to-morrow. I have no kindness for you, and know you have as little for me.
> I will not, therefore, take any pains upon your account; and should I labour
> with you upon my own account, in expectation of a return, I know I shou'd
> be disappointed, and that I shou'd in vain depend upon your gratitude. Here
> then I leave you to labour alone: You treat me in the same manner. The sea-
> sons change; and both of us lose our harvests for want of mutual confidence
> and security. (Hume 1739–1740/1978, pp. 520–521)

In an asynchronous game, the second player's strategy can be conditional on
what the first player does, so she has four strategies instead of two: *cooperate
regardless, defect regardless, cooperate if player one cooperates and defect if she
defects, defect if player one cooperates and cooperate if she defects*. In the interpersonal prisoner's dilemma *defect* is a *dominant strategy*: whatever the other
player does each player does best by defecting. In the asynchronous dilemma,
(*defect, defect regardless*) is the sole Nash equilibrium; however, it is not a
dominant strategy equilibrium since player two does equally well if she plays
the strategy *cooperate if player one cooperates and defect if she defects*. But
it is usual to expect Nash equilibrium strategies to be played and, as Hume
shows in the farmer example, backward induction also leads to both agents
defecting.

Smoking makes for a nice analogy with pollution, but the framework of costs
that are borne by the current transient agent for benefits that are, at least partly

---

7. For more on the asynchronous prisoner's dilemma in Hume see Vanderschraaf (1998) and
Skyrms (1998).

and maybe wholly, accrued by later agents can also accommodate other classic examples of self-control, such as dieting and studying for an exam.

It might be complained that, so far, I have assumed that each transient agent cares only about the here and now whereas, plausibly, they would also care about the past or future (i.e., they would exhibit some intrapersonal altruism). However, it is equally plausible that people exhibit some "present bias," with each transient agent giving herself relatively more weight than the other transient agents. Indeed, there is evidence of present bias (Ainslie, 1992; Thaler, 1981) and also of "hyperbolic discounting" (Frederick, Loewenstein, & O'Donoghue, 2002), which is closely related to present bias (Ainslie, 1991, 1992; Laibson, 1997). Even if there is some degree of intrapersonal altruism, if each transient agent gives herself more weight than the other agents, then the agents fail to take into account fully the positive externality. Hence, there is still likely to be an intrapersonal prisoner's dilemma—as can be seen in the model of decision making over time with some intrapersonal altruism provided by myself and Robert Sugden in our conclusion to Michael Bacharach's *Beyond Individual Choice* (Bacharach, 2006).

Further, displaying intrapersonal altruism is different from agency. Decision theory can accommodate altruism, or a concern for another agent's outcomes, which is usually modeled by a "payoff transformation" where the payoffs of the other agent appear in the altruistic agent's utility function (e.g., Collard, 1978). But agency involves planning (Bratman, 1987) and identity (Parfit, 1984, p. 319), neither of which appears in standard decision theory. Being altruistic does not necessarily solve problems of planning and agency, nor lead to cooperation in a prisoner's dilemma.[8] The payoff transformation involved in altruism is not enough; introducing "agency transformation" is also needed. In general, payoff transformations and agency transformations lead to different classes of results (Bacharach, 1999), hence the development of theories of team agency.

REASONING: TEAM AGENCY AND SELF-CONTROL

The prisoner's dilemma is one of the puzzles of game theory that motivated the development of theories of team agency. Since any individual player does better by choosing *defect* than by choosing *cooperate*, regardless of what other players do, game theory both predicts and prescribes *defect*. However, a substantial

---

8. Two *golden rule altruists* playing a prisoner's dilemma, who each give equal weight to self and others' payoffs in their utility functions, may transform the dilemma into a Hi-Lo game, which has two equilibria and, hence, an element of coordination (Gold & Sugden, 2007a). Standard game theory cannot prescribe a unique course of play where there is more than one equilibrium, even if one of the two equilibria gives a strictly higher payoff to both players. Hi-Lo is another of the "puzzles" that motivated the development of theories of team agency.

number of people *cooperate* in real life.[9] Further, there is a tension between individual and collective rationality because the players each do better by all choosing *cooperate* than by all choosing *defect*. While any individual player can reason to the conclusion that "The action that gives the best result *for me* is *defect*," it is also true that "The set of actions that gives the best result *for us* is not all *defect*." But reasoning about "our" outcomes has no status in standard game theory.

An analogous point can be made about the intrapersonal prisoner's dilemma. In the syntax of the theory of dynamic choice, each transient agent asks separately, "What should *I-now* do?" and, in the prisoner's dilemma, the answer is to *defect*. Intuitively, it seems reasonable for the players to ask a different question, "What should *I the person over time* do?" in which case the answer is surely not to *defect* in every time period. Indeed, this latter question seems more than reasonable; if anything, it is the standard model of dynamic choice that seems implausible, with its absence of intentions, plans, or any sense of agency that extends over time.

Theories of team agency try to reformulate game theory in such a way that "What should *we* do?" is a meaningful question. The basic idea of team reasoning is that, when an individual reasons as a member of a team, she considers which *combination* of actions by members of the team would best promote the team's objective, and then performs her part of that combination. Although the theory was originally developed with reference to individuals, it could equally be applied to the transient agents of dynamic choice theory, with the person being a team of transient agents over time.

We can follow Gold and Sugden (2007a, 2007b) in representing reasoning using schemas of practical reasoning, where agents infer conclusions about what they should do from premises that include propositions about what they are seeking to achieve and about the decision environment (which might respectively be thought of as analogs of Aristotle's general and particular premises). This is another way of representing the instrumental reasoning of game theory: the standard of success is taken as given and the conclusions tell the agent what s/he should do in order to be as successful as possible according to that standard.

There are four possible outcomes, O_i, corresponding to the four combinations of actions: O_1 from (*cooperate, defect*), O_2 from (*cooperate, cooperate*), O_3 from (*defect, defect*), and O_4 from (*defect, cooperate*). An "outcome" includes everything that the players want to achieve.

In the case of a two-period prisoner's dilemma, the backward induction reasoning of the second player could have the following form (the

9. In experiments in which people play the prisoner's dilemma for money, anonymously and without repetition, the proportion of participants choosing *cooperate* is typically between 40 and 50 percent (Sally, 1995).

propositions above the line are premises, while the proposition below the line is the conclusion):[10]

Schema 1: player 2's reasoning (individual agency)

(1) I must choose either to *cooperate* or *defect*.
(2) If the other player has chosen to *cooperate*, then the outcome will either be O_1 or O_2.
(3) If the other player has chosen to *defect*, then the outcome will either be O_3 or O_4.
(4) I prefer O_1 to O_2 and O_3 to O_4; that is, whatever player 1 has done, I prefer the outcome that results from my playing *defect*.

———————————————————————————————————

I should choose to *defect*.

The schema could be used by an individual playing an asynchronous prisoner's dilemma or by a transient agent playing a prisoner's dilemma over time with other transient agents. The reasoning is instrumental practical reasoning, and the "should" is the normativity of instrumental rationality.[11]

In an asynchronous dilemma, the first player can reason by backward induction, as follows:

Schema 2: player 1's reasoning (individual agency)

(1) I must choose either to *cooperate* or *defect*.
(2) If I choose to *cooperate* the outcome will be O_1.
(3) If I choose *defect* the outcome will be O_3.
(4) I prefer O_3 to O_1.

———————————————————————————————————

I should choose to *defect*.

10. I follow philosophical tradition in showing reasoning as the manipulation of propositions, which is also naturally interpreted as conscious manipulation. However, neither of these is necessary for my account. Decision theory is noncommittal about the mental processes underlying the choice. In cognitive science a broader definition of reasoning operates, where reasoning can refer to subconscious processes and algorithms. The schema presents a "rationalization" of the choice; that is, it shows how it could be the outcome of a rational process.

11. One might think that instrumental rationality provides only *prima facie* reasons and that what an agent all things considered ought to do is a question about ethics or morality. In some theories of team agency, team reasoning is required by morality (see the discussion in Gold & Sugden, 2007b). Under that interpretation of team reasoning, my analysis shows how reasoning as a transient agent (or as an individual, in the interpersonal case) can lead to deviations from ethically correct actions. This sort of lack of self-control is what Kennett and Smith (1996) label a failure of *orthonomy*, our capacity to act in accordance with our normative reasons.

These two schemas show how the two players in an asynchronous prisoner's dilemma can reason that they should defect. (In a synchronic prisoner's dilemma, both players will use a version of schema 1.) They are equivalent to individual rationality in standard game theory or to the reasoning of the transient agents in dynamic choice theory, where *I* may be understood as *I-now*.

If we allow, instead, that the players can ask, "What should *we* do?" and consider all possible plans, we get a schema with the following pattern:

Schema 3: collective rationality (team agency)

(1) We must choose one of *(defect, cooperate), (defect, defect), (cooperate, defect), (cooperate, cooperate).*
(2) If we choose *(cooperate, defect)* the outcome will be O_1.
(3) If we choose *(cooperate, cooperate)* the outcome will be O_2.
(4) If we choose *(defect, defect)* the outcome will be O_3.
(5) If we choose *(defect, cooperate)* the outcome will be O_4.
(6) We want to achieve O_a more than we want to achieve O_b, O_c, O_d.

——

We should choose *(x, y)*.

In the interpersonal case the *we* is a team of individuals; in the intrapersonal case the *we* is a team of transient agents that make up the agent over time. The actions that the team should take depend on how the team ranks the outcomes, that is, on the content of premise (6). We might think of O_a as the group goal. The question of how team goals should relate to the rankings of its members is complex (see Gold, 2012), but it seems clear that the team would rank the outcome of *(cooperate, cooperate)* above that of *(defect, defect)* as the former is ranked higher by every player.

In the interpersonal case, it seems reasonable to assume that the players will be treated symmetrically, and Gold and Sugden (2007a) suggest that it is natural to think that the group will rank *(cooperate, cooperate)* above *(defect, cooperate)* and *(cooperate, defect)*. In the intra-personal case, symmetry is a less obvious assumption.[12] However, whichever of the three remaining outcomes, *(cooperate, cooperate), (defect, cooperate),* and *(cooperate, defect),* the person over time ranks highest, it involves at least one transient agent taking an action that conflicts with her ranking as a person over time. If she follows team reasoning to its end and concludes that she should do her part in the best

12. With more than two players, it is possible to formulate more complicated *production functions*, which specify how combinations of cooperative contributions translate into benefits, where the optimal outcome for the team has some, but not all, team members cooperating. That might be a better model for examples like healthy eating and studying. In that case, it is the transient agents who are assigned to make a cooperative contribution that face a problem of self-control.

team plan, then that decision maker has an Aristotelian problem of self-control, with two conflicting reasoning schemas, depending on whether she reasons as a transient agent or as a team over time.

PERCEPTION: FRAMING AND SELF-CONTROL

Given that the agent has two conflicting reasoning schemas, what makes her use one over the other? In the Aristotelian account of self-control, the akrates does not use the second syllogism because of a failure of perception. Perception, in the form of "framing," also has an important role in team reasoning. As in the case of reasoning discussed above, we can apply insights from the interpersonal to the intrapersonal case.

A *frame* is the set of concepts a person uses when thinking about the world. Frames are notorious because of Kahneman and Tversky's work on *framing effects*, where changing the description of a choice problem affects the choices that people make (Tversky & Kahneman, 1981). In their classic example, subjects were told that the United States was threatened by a deadly disease, which is expected to kill 600 people, and asked to choose between two vaccination programs. Different groups of subjects received different presentations of the decision problem. One group received all the information in terms of how many of the 600 lives would be saved by each program, the other in terms of how many of the 600 would die. The modal choice of program differed between groups; the implication was that the presentation in terms of "saving" and "dying" influenced people's decisions.

Framing starts from the idea, familiar to philosophers, that seeing involves "seeing as." When you see the following marks, O Δ χ, you might see them as a circle, a triangle, and a cross. Or, if you know Greek, you might see them as an omicron, a delta, and a xi. If you do not know Greek, then the latter option is not a possibility. A larger set of descriptions is available to the linguist. However, the availability of a larger set of descriptions does not imply that they are all used. Someone reading Greek will tend to see the marks as letters, even though they could equally be described as shapes. She frames what she sees as letters, not as shapes. This is like the Aristotelian idea of having knowledge but not using it.

The standard agents of decision theory use all the knowledge that they have; they always see their world under all of the infinite number of descriptions available to them. However, real people are finite, so this is never a possibility for us. We have "bounded cognition."[13] At any time, we will be using only a small subset of the concepts that could describe our situation.

---

13. The allusion to Herbert Simon's "bounded rationality" is intentional (Simon, 1955). *Bounded rationality* is the idea that, unlike the ideal agents of decision theory, real agents are subject to cognitive limitations. Simon's research program emphasized limitations on information processing. Bounded cognition is (at least partly) a cognitive limitation. So, strictly

Framing is an important precursor to decision making. In order for something to feature in an agent's reasoning, she must have concepts related to it in her frame. Hence, in order to team reason, a player must have the concept "we" in her frame.

Many accounts of team agency emphasize the role of commitment in group identification, be it rational commitment, moral commitment, or simply the endorsement of a particular mode of reasoning by the agent (Gold & Sugden, 2007a, 2007b). But even accounts of group agency that do not give perception a prominent role have an implicit framing step, as seeing that a decision can be described as a problem for "us" is a necessary precondition for team reasoning.[14]

In contrast, Bacharach (2006) gives an account where team reasoning is purely the result of framing. For Bacharach, certain features of choice-problems may, when salient, promote group identity, which, in turn, primes team reasoning. In his model, these transitions are all the results of psychological processes, not of decisions. However, there is an implicit commitment to or pre-eminence of the *we*-frame. Team reasoners must have the *I*-concept in their frame, as they reason to conclusions about what individual actions they should take, and because team reasoning can be *circumspect*, taking into account the possibility that others do not group identify but act on individual reasoning instead. Nevertheless, there is an assumption that priming *we*-concepts tends to promote team reasoning.[15]

Bacharach elides the distinction between the noticing of *we*-concepts and their having what we might call "motivational grip" (Gold, 2012). Motivational grip has two components above and beyond merely noticing a feature or concept: noticing that it is choice relevant and, given that it has been noticed as choice relevant, deciding to act on the reason it provides. Hence, Bacharach's team reasoners must either not find *I*-reasons to be choice relevant or else they have decided not to act on them. In order to stay within a purely cognitive framework, Bacharach might say that the salience of the *we*-concepts outweighs that of the *I*-concepts. But, in order for framing the decision as a problem for "us" to affect behavior, *we*-reasons must have motivating power, which seems to presume an implicit commitment to the team agent.

speaking, bounded cognition is a species of bounded rationality, albeit not one that has come under much scrutiny. One advantage of the moniker "bounded cognition" is that it does not mention rationality, hopefully avoiding the increasing tendency to confuse bounded rationality with irrationality (Gigerenzer, 1997), when questions of rationality are really still up for debate.

14. See Gold (2012) for a more detailed examination of this point with respect to Sugden's account.

15. In an earlier presentation of his theory, Bacharach (1997) allows that there is an *I*-frame, a *we*-frame, and a *superordinate* frame, oscillating between the *I*- and *we*-perspectives. Smerilli (2012) explores this further, providing a simple model of vacillation between *I*- and *we*-modes of reasoning.

We can draw parallels with team reasoning at the intrapersonal level. In the same way that interpersonal team reasoning requires the decision maker to frame the decision as a problem for us, intrapersonal team reasoning requires the decision maker to frame it as a problem for herself over time. Of course, there is a sense in which everyone knows she is an extended self over time but, as we saw above, it is possible to have that knowledge without using it to frame a decision problem. Arguably, it is more natural for people to think of themselves as selves over time than as transient agents, so the team frame might be the default in the intrapersonal case. It certainly seems natural to think that people have an implicit commitment to their extended self over time. The lack of such a commitment is one reason why the pure transient agent model is impoverished.

When there is temptation, the divergence of interests between the transient agent and the person over time is salient. At the interpersonal level, social identity theorists say that awareness of common interest and a common fate promotes group identification, by raising awareness of a relevant basis for categorization into groups (Brewer, 1979). Conversely, awareness of divergent individual interests may inhibit group identification and obscure awareness of any basis for group categorization, and this may be true in both the interpersonal and the intrapersonal cases. Hence, akrasia may be associated with a lack of identification with the self over time.

The idea that akrasia involves a failure of perception is central to the Aristotelian account. For Aristotle, the akrates is unaware of a particular premise. However, in the team reasoning account, the concept of "we" is in every premise. Even the group goal is "our" ordering, from the point of view of the team, so perceiving it involves having the concept of the team in one's frame. Indeed, seeing the group goal may be more important in triggering team reasoning than any of the other premises if, as social identity theorists claim, recognizing a common interest can trigger group identity. Hence, it must be that the whole team reasoning schema is not used by the akrates.

PSYCHOLOGICAL EVIDENCE AND DISCRIMINATION BETWEEN THEORIES

The intrapersonal team reasoning account implies that we can improve self-control by increasing the salience of the self over time, and by increasing the salience of long-term goals relative to transient ones. The relative salience of long-term goals can be increased either by increasing the salience of the long term or by decreasing the salience of the short term, which can be done by focusing attention on the long-term goal or distracting oneself from the immediate temptation.

Here I present evidence that is compatible with the intrapersonal team reasoning account of self-control, explore why current evidence does not discriminate between the account and other explanations of self-control, and suggest a way in which the account might have increased explanatory power.

There is evidence that distraction from temptation, by engaging in other activities and even just by thinking about other activities, can increase self-control (Mischel & Baker, 1975; Mischel, Ebbesen, & Zeiss, 1972).[16] And, if directing attention is an effortful activity, then an account where self-control involves focusing attention is consistent with some of the psychological evidence on *ego depletion*, the idea that willpower is a limited resource. Being asked to exert self-control in a first task adversely affects subjects' performance in a second task that also requires self-control (Baumeister et al., 1998; Muraven, Tice, & Baumeister, 1998). Conversely, high glucose levels and consumption of calories can increase self-control (Gailliot et al., 2007). Muraven and Baumeister (2000) make an analogy between willpower and a muscle, whose strength gets depleted as you use it, but whose strength can be built up with exercise. If the analogy is correct, it implies that there is some unspecified effortful mechanism underlying self-control. Focusing attention plausibly requires effort, especially when one is trying to focus attention away from a salient stimulus. If we think that controlling attention can be learned, then the account can also explain why people can improve their self-control with practice (Muraven, Baumeister, & Tice, 1999).

However, while the efficacy of directing attention between outcomes is consistent with the intrapersonal team reasoning account, we can talk about framing the options without introducing levels of agency. The idea that we can solve problems of self-control by redescribing the options is already present in the philosophical literature (Kennett& Smith, 1996; Mele, 2012), and there are models that explain akrasia as a conflict of reasons (Kavka, 1991; Pettit, 2003) and as conflicting perceptions of reasons (Gold, 2005; Schick, 1991).

The model of intrapersonal team reasoning suggests that, in addition to reframing the options, we should be able to improve self-control by reframing the agent. This hypothesis needs further research. Here are two reasons for thinking that it might be fruitful.

First, there is some evidence on the self over time and delayed gratification, from the work of Dan Bartels and colleagues (Bartels & Rips, 2010; Bartels & Urminsky, 2011). This starts from Derek Parfit's (1984) argument that personal identity depends on *psychological connectedness*, having psychological

---

16. Mischel's experimental paradigm involves a child who can obtain a less preferred food reward immediately or wait for a more preferred food reward. Since the temptation and the reward are in the same currency, distractions are distractions both from the temptation and the more preferred reward, which is the long-term goal.

connections with our future selves such as sharing memories, intentions, beliefs, and desires. Bartels wanted to see if there is a correlation between connectedness and the "discount rate," which leads us to choose sooner smaller rewards over larger later ones. In fact, he tested the relation between *perceived* connectedness and the discount rate, finding that subjects who rated themselves as more connected to later selves were more patient (Bartels & Rips, 2010) and that connectedness can be manipulated, resulting in increased patience (Bartels & Urminsky, 2011).

Bartels' work involves the perception of psychological connectedness. This is not the same as the perception of shared agency, but it is plausible that they are related. At the interpersonal level, identification with other members of a group enhances the accessibility of shared characteristics (Smith & Henry, 1996). Perceived similarities may also increase the likelihood of group identification. It is likely that the causality runs in both directions. At the intrapersonal level, we might hope that future research will attempt to discriminate between the effects of psychological connectedness and those of team agency or, alternatively (should discrimination not be possible), to explore the connections between the two.

A further confound is that the perception of psychological connectedness might increase intrapersonal altruism as well as or instead of increasing the perception of the self as an agent over time. Again, intrapersonal altruism and sense of agency may be related: framing a decision as a problem for us may also encourage a concern for the welfare of the other transient agents that belong to the self over time. The same issue occurs at the interpersonal level, where the question becomes how to discriminate between interventions that increase interpersonal altruism and those that make salient team agency. Bacharach (2006) claims that a test that discriminates team reasoning can be constructed by using the fact that team reasoners take actions that lead to the group utility maximizing outcome, whereas individual reasoners will sometimes end up at an outcome with lower payoffs, if it is salient and solves a coordination problem. More work remains to be done, at both the interpersonal and intrapersonal level.

A second reason favoring the intrapersonal team reasoning account is that it has increased explanatory power. There is a datum that cannot be explained by a simple framing of the object account: the relation between borderline personality disorder (BPD) and self-control. A personality disorder occurs when the way that a person is inclined to think, feel, and act causes that person severe psychological distress, impairs her in important contexts, and does her harm (Pickhard, 2011). BPD is defined by instability of interpersonal relationships, self-image, and affects, and a marked impulsivity. A person is diagnosed with

BPD when she displays at least five of a list of diagnostic traits, which include "identity disturbance: markedly and persistently unstable self-image or sense of self" and "impulsivity in at least two areas that are potentially self-damaging" (American Psychiatric Association, 2000, p. 706).

BPD patients have a fractured sense of self. They do not identify with their later selves and they do not think through the consequences of their actions on either themselves or others. The amount of impulsivity displayed by BPD patients can be extreme, and their inability to carry through plans causes severe detriment to their lives. They cannot hold down jobs and they have impoverished relationships. However, although impulsivity is a diagnostic criterion for BPD, there is currently no theoretical explanation of the co-occurrence of impulsivity and identity disturbance.

BPD is also characterized by "affective instability," with intense emotions and mood swings (American Psychiatric Association, 2000). Current treatments for BPD, such as therapies involving "mindfulness" (Breslin, Zack, & McMain, 2002) and "mentalizing" (Fonagy & Bateman, 2007), focus on patients' emotional shifts, helping them to take a more detached perspective on intense emotions, especially negative ones, and teaching them how to focus their attention. There is evidence that BPD patients have difficulty in controlling their attention (Hoermann et al., 2005; Lenzenweger et al., 2004; Posner et al., 2002) and that negative affective cues activate alcohol cognitions in problem drinkers with psychiatric disorders (Zack, Toneatto, & MacLeod, 1999, 2002). As with other evidence cited above, this could be explained by an account of self-control as involving reframing options. However, in this case, that account leaves a feature of the condition unexplained, namely, the connection between unstable self-identity and impulsivity—exactly the extra component that the intrapersonal team reasoning theory can provide.

The theory of intrapersonal team reasoning is not the only account of self-control that invokes a division of agency and a diachronic perspective. There are models involving a long- and a short-sighted self (Schelling, 1984), a planner and a doer (Thaler & Shefrin, 1981), global and local choice (Heyman, 2009), and short-range and long-range interests (Ainslie, 1992). Intrapersonal team reasoning is compatible with some of these accounts, providing more detail about what the long-sighted or global perspective involves, and explicit modeling of the interaction of successive transient agents. However, it is not obviously compatible with accounts where the long-range interest is constrained to always take the same action in every period (e.g., Ainslie, 1992). In the team reasoning account, it is possible that the optimal team plan involves occasional lapses, if that produces the best outcome for the self over time.

CONCLUSION

Aristotle examined the reasoning of the akratic agent but did not specify the reasoning of the agent who exhibits self-control. Similarly, the framework of decision theory explains why people would give in to temptations but not how people can use willpower to exert self-control. I introduced the idea of levels of agency, with the self as a team over time that makes and follows plans, and showed how intrapersonal team reasoning can lead to self-control. The account is Aristotelian in that it involves reasoning schema and a lack of perception on the part of the akratic agent, who does not see her decision problem as a problem for her self over time. It suggests a role not just for framing of the options, but also for framing of the agent. This would merit further investigation in future research.

ACKNOWLEDGMENT

I thank John Broome, Dan Hausman, Steve Pearce, and Hanna Pickard for helpful comments on early presentations of this material, and Neil Levy and an anonymous referee, whose identity was later revealed as Jeanette Kennett, for helpful input on the paper.

This research received funding from the European Research Council under the European Union's Seventh Framework Programme (FP/2007-2013)/ERC Grant Agreement n. 283849.

REFERENCES

Ainslie, G. (1991). Derivation of "rational" economic behavior from hyperbolic discount curves. *American Economic Review* 81: 134–140.

Ainslie, G. (1992). *Picoeconomics*. Cambridge: Cambridge University Press.

American Psychiatric Association. (2000). *Diagnostic and Statistical Manual of Mental Disorders Revised 4th ed.* Washington, DC: Author.

Austin, J. L. (1956-1957). A plea for excuses. *Proceedings of the Aristotelian Society* 57: 1–30.

Bacharach, M. (1997). 'We' equilibria: A variable frame theory of cooperation. Working paper, Institute of Economics and Statistics, University of Oxford. Oxford, England.

Bacharach, M. (1999). Interactive team reasoning: A contribution to the theory of cooperation. *Research in Economics* 53, 117–147.

Bacharach, M. (2006). *Beyond Individual Choice*. N. Gold & R. Sugden (eds.). Princeton, NJ: Princeton University Press.

Barnes, J. (1984). *The Complete Works of Aristotle Volume II*. Princeton, NJ: Princeton University Press.

Bartels, D., & Rips, L. (2010). Psychological connectedness and intertemporal choice. *Journal of Experimental Psychology: General* 139: 49–69.

Bartels, D., & Urminsky, O. (2011). On intertemporal selfishness: How the perceived instability of identity underlies impatient consumption. *Journal of Consumer Research* 38: 182–198.

Baumeister, R. F., Bratslavsky, E., Muraven, M., & Tice, D. M. (1998). Ego depletion: Is the active self a limited resource? *Journal of Personality and Social Psychology* 74, 1252–1265.

Bostock, D. (2000). *Aristotle's Ethics*. Oxford: Oxford University Press.

Bratman, M. (1987). *Intention, Plans and Practical Reason*. Cambridge, MA: Harvard University Press.

Breslin, F. C., Zack, M., & McMain, S. (2002). An information-processing analysis of mindfulness: Implications for relapse prevention in the treatment of substance abuse. *Clinical Psychology: Science and Practice* 9(3), 275–99.

Brewer, M. B. (1979). In-group bias in the minimal intergroup situation: A cognitive-motivational analysis. *Psychological Bulletin* 86, 307–324.

Charles, D. (1984). *Aristotle's Philosophy of Action*. London: Duckworth.

Collard, D. (1978). *Altruism and Economy: A Study in Non-Selfish Economics*. Oxford: Martin Robertson.

Fonagy, P., & Bateman, A. W. (2007). Mentalizing and borderline personality disorder. *Journal of Mental Health* 16(1), 83–101.

Frederick, S., Loewenstein, G., & O'Donoghue, T. (2002). Time discounting and time preference: A critical review. *Journal of Economic Literature* 40(2), 351–401.

Gailliot, M. T., Baumeister, R. F., DeWall, C. N., Maner, J. K., Plant, E. A., Tice, D. M., Brewer, L. E., & Schmeichel, B. J. (2007). Self-control relies on glucose as a limited energy source: Willpower is more than a metaphor. *Journal of Personality and Social Psychology* 92, 325–336.

Gigerenzer, G. (1997). Bounded rationality: Models of fast and frugal inference. *Swiss Journal of Economics and Statistics* 133 (2/2), 201–218.

Gold, N. (2005). Framing and decision making: A reason-based approach. Unpublished D.Phil thesis, University of Oxford.

Gold, N. (2012). Team reasoning and cooperation. In S. Okasha & K. Binmore (eds.), *Evolution and Rationality: Decisions, Cooperation and Strategic Behaviour* (pp. 185– 212). Cambridge: Cambridge University Press.

Gold, N., & Sugden, R. (2007a). Theories of team agency. In F. Peter & S. Schmidt (eds.), *Rationality and Commitment* (pp. 280–312) Oxford: Oxford University Press.

Gold, N., & Sugden, R. (2007b). Collective intentions and team agency. *Journal of Philosophy* 104(3), 109–137.

Heyman, G. M. (2009). *Addiction: A Disorder of Choice*. Cambridge, MA: Harvard University Press.

Hoermann, S., Clarkin, J. F., Hull, J. W., & Levy, K. N. (2005). The construct of effortful control: An approach to borderline personality disorder heterogeneity. *Psychopathology* 38, 82–86.

Hume, D. (1739–1740/1978). *A Treatise of Human Nature*. Oxford: Clarendon Press.

Kavka, G. (1991). Is individual choice less problematic than collective choice? *Economics and Philosophy* 7: 291–310.

Kennett, J., & Smith, M. (1996). Frog and toad lose control. *Analysis* 56: 63–72.

Laibson, D. (1997). Golden eggs and hyperbolic discounting. *Quarterly Journal of Economics* 112: 443–477.

Ledyard, J. O. (1995). Public goods: A survey of experimental research. In J. H. Kagel & A. E. Roth (eds.), *Handbook of Experimental Economics* (pp. 111–194). Princeton, NJ: Princeton University Press.

Lenzenweger, M. F., Clarkin, J. F., Fertuck, E. A., & Kernberg, O. F. (2004). Executive neurocognitive functioning and neurobehavioral systems indicators in borderline personality disorder: A preliminary study. *Journal of Personality Disorders* 18, 421–438.

McCarthy, D., & Arntzenius, F. (1997). Self torture and group beneficence. *Erkenntnis* 47: 129–144.

Mele, A. R. (2012). *Backsliding: Understanding Weakness of Will*. Oxford: Oxford University Press.

Mischel, W., & Baker, N. (1975). Cognitive appraisals and transformations in delay behavior. *Journal of Personality and Social Psychology* 31(2), 254–261.

Mischel, W., Ebbesen, E. B., & Zeiss, A. R. (1972). Cognitive and attentional mechanisms in delay of gratification. *Journal of Personality and Social Psychology* 21(2), 204–218.

Moss, J. (2009). Akrasia and perceptual illusion. *Archiv fur Geschichte der Philosophie* 91, 119–156.

Muraven, M., & Baumeister, R. F. (2000). Self-regulation and depletion of limited resources: Does self-control resemble a muscle? *Psychological Bulletin* 126, 247–259.

Muraven, M., Baumeister, R. F., & Tice, D. M. (1999). Longitudinal improvement of self-regulation through practice: Building self-control strength through repeated exercise. *Journal of Social Psychology* 139, 446–457.

Muraven, M., Tice, D. M., & Baumeister, R. F. (1998). Self-control as a limited resource: Regulatory depletion patterns. *Journal of Personality and Social Psychology* 74, 774–789.

Parfit, D. (1984). *Reasons and Persons*. Oxford: Clarendon Press.

Pettit, P. (2003). Akrasia, collective and individual. In Sarah Stroud & Christine Tappolet (eds.), *Weakness of Will and Practical Irrationality* (pp. 68–96). Oxford: Oxford University Press.

Pickard, H. (2011). What is personality disorder? *Philosophy, Psychiatry, and Psychology* 18(3), 181–184.

Posner, M. I., Rothbart, M. K., Vizueta, N., Levy, K. N., Evans, D. E., Thomas, K. M., & Clarkin, J. (2002). Attentional mechanisms of borderline personality disorder. *Proceedings of the National Academy of Sciences of the USA* 99, 16366–16370.

Sally, D. (1995). Conversation and cooperation in social dilemmas: A meta-analysis of experiments from 1958 to 1992. *Rationality and Society* 7, 58–92.

Schelling, T. (1984). Self-command in practice, in policy, and in a theory of rational choice. *American Economic Review* 74, 1–11.

Schick, F. (1991). *Understanding Action*. Cambridge: Cambridge University Press.

Simon, H. A. (1955). A behavioral model of rational choice. *Quarterly Journal of Economics* 69, 99–118.

Skyrms, B. (1998). The shadow of the future. In Coleman & Morris (eds.), *Rational Commitment and Social Justice: Essays for Gregory Kavka*. New York: Cambridge University Press.

Smerilli, A. (2012). We-thinking and vacillation between frames: Filling a gap in Bacharach's theory. *Theory and Decision*. Online first publication.

Smith, E. R., & Henry, S. (1996). An in-group becomes part of the self: Response time evidence. *Personality and Social Psychology Bulletin* 22, 635–642.

Strotz, R. H. (1955–1956). Myopia and inconsistency in dynamic utility maximization. *Review of Economic Studies* 23, 165–180.

Sugden, R. (1993). Thinking as a team: Toward an explanation of nonselfish behavior. *Social Philosophy and Policy* 10, 69–89.

Thaler, R. (1981). Some empirical evidence on dynamic inconsistency. *Economics Letters* 8(3), 201–207.

Thaler, R. H., & Shefrin, H. M. (1981). Temporal construal. *Psychological Review* 110, 403–421.

Tversky, A., & Kahneman, D. (1981). The framing of decisions and the psychology of choice. *Science* 211, 453–458.

Urmson, J. O. (1988). *Aristotle's Ethics*. Oxford: Basil Blackwell.

Vanderschraaf, P. (1998). The informal game theory in Hume's account of convention. *Economics and Philosophy* 14, 215–247.

Wiggins, D. (1980). Weakness of the will, commensurability, and the objects of deliberation and desire. In A. Oksenberg Rorty (ed.), *Essays on Aristotle's Ethics* (pp. 221–240) Berkeley: University of California Press.

Zack, M., Toneatto, T., & MacLeod, C. M. (2002). Anxiety and explicit alcohol-related memory in problem drinkers. *Addictive Behaviors* 27, 331–343.

Zack, M., Toneatto, T., & MacLeod, C. M. (1999). Implicit activation of alcohol concepts by negative affective cues distinguishes between problem drinkers with high and low psychiatric distress. *Journal of Abnormal Psychology* 108, 518–531.

5

Phenomenal Authority

The Epistemic Authority of Alcoholics Anonymous

OWEN FLANAGAN

GETTING ADDICTION RIGHT

To understand a complicated psycho-bio-social phenomenon such as addiction to alcohol, one wants ideally a phenomenology, a behavioral and cognitive psychology, a physiology, and a neurobiology—all embedded in a sociology. One wants to know what it is like to be alcoholic—if, that is, there is any commonality to the experiences of alcoholics (Flanagan, 1992, 2011, in press). One wants to know about such things as whether and if so what kind of loss of control alcoholics experience in relation to alcohol (as well as any and all affective and cognitive deficits). One wants to know what the brain is doing and how it contributes to the production of the characteristic phenomenologies and control (and other cognitive and affective) problems. One wants to know what effect heavy drinking has on vulnerable organ systems (e.g., the brain, the heart, and the liver). And, of course, all along the way, one should want to know how the sociomoral-cultural-political ecology normalizes, romanticizes, pathologizes (and so forth) alcoholism and its relations, heavy drinking, recklessness under the influence, and so on. Some scientists and philosophers worry that the program of Alcoholics Anonymous (A.A.) biases our understanding of the phenomenology, psychology, physiology, and neurobiology of addiction and prevents a unified, or at least a consilient, account of the nature, causes, and treatment of alcoholism from emerging. I have experience in the rooms of A.A., as well as in seminar and conference rooms with experts on addiction. From this perspective, I assess this claim that A.A. is part of the problem, not of the solution, and suggest some ways to increase mutual understanding between the various modes of understanding alcoholism, which if abided by would yield sensitive and sensible interaction among the practical program of A.A. and the sciences of addiction. One consequence is that A.A. would need to acknowledge that as a therapeutic social institution it is a repository of some practical knowledge about what works to help some people recover and stay abstinent, but has no expertise on alcoholism or even on "how it works" if, that is, it does work.

THE TWIN DISCIPLINES OF A.A.

A.A. is a discipline, actually two disciplines. A.A. offers hope to alcoholics in the form of a program, what it insists is a "spiritual program," which if followed in a rigorous way promises recovery through lifelong abstention, one day at a time. A.A. also offers a form of intellectual discipline, a cognitive framework that discourse about alcoholism and recovery from alcoholism is encouraged and expected to abide. This latter, disciplinary discipline has two audiences. First, individuals who get better inside the program are encouraged to speak— even as they work through the program—in a certain way about the nature of alcoholism and what brings recovery; second, workers in the field of alcohol addiction are encouraged to speak and write in a way that conforms to what A.A. says about alcoholism and recovery. A.A. is alleged to work so, at a minimum, experts on alcoholism ought not say anything about alcoholism that is inconsistent with what A.A. says.

These two ways in which A.A. is a discipline, or disciplines, first as a spiritual regimen for recovery, and second as the dominant theory of alcoholism and the most well-known therapeutic technique for recovery, are both indices of its status and power as a social institution. This high social status supports a certain ubiquity of "A.A. speak," which gives the impression that what the program says about the nature of alcoholism and recovery is legitimate and well confirmed. But this is not obvious. Indeed, some of what A.A. says about the nature of the disease and about recovery is now known to be either superficial or false. One problem is to explain how a theory with these characteristics, being superficial or false, could nonetheless work.

The suspicion that A.A. claims more legitimacy for what it teaches than it deserves rests on two worries: first, A.A. originates in a program that, in addition to promoting abstention, which will, if anything will, support not drinking (abstention *is* after all not drinking), has its roots in a variety of Christian perfectionism that has nothing to do with drinking; second, there are worries about the confirmation bias and self-fulfilling prophesy in the face of competing hypotheses about the nature of alcoholism and recovery from it.

The ways in which A.A. disciplines speech in conformity with how it conceives of alcoholism guarantees that its way of speaking will be repeated. This can seem like confirmation. But the fact that people who recover in A.A. attribute their recovery to A.A. is an effect that the discipline of A.A. seeks, intends, and encourages. And for that very reason, it does not count as independent, or further or additional, support for its truth or validity, that is, of neutral evidence that shows that the program has such causal power. I'll explain and try to reconcile the superficiality and possibility of the falsehood of some of what A.A. says about the nature of alcoholism and recovery from alcoholism with a theory of how, despite this, it could, indeed does, work.

A.A. AS AN *EPISTEME*

In the *Order of Things* (1966), Michel Foucault introduces the idea of an *episteme* to depict a normative community within which certain ways of speaking are accepted as authoritative, as based on justified true beliefs, often with the imprimatur of experts. Foucault allows, and even if he didn't, we should allow, that there can be competing epistemes, competing ways of speaking and conceptualizing a set of phenomena. Methodist and Muslim theologians both speak authoritatively about the nature and will of God. Libertarians and liberals speak authoritatively about the nature of justice and rights. Furthermore, competing theological and philosophical epistemes claim to warrant different ways of acting. And so it is with addiction. Some say it is a disease, some not. Some say addiction diminishes responsibility, some not. Some say addiction should not be moralized, others that it is a moral failing.

A.A. is an episteme that speaks with considerable authority and confidence about the nature, causes, and cure, such as there is one, of alcoholism (and, in its progeny, N.A., etc., for other substance addictions). But many members of the scientific community—a different episteme—think A.A., at least as far as its pronouncements on the nature and causes of alcoholism, is wrong (alcoholism is not an allergy), superficial (alcoholism does not involve "powerlessness over alcohol"), and cult-like (alcoholism is not a symptom of a deeper disease of the soul to be cured by practices—yielding to a "Higher Power"—that have nothing to do with drinking but carry all the trappings of confessional Christian practices).

Paradoxically, but not incoherently, many of these same scientists who think that A.A. is hocus pocus on the nature and causes of alcoholism believe that A.A. works despite this. There is a long tradition of careful work in psychology on "positive illusions" (even "delusions")—what look like unwarranted, typically self-serving beliefs (although see Flanagan 2007, 2009, for the possibility that these so-called illusions may be hopes, not beliefs), for example, lowballing probabilities of common bad things happening to oneself—that nonetheless produce good effects, such things as personal happiness or caring behavior toward others. Relatedly, the history and philosophy of science calls our attention to the possibility, because it is actual, of making, for example, accurate astronomical predictions based on a false theory, a geocentric theory or a theory of celestial spheres say, rather than a true heliocentric theory or expanding universe model.

Among philosophers who are interested in addiction and who focus on matters such as weakness of will, the unity and disunity of the self, self-control, responsibility, and the like, there are related worries and suspicions about A.A. Overcoming addiction involves exerting self-control. At least among naturalists, the power of overcoming addiction does not come from a "Higher Power," even from "God, as we understand Him." It comes from a person, in a community perhaps, who regains control or leverages control over his or her own behavior, transforming eventually his or her wants, desires, and needs, as well as his or her behavior. Recovery cannot involve nonphysical processes, genuine miracles, any more than the winning shot in a basketball game can. Of course, it remains possible even on naturalistic principles that the *belief* in a higher power can do genuine causal work even if a higher power can't and thus that one can think that God gets the assist on the winning shot, even though this is false. So from the point of view of the episteme constituted by philosophers who work on the nature of human action, agency, control, and responsibility, A.A. is similarly seen, or better, suspected of being, a secret society of people who do about as well as any group in staying sober—which is not all that well—but who speak in tongues and utter gobbledygook.

So there is a problem in social epistemology: what can be done to correct this predicament where there is competition of epistemes, specifically where many of the experts, first and foremost, the scientists of addiction, think that A.A.'s description of the nature and causes of alcoholism is at best superficial, at worst false, and where many of the experts on how to conceive of alcoholics' responsibility and control capacities, the cognitive scientists and philosophers, think the same, while at the same time, all parties think that A.A. works?

Or better: there are some who think that A.A. doesn't actually work. But the data are now finally in and all the evidence suggests that A.A. works as well as, probably better than, any other program, medical, psychiatric, and so on (Heyman 2009; Vaillant 1995). Heyman speaks for the mainstream scientific consensus when he writes:

> In research circles A.A. has been notorious for not evaluating itself and for not supporting studies of its effectiveness. However, several recent studies provide evidence that A.A. works. The most convincing report... (McKellar

et al., 2003) …indicated that the correlation between sobriety and A.A. membership was a function of engaging in the A.A. programs. The idea that A.A. success is really a function of the individual characteristics of those who choose to stay in A.A. (and not what they do in A.A.) was not supported by the data. (2009, pp. 169–170)

The situation then looks as follows: the evidence suggests that A.A. works and that it works because of something "it" does, not because of some feature of the kinds of alcoholics who go to A.A. And indeed, this is exactly what alcoholics say of their program—"it works if you work it." But even if it is true that A.A. causally contributes to recovery, without controlled experiments, we do know what aspect or aspects of A.A. help produce recovery, or by what mechanism.

TWO DISEASES THAT ALCOHOLISM ISN'T

In 1988, Herbert Fingarette, a philosopher, published an important book, *Heavy Drinking*, that starts with this bravado: "Almost everything that the American public believes to be the scientific truth about alcoholism is false." What most every American believes is the scientific truth is "the great myth: the classic disease concept," a concept that "no leading researcher accepts" (1988, p. 3). The myth is that alcoholism is a "specific disease" and that "those afflicted by the disease inevitably progress to uncontrolled drinking because the disease produces a distinctive disability—'loss of control,' a loss of the power of choice in the matter of drinking" (1988, p. 3).

According to Fingarette, various elements of the myth were widely endorsed in the first part of the 20th century and the myth was instrumental in passing the 18th amendment prohibiting the manufacture and use of alcohol.[1] Fingarette writes that the myth was resurrected, after its constitutional demise with the repeal of the 18th amendment by the 21st amendment, when in "1935 the old doctrine was given new life by the founders of Alcoholics Anonymous (A.A.). Inspired by the teachings of the popular religious sect, the Oxford

1. A common view, not questioned by Fingarette, is that widespread acceptance of the myth explains how the 18th amendment could have been ratified in 1919, and that furthermore its repeal in 1933 by the 21st amendment was not due to denial of the myth so much as by concerns for respect for the law and respect for freedom. The truth is that prohibition was about much more than alcohol. According to Okrent (2010), prohibition served as a unifying cause that brought together the Protestant culture of the heartland (especially Baptists and Methodists) with women's suffrage groups who abhorred saloon culture, and the KKK who fear mongered the horror of freed blacks with whiskey, into a coalition aimed at the alleged habits of urban immigrants, mostly Catholics, Jews, and African Americans.

movement [*sic*], two reformed heavy drinkers, a stockbroker and a physician proposed a less extreme version of the temperance thesis. Their new approach was in essence a mixture of pseudomedical, psychological, and religious ideas" (1988, p. 18).

There are three features of the disease model as depicted by Fingarette, call it Alcoholism[Fingarette], that he claims ground the model and that are dubious: the idea that the disease is specific in the sense that its cause lies in a well-defined functional system, some set of genes, say, or that it unfolds in a specific organ (e.g., the brain or the liver); that people have the disease even if they never display it (presumably because all it takes is activation by drinking); and that it involves "'loss of control,' a loss of the power of choice in the matter of drinking." All three features are dubious, but consider only the third.

The evidence is pretty unambiguous that there is never, or almost never, a complete "loss of the power of choice in the matter of drinking." Many people who self-identify as addicts, specifically as "alcoholic," and who are identified by others as addicts, specifically as "alcoholics," stop using the substance that they claim to be addicted to, specifically alcohol, and they do so without being tied to the mast like Ulysses before the Sirens. According to Vaillant's (1995) longitudinal study of male drinking patterns, now in its sixth decade, many such people stop using (some only moderate significantly) between the ages of 30 and 50 when they marry or start a career. The heavy drinking, the problem drinking, the addiction yields or abates without anything like standard physical compulsion or coercion. Or perhaps if, or insofar as, the situation is sometimes like Ulysses and the Sirens, the agent participates in tying himself to the mast and untying himself when he is ready; for example, he goes to see a therapist, psychiatrist, or M.D., or voluntarily chooses to go into detox or rehab. Some recuperated souls go to support groups for help, A.A. and the like; others do not. Some alcoholics take other kinds of potentially addictive drugs under an M.D.'s supervision (e.g., benzodiazepines) to cut the craving and control the dangerous features of physical withdrawal during the early stages of recuperation (alcohol withdrawal is much more dangerous than heroin or cocaine withdrawal). But—incarcerated addicts aside—most every case of recuperation from alcohol addiction ever seen involves the addict's own agency, typically where the person wants to stop and experiences some difficulty, but almost never impossibility, in so doing. Those who fail, those who try again and again and die as alcoholics—often from organ damage to the brain, heart, and liver—don't recuperate. But there is rarely—cases of alcoholic-induced dementia aside—reason to think that they could not have recuperated. Such people failed to recover, to recuperate, but they could have. Cases of self-cure, by which I mean recuperation where the alcoholic stops using and plays a crucial causal role in his or her own recovery, are ubiquitous. But self-cure that takes the form of regaining self-control, sufficient self-control to stop using, is more than paradoxical—it should not be possible if Alcoholism^{Fingarette} is the right model. But people do get better and they do so by using agentic powers they possess, so Alcoholism^{Fingarette} is not the right model, but is just, as he says, a "myth."

Alcoholism^{Fingarette} might be a myth while it is still true that alcohol addiction involves diminished control, sometimes, perhaps often, big control problems. In any case, without deciding the matter of whether alcoholism is a disease or not, one can on the evidence say that it is not the disease defined as Alcoholism^{Fingarette}. Perhaps it is a disease defined in some other way.

A second model that defines alcoholism as a disease but as a somewhat different disease from Alcoholism^{Fingarette} is Alcoholism$^{A.A.}$. Both conceptions share the view that alcoholism is an organic disease. The differences between the two disease concepts are subtle. Alcoholism^{Fingarette} emphasizes the idea that the disease is innate in a way Alcoholism$^{A.A}$ does not or need not; and Alcoholism$^{A.A}$ insists in a way that Alcoholism^{Fingarette} does not or need not that alcoholism is not a moral failing nor a kind of "mental imbalance." Here I take no general position on whether alcoholism is best thought of as a disease or not, although I am skeptical that that discussion or debate is useful. I only provide reasons to doubt that it is best conceived as either Alcoholism^{Fingarette} or Alcoholism$^{A.A.}$. It is possible that alcoholism could be a disease of some sort. Arguments that it is a disease are always, in my experience, arguments from analogy: x is a disease; alcoholism is like x in these respects; therefore, alcoholism is a disease. It might be that some concept of alcoholism as a disease is a myth, e.g., that it is an allergy, but that it is not necessarily a myth that alcoholism is some sort other sort of disease, possibly still unidentified. Regardless, it seems enough to say that being an alcoholic or addict is not among the ways of living well; it is not wholesome; it is a disorder, a mode of ill-being.

Alcoholism$^{A.A.}$ is defined nicely in a pamphlet available to all newcomers at A.A. meetings, which asks the pressing question: *What is alcoholism?* Like a good catechism, it answers:

> The explanation that seems to make sense to most A.A. members is that alcoholism is an illness, a *progressive* illness, which can never be cured but which, like some other diseases, *can* be arrested. Going one step further, many A.A.'s feel that the illness represents the combination of a physical sensitivity to alcohol and a mental obsession with drinking, which, regardless of consequences, cannot be broken by willpower alone. [B]efore they are exposed to A.A., many alcoholics who are unable to stop drinking, think of themselves as morally weak, or possibly, mentally unbalanced. The A.A. concept is that alcoholics are sick people who can recover if they will follow a

simple program that has proven successful for more than two million men and women. (*Frequently Asked Questions About A.A.* 1952, p. 7)

This influential answer, which depicts alcoholism—or, as the medical and psychiatric communities now prefer to call it, "alcohol dependence" or "alcohol dependence syndrome"—as a sickness or disease in some standard medical sense, but not a moral weakness or a kind of mental imbalance, is increasingly implausible. Alcoholism is a disorder. It is a complex psycho-biological-social disorder, not a specific disease of the body or the brain, despite involving both (Graham 2010). The A.A. definition in the pamphlet, Alcoholism[A.A.], characterizes the alleged disease as a syndrome largely inside a person (or extending as far as the hand-mouth connection) —it involves mainly a special sensitivity to alcohol and a mental obsession, which yield ballistically drinking. But in the actual world alcoholism involves all sorts of doings and deeds that are not in the alcoholic (e.g., dishonest, unreliable, and dangerous behavior in the service of using). Alcoholics commonly display some character weaknesses—they make but do not keep resolutions, and they often have some cognitive and affective abnormalities (e.g., forgetfulness, emotional unpredictability). Furthermore, whereas we do not know for sure whether genes causally contribute to alcohol addiction (although twin studies suggest there is some influence on susceptibility, Heyman 2009, p. 90; also see W. Liedke et al. (2011) that indicates that the brains of animals that are most susceptible to cocaine addiction activate genes associated with the salt instinct when they use), which if we did know would allow us to say that there is a component that is "inside the person" (and which he did not choose), we do know for sure that being a member of a family, ethnic group, or institution that tolerates or jokes about adult drunkenness is a causal contributor. But this property, being a member of a normative community that tolerates or jokes about adult drunkenness, is not inside the person (although fraternal organizations aside, one's family, ethnic group, and socioeconomic status are also not chosen).

But, most importantly for my purposes, whether alcoholism is a progressive disease or illness or, what is different, whether it is a disease or illness essentially characterized by a mental obsession and physical crazing is not something the phenomenological reports of small groups of patients, early members of A.A., for example, have any bearing on. Alcoholism[A.A.] speaks about what "makes sense," or what did make sense, to people with drinking problems in the 1930s to 1950s. These early members of A.A. were problem drinkers, drunks, alcohol addicts, not experts on the nature and causes of problem drinking. No one would trust cancer patients or schizophrenics to define their illness, although one ought to listen carefully to how things seem to them.

What sort of evidence did or does A.A. have that there is a disease characterized by "physical sensitivity" to alcohol and a "mental obsession" that "cannot be broken by willpower alone"?[2] My answer is that the evidence, then and now, for the view that alcoholism is best defined as Alcoholism[A.A.] is weak. There are several reasons. First, the science of addiction points to the idea that alcoholism is a spectrum disorder—it comes in a great variety. There is strong reason to believe that the early members of A.A. were in fact unrepresentative of most alcoholics, that they made up an extreme type at one end of the spectrum, who suffered perhaps from mental obsession and the phenomenon of craving. But the evidence suggests that not all problem drinkers suffer from these psychological symptoms or, most importantly, from "impotence" or "powerlessness" over alcohol. At the end of the day, what the word "alcoholism" means, or comes to mean, is a matter that will be determined at least in part by a complex process in which science, ethics, politics, and the law will have a say. Maybe we will say it is some kind of disease, maybe not. But what definition "seems" best or "makes sense" to alcoholics (over 75 years ago or now) will not and should not carry much weight.

To sum up: Alcoholism is a problem. Alcoholics think or say they have a problem and those with whom they interact—loved ones, family, employers— say they have a problem. Whether alcoholism is also a disease or not is not for me to say. But if it is a disease, it is not the disease defined by either Alcoholism[Fingarette] or Alcoholism[A.A.].

THE CONSENSUS: ALCOHOLISM IS A DISEASE

Fingarette's aim was to get rid of the unhelpful disease myth and replace it with something like a spectrum disorder idea. Alcoholism comes in degrees. There is an emerging consensus this is so.[3] There are those who experience tremendous difficulty in stopping and those who experience less difficulty (Vaillant 1995; Heyman 2009). Fingarette writes:

> Because there are so many different patterns of chronic alcohol abuse, I use the phrase *heavy drinking* as the general label for all forms of excessive consumption—and most importantly to get rid of the idea that heavy drinkers suffer from "loss of control." The classic disease concept proposes a simple

2. See Ainsle 2001, Bayne and Levy 2006, Holton 2009, Wallace 1999; Watson 1999; and Yaffe 2001 for high quality work on addiction, compulsion, control, responsibility, will and willpower.

3 Actually Jellinek (1946), and especially in his important and influential *The Disease Concept of Alcoholism* (1960), who Fingarette rails against because he pushes the disease concept, distinguishes among five kinds of alcoholics, not all of whom have loss of control, although sometimes they have organ damage from drinking. In general, Fingarette's somewhat mythic target—Alcoholism[Fingarette]—is not equivalent to Alcoholism[A.A.] or to Alcoholism[Jellinek] and thus one might be skeptical that the myth as he defines it is what most every American circa 1988 believed.

hypothesis: Chronic heavy drinkers do not stop or limit their drinking—despite the medical, emotional, social, and financial problems they may encounter—because they cannot control their drinking, even when they realize that it would be prudent or preferable for them to do so. (1988, p. 31)

As we have seen, Fingarette's argument is multipronged, taking aim at the ideas that all heavy drinkers suffer a specific, chronic, progressive disease that is characterized essentially by loss of control. His argument is still spot on because every study with incentives (Heyman 2009) shows that heavy drinkers do respond to incentives. Indeed, most alcoholics control the when, where, and how of their drinking each and every day. There are now also explanations of why, brain-wise, it is so hard for heavy drinkers to stop drinking completely and for good, and why they must be on guard to the charms of drink long after they feel that they have overcome the desire (Ainslie, Holton and Berridge this volume; Lowenstein 1996, Elster 1991). All the research shows that although it is hard, sometimes very hard for heavy drinkers to control their drinking, it is not impossible. No research shows complete "loss of control."

What is peculiar, ironic may be a better word, is that the disease myth that Fingarette lamented in 1988, but which he thought was not given any credibility by any expert, is now the mainstream view among the experts. Gene Heyman, in his important *Addiction: A Disorder of Choice* (2009), writes that "The idea that addiction is a disease is now the prevailing view among researchers, clinicians, and the media. In clinical texts and articles, addiction is introduced as a 'chronic illness' that should be classified with diseases like diabetes and asthma" (2009, p. 17). He writes that most clinicians now think that the "disease interpretation" is "the scientific, enlightened and humane perspective."[4] George Vaillant, psychiatrist and author of *The Natural History of Alcoholism Revisited* (1995), by far the best longitudinal study (now into its sixth decade) of drinking patterns among men, also thinks that alcoholism is a disease. But he thinks it is voluntary.[5] So even if Fingarette's aim to get rid of the disease concept has not succeeded, it may be that his desire to return the idea of agency, control, voluntariness, and responsibility to the alcoholic is winning. Or, to put it another way: although very few

4. It is interesting that Heyman does not help himself to the better idea contained in his title, *Addiction: A Disorder of Choice,* that addiction is a disorder but not necessarily a disease.

5. When people wonder whether alcoholism is voluntary or not, there is almost always this ambiguity. They might wonder about etiology. If so, the situation looks this way: surely, no one intends to become an alcoholic, although it requires a large number of voluntary actions to become one. So becoming an alcoholic is voluntary but not intentional. Alternatively, the issue might be whether a person in the grip can stop herself. Here the answer is a bit more complicated. It will take a host of voluntary actions on her part to stop. She might need help and it is likely to be very hard.

hold that alcoholism is the disease defined as Alcoholism[Fingarette], many, perhaps most, experts think that alcoholism is a disease of some sort or another, perhaps it is Alcoholism[A.A.] or something in its vicinity, or more likely, the kind of disease alcoholism is depends on some interest-relative features of what a particular *episteme* finds most salient.[6] My view is this: it would be best to simply stop discussing the disease concept of alcoholism and get down to describing the mechanisms of alcoholism, its genetics, psychology, neurobiology, and sociology. One important element in bringing that about is undermining the idea that alcoholism is involuntary and involves a "loss of control." The facts suggest this: no one plans or intends to become an alcoholic, but becoming one requires a large number of voluntary actions. Undoing alcoholism also requires a large number of voluntary actions. Alcoholics are agents. It is no use whatsoever—except perhaps to unimaginative insurance underwriters—to consider alcoholism as a disease and the alcoholic as a victim. Alcoholism is a problem, a disorder, a complex dysfunctional syndrome, which the alcoholic contributes to bringing about by his own actions, and will, if he overcomes, also be the primary agent, thereby displaying willpower in so doing. Alcoholics deserve compassion, not because they are victims of forces beyond their control, but because they suffer and cause others to suffer.

HISTORY: A.A.'S "TALKING CURE"

A.A. began in 1935 when a stockbroker and a surgeon found that talking to each other helped them abstain from drinking, which in their cases always led to getting drunk. Just as Freud and Breuer stumbled upon psychoanalysis, "the talking cure," by watching Anna O.'s symptoms of hysterical paralysis yield to her narrating the memories of what it was like to experience her father's death, Bill W. and Dr. Bob found that talking about their drinking lifted the desire to drink, diverted the desire to drink, or some such, which resulted in periods of abstention—eventually, in both cases, that were lifelong (unless one counts Bill W.'s 1970s dalliance with LSD as a fast-track "spiritual awakener" and relapse preventer)—that were longer than either was able to maintain on his own, without talking to another alcoholic. The experience of these two well-educated men was quickly packaged in the institutional garb of the Oxford Group, a then-popular perfectionist confessional Protestant movement, founded by an American Lutheran of Swiss decent who had his own moment on the road to Damascus near Oxford, UK, thus the name "Oxford Group." Bill W. was clear that the emphasis in A.A.'s twelve steps on self-examination,

---

6. Vaillant (1995) and Heyman (2009) get that the concept of disease is polysemous, ambiguous, etc., but believe that it, as applied to alcoholism, has helped to remove a certain stigma. This might be an effect, perhaps even a good effect, of adopting disease talk. But it would leave open the question of how alcoholism ought to be scientifically classified.

acknowledgment of character defects, restitution for harm done, and working with others came straight from the Oxford Group, although anyone familiar with any variety of Christian confessional practices will find many of the steps familiar, and utterly independent of any other malady than being human, fallible, fallen (Kurtz 1991).

In 1939, only four years after Bill and Bob's initial meeting, the *Big Book* of A.A. was published. The *Big Book* is the basic text, and to this day, the world over, most meetings begin with a reading of the "Preamble" and the "Twelve Steps" (often the "Twelve Traditions" as well).[7]

A.A. Preamble

Alcoholics Anonymous is a fellowship of men and women who share their experience, strength and hope with each other that they may solve their common problem and help others to recover from alcoholism. The only requirement for membership is a desire to stop drinking. There are no dues or fees for A.A. membership; we are self-supporting through our own contributions. A.A. is not allied with any sect, denomination, politics, organization or institution; does not wish to engage in any controversy, neither endorses nor opposes any causes. Our primary purpose is to stay sober and help other alcoholics to achieve sobriety.

Twelve Steps

1. We admitted we were powerless over alcohol—that our lives had become unmanageable.
2. Came to believe that a Power greater than ourselves could restore us to sanity.
3. Made a decision to turn our will and our lives over to the care of God as we understood Him.
4. Made a searching and fearless moral inventory of ourselves.
5. Admitted to God, to ourselves and to another human being the exact nature of our wrongs.
6. Were entirely ready to have God remove all these defects of character.
7. Humbly asked Him to remove our shortcomings.
8. Made a list of all persons we had harmed, and became willing to make amends to them all.
9. Made direct amends to such people wherever possible, except when to do so would injure them or others.

---

7. The Twelve Steps were in place in 1939 when the first edition of the *Big Book* was published; the Twelve Traditions were published in 1950. The Preamble dates from 1947 and was based on the Forward to the first edition of the *Big Book*. In 1958, its wording was changed from "honest desire to stop drinking" to "desire to stop drinking" in order to conform to the third Tradition in the *Big Book*.

10. Continued to take personal inventory and when we were wrong promptly admitted it.

11. Sought through prayer and meditation to improve our conscious contact with God, as we understood Him, praying only for knowledge of His will for us and the power to carry that out.

12. Having had a spiritual awakening as the result of these steps, we tried to carry this message to alcoholics, and to practice these principles in all our affairs. (pp. 59–60)

The 12 Steps and 12 Traditions plus the first 168 pages of the *Big Book* are the core of what is called "the program." The *Big Book* begins with a "Foreword" and two letters, the equivalent of blurbs, called "The Doctor's Opinion," by Dr. William Duncan Silkworth, M.D. (1873–1951). Silkworth was a leading specialist in the treatment of alcoholism and director of the Charles B. Towns Hospital for Drug and Alcohol Addictions in New York City in the 1930s, during which time Bill W. was admitted on three separate occasions for treatment. Silkworth encouraged Bill W. to believe that alcoholism was more than just a matter of moral weakness (which is compatible with it being in part a "moral weakness"), and he introduced Bill Wilson to the idea that alcoholism had a pathological, disease-like basis. Silkworth's sensitive and compassionate letters rehearse his view that alcoholism is an illness, specifically an allergy, which causes the phenomenon of craving in susceptible persons, and is incurable unless the alcoholic undergoes a wholesale, psychic and spiritual makeover.[8] Bill's own highbrow "psychic change" occurred during his third detox at Towns after or while reading William James's *Varieties of Religious Experience* (1902)![9]

C. G. Jung had endorsed this idea of the requirement of wholesale psychic change—something beyond abstention—antecedently and independently. And both Bill W. and Silkworth knew of Jung's opinion.[10]

After Silkworth's short letters, the first 168 pages consist of "Bill's Story" followed by chapters that outline the normal trajectory and psychology of a certain ideal type, "the alcoholic," followed by a chapter offering hope—"There is

8. Note that the allergy idea and the requirement of a wholesale psychic and spiritual change are not part of the definition Alcoholism[A.A.].

9. Bill was being encouraged to have such an awakening in Towns and was on a belladonna regimen—known to produce hallucinations—at the time. http://www.nytimes.com/2010/04/20/health/20drunk.html

10. Here is a letter that Jung wrote to Bill W. in 1961, after Bill W. had written him about Rowland H., a friend of Bill's and a former patient of Jung's in Zurich, who Bill W. had met in the Oxford Groups in the early 1930s and who had told him of Jung's longstanding conviction that total psychic change was required for recovery.

a Solution"—and another, called "How It Works," that provides an overview of the steps, along with promises that doing them leads to the lifting of the mental obsession, physical craving, and loss of control that are constitutive of the disease of alcoholism, Alcoholism[A.A.]. There is a chapter called "We Agnostics" that reassures the agnostic and atheist that he can recover if he "makes believe" that he turns his life and will over to the care of a Higher Power, who (in a classic bait and switch) will eventually reveal himself by curing his disease and thereby dissolving his agnosticism.[11] There are chapters "To Wives," "To Employers,"

Dear Mr. W.
Your letter has been very welcome indeed.

I had no news from Rowland H. anymore and often wondered what has been his fate. Our conversation which he has adequately reported to you had an aspect of which he did not know. The reason that I could not tell him everything was that those days I had to be exceedingly careful of what I said. I had found out that I was misunderstood in every possible way. Thus I was very careful when I talked to Rowland H. But what I really thought about was the result of many experiences with men of his kind.

His craving for alcohol was the equivalent, on a low level, of the spiritual thirst of our being for wholeness, expressed in medieval language: the union with God.*

How could one formulate such an insight in a language that is not misunderstood in our days?

The only right and legitimate way to such an experience is that it happens to you in reality and it can only happen to you when you walk on a path which leads you to higher understanding. You might be led to that goal by an act of grace or through a personal and honest contact with friends, or through a higher education of the mind beyond the confines of mere rationalism. I see from your letter that Rowland H. has chosen the second way, which was, under the circumstances, obviously the best one.

I am strongly convinced that the evil principle prevailing in this world leads the unrecognized spiritual need into perdition, if it is not counteracted either by real religious insight or by the protective wall of human community. An ordinary man, not protected by an action from above and isolated in society, cannot resist the power of evil, which is called very aptly the Devil. But the use of such words arouses so many mistakes that one can only keep aloof from them as much as possible.

These are the reasons why I could not give a full and sufficient explanation to Rowland H., but I am risking it with you because I conclude from your very decent and honest letter that you have acquired a point of view above the misleading platitudes one usually hears about alcoholism.

You see, "alcohol" in Latin is "spiritus" and you use the same word for the highest religious experience as well as for the most depraving poison. The helpful formula therefore is: *spiritus contra spiritum.*

Thanking you again for your kind letter

I remain
Yours sincerely
C. G. Jung*
"As the hart panteth after the water brooks, so panteth my soul after thee, O God." (Psalms 42:1)

11. To be fair many, perhaps most, members believe that the agency works from the belief in something greater to gaining control, not by direct intervention of this power once one believes in Him. I say more about this issue later.

and to "The Family Afterwards," which taken together articulate the A.A. way of thinking about alcoholism as a disease and an illness, and the alcoholic as sick and ill, and offers help to the alcoholic and those who are affected or suffer also from his alcoholism.

But there is a disconnect, an epistemically significant disconnect between a single "Doctor's Opinion" and what follows. The book begins with the claim that alcoholism is a disease, a sickness, an illness, but then proceeds to offer a two-part prescription, a fellowship ("whenever two or more are gathered," etc.) and a program (the 12 steps), which are entirely nonmedical. Furthermore, in both the *Big Book* and in many church basements where A.A. meetings are held, there is the view that the primary disease is a "soul sickness," and that drinking is only a symptom, perhaps the main symptom, but a symptom nonetheless of this soul sickness. The steps promise by the 12th step that the alcoholic will have had a "spiritual awakening." This Rx is what is needed if the Jung-Silkworth impression of what works with "real alcoholics" is accepted. But conceived as a treatment for a disease, this is, to be polite, very odd.

Fingarette puts his finger on the oddity, the source of the disconnect, when he writes this: "It deserves note...that while the group's doctrine holds that alcoholism is a disease, the practice of A.A. is entirely nonmedical. A.A. is not a treatment, but a new way of life for those who choose to become involved" (1988, p. 89). Two decades later, Heyman (2009, p. 20) says essentially the same thing, pointing out correctly that whatever abstention A.A. helps bring about comes from neither a medical nor a penal treatment since A.A. offers neither. A.A. requires choice and compliance with a regimen of abstention. Common advice is "Don't drink, come to meetings." Those who succeed do so.

Whatever alcoholism is, it is a problem that essentially involves drinking. It follows that if you don't drink, you don't get drunk. It might be true that going to A.A. helps (i.e., causally contributes to) abstention. But abstention doesn't then cause the drinking to stop. Abstention is not drinking. Many people find ways to leverage themselves out of drinking. To change a flat tire, most of us need a jack. Even if you used a jack to change the flat, you changed the tire. So it seems with alcoholism: even if you needed to hear "the experience, strength, and hope" of others before you could figure out how to stop, you stopped. If alcoholism is a disease, it is a very unusual one if choosing not to use and figuring out a way to keep that resolution typically stop it.

A.A. and Who Is and Is Not a *Real* Alcoholic

As I mentioned above, one of Fingarette's prescient points is that alcoholism is what we would now call a spectrum disorder. It comes in degrees. There is an emerging consensus this is so.[12] There are those who experience tremendous difficulty in stopping and those who experience less difficulty (Vaillant 1995; Heyman 2009). This is something A.A. could claim to have noticed itself right from the start when it reserved the designation "alcoholic" only for drinkers who have the following profile: They are mentally obsessed with drinking; when they drink craving sets in for more and they cannot stop, often until they go unconscious. They have bargained and tried to moderate, but they always fail. No normal incentives—health, love, and professional success—are sufficient to keep the "true alcoholic" from using. Often they drink themselves to death.

If one were asked for a hermeneutic of what "powerlessness" means in the first step of the 12 steps, most alcoholics would say it refers to something like this latter sort of relationship to alcohol. In Chapter 2, "There is a Solution," we read of another type of drinker: "Then we have a certain type of hard drinker. He may have the habit badly enough to gradually impair him physically and mentally. It may cause him to die a few years before his time. If a sufficiently strong reason, ill health, falling in love, change of environment, or the warning of a doctor becomes operative, this man can also stop or moderate, although he may find it difficult and troublesome and may even need medical attention." This much sounds exactly right. And I know many people who fit the latter description from the rooms of A.A. What I do not know—for the curious—are any people who showed up in an A.A. room and were able to find a way back to normal or moderate social drinking. I know many, including myself, who have tried and failed. And there may be some who I don't know.

But then we are immediately told that this type of person is not a "real alcoholic." But this is stipulative, and carves the natural phenomena in an odd way, although it does—as I said above—pretty well mark the early clientele of A.A. One reason the designation is stipulative is that most every "real alcoholic" was once a "certain type of hard drinker." It also means that many members of A.A. nowadays who identify as alcoholics, who have a desire not to drink, and who achieve abstention are not alcoholics, at least not "real" ones.

Whereas most of the early A.A. members had "low bottoms"—they repeatedly chose alcohol over relationships, jobs, health, and so forth—many newcomers nowadays come into the rooms with "high bottoms" (e.g., they find themselves drinking more than they wish and are having trouble cutting back). They look very much like that "certain type of hard drinker," who, as far as the *Big Book* goes, are not (at least not yet) in the grip of a chronic, progressive, fatal disease.

12. Jellinek in his important and influential *The Disease Concept of Alcoholism* (1960), who Fingarette rails against because he pushes the disease concept, did himself distinguish among five kinds of alcoholics, many of whom have no loss of control.

They are not (at least not yet) gripped by a mental obsession or physical craving. And they are not "real alcoholics," and thus they are not, as far as the program of A.A. is concerned, in need of a "spiritual transformation."

The key leap, the odd piece of logic is this: there are certain kinds of heavy drinkers who can stop and stay stopped, although it is difficult. These folk are not in need of a Jung-Silkworth style of "spiritual transformation" or "wholesale psychic change." But the true or "real" alcoholic who was formerly this kind of heavy drinker (one who could of stopped but who can't any longer) requires this kind of cure.

The first thing to say is that the idea is not completely crazy. There are many bona fide diseases that call for different treatments depending on how far along the disease is. But here, with diabetes and cancer, say, we are talking about such things as different doses of medicines and whether surgery is necessary or not. If A.A. is a medical treatment, the most charitable interpretation is that it is some kind cognitive-behavioral therapy. And that seems like the right view, better than saying less politely, as some critics do, that it is akin to brainwashing and voodoo than to ordinary medicine or ordinary therapy. But still, if it is that, a therapy to change thinking and behavior primarily in terms of the relation of the person to alcohol, why the spiritual transformation Rx? A reasoned answer is not provided inside the *Big Book*, although it is repeatedly said that such a wholesale transformation is necessary for the "real" alcoholic. The second thing to say, and it sheds some light on the latter issue, is that, of course, the whole-sale psychic change is not in fact wholesale. An individual in recovery does not change his personality or values. Indeed, the key is normally to realign the person's personality traits and his behavior with his values. A conscientious father controls his anger, goes to work, pays the bills, and does not drive the children to soccer practice drunk. What this suggests is that the claim that A.A. offers or delivers wholesale psychological transformation and that it delivers such transformation is a form of boastful advertising. It doesn't happen. What does happen is that many people who are seriously messing themselves and their lives up stop drinking, heal, and become better, more the person they once were, or want to be.

One finding in the literature, dubbed the "Berkson Effect," suggests that those individuals who show up in A.A. or in A.A. by way of various drying-out periods in jail, detox, psych wards, or 28-day programs are unrepresentative. They have crossed a line (perhaps their brains have changed in ways studied by Berridge or Koob) and are the really hard nuts to crack. One doesn't see the many heavy drinkers or alcoholics who moderated or stopped drinking without these forms of treatment. Did these other folk who one does not see stop on their own? Some did, but in the sorts of people whose family and work life was influential in their moderating or stopping drinking (before, as we say, it is too late and the "off switch" stopped working, is broken, etc.), these people, these relations, and these ever-present institutions played a role. Normally, a community, a significant social ecology, is in play in habit change that many heavy drinkers undergo in finding an equilibrium as a normal social drinker or a teetotaler.

MEETERS AND STEPPERS

Many A.A.'s distinguish nowadays between the *fellowship* and the *program*. The fellowship consists of the meetings and the interactions that take place in them (as well as, to some extent, before and after meetings). All meetings have a chair, whose role is to provide or enforce a structure so that those congregated can share their "experience, strength, and hope," so that they can "solve their common problem," typically by telling stories or snippets of stories about "what it was like, what happened, and what it is like now." It is common to tell newcomers "Don't drink, come to meetings."

The *program* is the Twelve Steps. For many, perhaps most, members of A.A., doing the 12 steps in order, normally in a formal manner with a sponsor, is considered to be what it takes to be assured, as best one can be assured, that one might "have a spiritual awakening" and experience relief from the "mental obsession and physical craving." Some people believe that doing the program, becoming a true A.A. Eagle Scout, involves working through and understanding the 12 traditions, as well as the 12 steps. The most important tradition for our purposes, and also the one most commonly cited and used to settle disputes at meetings, is the third tradition: "the only requirement for membership is a desire to stop drinking," which is also incorporated into the "Preamble" and which again, it is worth noting, says nothing, exactly zero, about alcoholism.[13]

A.A. is composed, then, of a basic text, the *Big Book*; a small number of additional authorized texts and pamphlets given an imprimatur by the General Service Offices in New York City; plus an oral tradition of do's and don'ts, fables and lore, mottoes and maxims that incorporate all sorts of variable customs and habits. Part of the lore involves claims that attribute causal powers to A.A., sometimes to meetings and the example of others;

---

13. At meetings it is customary for people to "introduce and qualify." "I am Owen and I am an alcoholic" is most common. "I am Owen and I have a desire not to drink today" is acceptable because of the third tradition. "I am Owen and I am powerless over alcohol" is rare, but not extremely so, and is acceptable because it substitutes the first half of the first step, "We admitted we were powerless over alcohol," for the word "alcoholic." The word "alcoholic" does not appear in the 12 steps. Depending on local rules, if a person at a closed meeting (members only) introduces himself as "I am Owen, I am a drug addict" or "I am Owen, I am here to find out about the program," the person will be asked if he is an alcoholic. If he says he is not sure, he will be asked if he has a desire not to drink, which is, according to the third tradition, the sole requirement for membership.

sometimes to the steps; sometimes to admixtures, like the steps and one's wise sponsor; and sometimes to little gems, like HALT—don't get hungry, angry, lonely, tired.[14]

One reason for worrying that the ways A.A. members speak is colored by how A.A. describes alcoholism rather than serving as evidence for the way A.A. describes alcoholism and recovery is because new members are told to "identify" with the stories and not to look for differences. Old timers typically say that the first 168 pages of the *Big Book* pretty well describe what alcoholics are like.[15] Such commonplaces, as that alcoholics try to moderate or stop, but can't, and that this leads to bewilderment, shame, and guilt, become elements in a social phenomenology, a social epistemology. The discipline is powerful enough so that members who think, say, or point out that they have not lost their health, or jobs, or loved ones, or self-respect, or self-control are said to suffer from the "YETS," as in the "*not*-yets," since these eventualities are what is to be expected, the normal progression of heavy drinking or, what is different, of feeding the chronic disease of alcoholism (if there is such a thing). So A.A. meetings encourage a kind of normative conformity in how members are encouraged to speak and think about our "common problem," and in this way meetings discipline how alcoholism is conceptualized.

True believers in A.A. think that not only does A.A. work but also A.A. speaks truthfully about the phenomenon of alcoholism. But, of course, there is no necessary connection. One can be a member of the fellowship,

---

14. I have been to meetings on several continents. Local rules govern such things as the speed at which one does the steps (a week, a month, a year); whether the steps are absolutely required; how many meetings a newcomer should initially attend (some think "30 meetings in 30 days," some "90 meetings in 90 days," others fewer; how fundamentalist or liberal/historicist the interpretation of the *Big Book* is; how people interpret A.A.'s being "a spiritual, but not religious" program; how close to drinking vs. general life improvement shares at meetings should be; how anonymity is interpreted—most think it is OK for me to tell you I am a member, but some think even that should not be shared, especially with media. One example of local customs and habits: In America, especially in the South, people end meetings with a prayer. Often this is the "Our Father." Early in recovery I mentioned to the matriarch of my local group that this might put off Jews and Muslims. She was surprised, saying she did not know it was a Christian prayer. In the United Kingdom, in my experience, the "Our Father" would not be said. But the serenity prayer would: "God, grant me the serenity to accept the things I cannot change, the courage to change the things I can, and the wisdom to know the difference." This prayer is considered nondenominational, spiritual not religious. *Aside*: The 14th Dalai Lama told me in Dharamsala, India, in 2000 that he thought this prayer was written by Buddha! (Reinhold Niebuhr is the most likely suspect.)

15. The rest of the *Big Book*—after the first 168 pages—consists of stories of recovery of all sorts of folk, the founders and early members, and in new editions of contemporary men, women, gay, straight, all colors of the rainbow, who tell their story and thereby, as we say, "share their experience, strength, and hope with each other" so that they can solve "a common problem."

enjoy an hour among people who also don't drink (although many still smoke a lot), and find that doing this helps break the habit of drinking. Call people who say that coming to meetings for a while did this—helped them stop drinking—"meeters." Meeters think that the fellowship causally contributed to their regaining control and stopping drinking. Meeters might or might not go to meetings for life.

"Steppers" think that meetings, the fellowship, is a temporary fix, and that it is doing (and redoing) the 12 steps of A.A. that fixed their drinking problem. "What we really have is a daily reprieve contingent on the maintenance of our spiritual condition" (*Big Book* 2001, p. 85). Meeters might think, and think truthfully, that any regular gregarious social activity (playing basketball, knitting, meet-ups, etc.)—perhaps with other nondrinkers, perhaps not—might have helped break the grip of their drinking problem, even if this involved the full-blown mental obsession, physical craving, and loss of control. One stops drinking when one adopts a lifestyle that involves putting "the plug in the jug."

"Steppers" think that the fellowship is only a temporary fix, or, as they sometimes say, one will be a dry drunk or still suffer the disease even if one never drinks again *unless* one does the 12 steps.[16] The "spiritual" program of the 12 steps is causally required for true recovery. This is so either because drinking is only a symptom of some other kind of soul sickness or because it isn't only a symptom, but one will continue to be prone to reactivating the disease if one doesn't take care of one's overall spiritual well-being, for example, by avoiding negative emotional states (fear, anxiety, shame, guilt) that alcohol is (known to be) effective against.

Now this view—really these views—of the steppers is really interesting IF true. The steps mention admitting that one has a problem with alcohol in the first half of the first step, and then alcohol and alcoholism are neither mentioned, implied, nor even hinted at in the next 10 steps, until, that is, we hear in the 12th: "Having had a spiritual awakening as a result of these steps, we tried to carry this message to alcoholics, and to practice these principles in all our affairs." What happened in between? And what are *these* principles? Answer: one is told to turn over one's will and one's life over to a "power greater than oneself," to "God, as we understand him," (steps 2 and 3); to do a life-long inventory (step 4); to confess one's sins and identify one's main character defects to God and another person (step 5); to will that these are lifted (steps 6 and 7); to make amends to those one has harmed (steps 8 and 9); to continue to

---

16. A dry drunk is someone who still displays the character defects that were causes or effects of his drinking (e.g., anger) or who has not been relieved of the mental obsession but abstains. This causes him to be not very nice, not present, angry, resentful, and so on.

take inventory on a daily basis (step 10); to pray and meditate (step 11); and, in general, to be a good, honest, reliable person.

I want to be fair here. I do not think it is preposterous to think that doing *this* program in *this* way might causally contribute to recovery. One reason is that many alcoholics claim to have first learned to use to produce pleasant effects, and what is different, as a shield from negative emotions (fear, social anxiety and awkwardness, and the like), exactly as normal social drinkers do, but to have eventually experienced great shame, guilt, remorse, or bewilderment as they lost control, creating a self-reinforcing cycle. Thus, doing anything that helps a person regain a sense of his or her own worth and agency might serve as a prophylactic for one common occasion of using, namely, shame, guilt, self-disappointment, or self-loathing. It isn't that alcoholics start as self-loathers. But many end up that way, and a recalibration to a way of living and being that is normatively endorsed as acceptable, even good or worthy, could help end that cycle.

HOW COULD A.A. WORK?

Bill W.—seemingly with approval—relates a story about Asian Buddhists, who do not believe in God, nonetheless finding a way to do the 12 steps by replacing "God" throughout the steps by "Good" (*A.A. Comes of Age* 1957, p. 81). This is interesting and important, and it suggests that the 12 steps are adaptable to any moral life form and do not require belief in any divinity, and that the goal of the steps is to create or re-create the psychological conditions for compliance with the norms of moral decency or conformity as conceived inside a tradition, where norms are a condition of self-respect inside that tradition. Why does or might this—conventional moral decency—matter? The answer need not be because alcoholism is caused in the first place by being bad, or soul sick, but because many—including normal drinkers—do some not-so-good things (e.g., not living up to one's own standards when using), and many learn to use alcohol as a shield against negative emotional states; thus, re-equilibrating a life is helpful to maintaining a regimen of self-control in the matter of drinking.

Another possibility—there really are numerous ones—is that "steppers" are right in the sense that they have had a conversion to a form of life and way of being that, as described in the first 168 pages of the *Big Book*, is inconsistent with them drinking again. If this is right, then becoming a Buddhist (or a Muslim) and abiding by the five universal precepts (often compared to the 10 commandments), and which include at step 5 the imperative to abstain from "intoxicating drinks and drugs causing heedlessness," would be the kind of conversion that would support sobriety without, again, requiring one to become an altogether different person or without requiring a Nietzschean-like "transvalu-ation" of all values.[17]

Not surprising, it is common to find all sorts of mixed views from pure meeters (the meetings are the key), to pure steppers (the 12 steps are the *sine qua non*), to all sorts of hybrid views. Even if it is sometimes true that A.A.—the fellowship or the program or some admixture—plays a causal role that meeters or steppers say it does, it is implausible to think that it is necessary. Indeed, there is abundant evidence that it is not necessary.

CONCLUSION: PHENOMENOLOGICAL AUTHORITY AND HOW A.A. WORKS

Psychology and cognitive science have pretty much established that we ought to beware any simple confidence in first-person psychological reports. Cautions abound and relate to a disconnect between confidence in and accuracy of reports, the lack of checks on sameness of meanings for psychological terms ("obsession," "craving") across persons, the theory-ladenness of first-person reports, which in the case of A.A. has to do with its extraordinary social power, and ideological contagion.

And thus there is an objection to claiming the truth of the *episteme* that is A.A., which involves raising the suspicion that the phenomenology of members of A.A. conforms to what A.A. says because it is the episteme imposed, often retrospectively, on experience, but not because it really fits and thereby supports that episteme, had that same experience been seen with a clear, untutored eye.

Here is how Fingarette describes the way A.A., like any episteme, disciplines its members to experience or recall the shape of their own problem drinking in the terms favored by its way of conceiving alcoholism:

A.A. groups provide individual members with powerful moral and emo-tional support, as well as practical aid and advice—provided the member conforms to the key expectations of the group....Members are encouraged to search their souls and their memories, and they are expected to gradu-ally discover therein a personal history that by and large conforms to the A.A. picture of the course of alcoholism. Members whose memories or

17. William James is often quoted as saying "the only radical remedy I know for dipsomania is religiomania." This quote (1902, p. 200) is in a footnote and James does not endorse it. He writes that "it is a saying I have heard quoted from some medical men." And indeed it was a commonplace view in the temperance movement that started in the 1890's. In South America, specifically in Peru and Ecuador at present, Christian evangelical churches are doing well con-verting former Roman Catholic families because they are opposed to drinking, and women in particular see that drinking (about which Catholicism is technically neutral) causes trouble.

understanding of their experiences are inconsistent with A.A. doctrine may be confronted and charged with denial. The group exerts a powerful form of peer pressure on new members to see themselves and explain themselves in terms of the A.A. picture of an alcoholic.... [M]embers who would fully participate must therefore acknowledge that they have an incurable, progressive disease, which they are powerless as individuals to overcome. They must accept total abstention as their only hope. They must confess their reliance on a Higher Power and commit themselves to helping fellow members discover these truths and fight off drink. The emotional pitch and sense of comradeship, in both despair and hope, can be intense. *Not surprisingly, those who become regular A.A. members do learn to believe in an autobiography that exemplifies A.A. teaching and to gloss over or ignore experiences and feelings that are contradicted by the teaching....* It is rather like...ideological re-education or a modest form of elective brainwashing. (1988, pp. 87–88)

What Fingarette writes here is fairly accurate, if slightly exaggerated. There is considerable variation, for example, in what the confession of faith in a Higher Power amounts to. Some think that the key is to give up the hope that one can regain control without help from God, where God is explicitly said by some to be a "Group Of Drunks." Not surprisingly, some alcoholics nowadays are agnostics or atheists, so words like "God" and "Higher Power" are sometimes given a social meaning or an aspirational meaning (wanting to be a better version of oneself, Me* rather than Me), and there are reminders to members who resist A.A. because it looks "religious" that the third step does not refer to "God" but to "God, as we understand Him."[18] The emphasis to resisters, and it may be part of the seduction into the episteme, is on the fairly obvious fact that one needs the support of others to break the cycle of drinking, getting drunk, shame, guilt, drinking, getting drunk, shame, guilt.

The key to any cognitive-behavioral therapy is that it provides techniques or skills that realign, restructure, or remake some problematic patterns of thought, feeling, and action. One puzzle for how cognitive-behavioral therapy might work in the case of alcoholism is that it is so recalcitrant to cognition. The alcoholic knows drinking is harmful to his mind and his body, his social and work relations. He determines that he will stop and yet he drinks. Again and again. He is a performative inconsistency. So how does it work, assuming it does?

18. Of interest to philosophers only: I have never at a meeting (and I have been listening) ever heard any A.A. member make a use-mention, object language-metalanguage distinction or the distinction between meaning and reference. That is, God (The Guy) is not distinguished from belief in God (The Guy) Failure to make the distinction may be why some members who start as agnostics and who get better attribute their recovery to God (The Guy) and not simply to their belief in God (The Guy).

Heyman (2009) give this plausible account of why and how A.A. works:

First, all new members have a sponsor or mentor to whom they can turn when they feel that they need to have a drink. The contact functions as an alternative or distraction, reorienting attention to something other than alcohol. Similarly, people learn to cope with discomfort or even pain by finding a distracting activity to occupy their thoughts. Second, at the meetings, new A.A. members meet people who had drinking problems similar to theirs but are now sober. The meetings demonstrate that it is possible to quit and that quitting leads to better overall existence.... Third, A.A.'s emphasis on faith in higher powers can be seen as a mechanism for instilling hope. A.A. claims that if an alcoholic has faith, he or she can become sober. For some, the statement itself is reassuring, and for all the statement is reinforced by the successes of sober A.A. members. Fourth, A.A. offers its members opportunities for successful and meaningful social relations...support, guidance, and friendship.... [B]oth hope and alternatives to drugs are what is needed. A.A. offers both. (p. 179).

There are several key claims here: One is the importance of the group functioning as a distraction, a place where attention is reoriented.[19] Another is that the group and its members offer both hope that recovery is possible and gregarious social activity that does not involve drinking. Some alcoholics drink in isolation, but many don't. But alcoholism is often lonely because "earth people" do not get why we alcoholics don't just stop and stay stopped. When you go to meetings you are around people from all walks of life who get it, get you, and who don't drink. Many of them are "happy, joyous, and free."

---

19. As I have written elsewhere (2011), my own drinking career was a "low bottom" one. For the first three months of sobriety I could not shake the mental obsession. I sat on my hands, talked to A.A. friends, and went to many meetings, sometimes two to three a day. I'd make it home relieved that I hadn't had a drink, but I was still obsessed (but at least not ashamed). One day I realized I had not thought about using for a few hours. After about six months, I started to have full days without intrusive thoughts/desires. Now, years later, I rarely have a desire, but sometimes I do and when I do it is not an intrusive one, more a "that beer/martini looks good" or "wouldn't it be nice to have that wine with this meal." I do not act upon these desires, having resolved that my life goes very much better without alcohol. If I had to guess what psychological or neurobiological models fit my kind of alcoholism I'd say this: I get hyperbolic discounting (Ainsle, 2001). I get ego-depletion (Levy) in trying to keep resolutions. I often felt as if I gave in to drinking for no better reason than that I was exhausted not drinking. I get intrusive, obsessive thoughts. I had them whenever I was awake. I suspect (maybe an autopsy can reveal) that I used so much that I crossed the line that Berridge and Koob write about so that my wanting-liking systems and my dopaminergic system were messed up. These features of alcoholism, on the view I am inclined to, are effects of drinking too much, not causes of drinking too much, although they each seem like obstacles to stopping once they are in play. Whether I am right is of course not a matter of what I think or guess.

I have tried to say some helpful things about how A.A. might work despite speaking superficially or falsely about the nature of alcoholism, for example, by counting too much on the phenomenology of early members with low bottoms in characterizing the phenomenon, or by requiring a "spiritual transformation" for recovery from alcoholism, given that such transformation is more part of lore than of fact. Alcoholics in A.A. sometimes stop drinking. Some also become better versions of themselves. Sometimes this is a version of who they once were, what they were like before; sometimes it is who they mostly were while drinking minus the drinking and the associated poor thinking and behavior. Occasionally, it is a new and improved version of oneself who does not drink. In every case, it is the not-drinking part that is the necessary condition for whatever additional or collateral self-help and self-improvement is on offer and/or attained. A.A. provides a comfortable place for people, especially those who have a dose of Christian confessional religion in their blood and bones,[20] to regain self-control in a zone of life (around booze) where they are weak, where they lack the ability on their own to stop doing something that is bad for them, and for others. If I am right, then A.A. is a kind of cognitive-behavioral therapy. It employs a host of techniques to change the alcoholics' economy of desire, to distract and re-orient, to re-learn how to behave in the zones of life where booze is an option, and to find a vibrant and loving community that supports the entire re-construction project. In many cases, especially ones in which the alcoholic deeply identifies with a drinking life, the reconstruction required can be massive (Flanagan in press). There is reason to think that it can and does work while its underlying theory of what alcoholism is and what it takes to get better is false or, at best, superficial. One can do controlled experiments in clinical settings where cognitive-behavioral therapy modeled on A.A. is done (such programs are abundant) and over time discover what aspects of the program are doing the mother lode of the causal work. What early members of A.A. or what current members say caused their recovery is worth listening to as a form of hypothesis generation. It is not worth listening to for evidence of what in fact caused recovery or even of what exactly ailed them in the first place.

In the meantime, it seems fair to say this much: Alcoholism is a psycho-bio-social syndrome; it is a disorder in the straightforward normative

---

20. But one might say, and say truthfully, that the steps are a platform that any of the Abrahamic traditions (all brands of Christianity, Islam, and Judaism) will find congenial because much of the talk of a Higher Power invokes images of the all-powerful God of these monotheistic traditions. Many have also noticed the ways in which the steps are Buddhist-friendly, requiring less willful fighting and more acquiescence as a way of leveraging self-control. So it may be that the steps can be viewed as composed of general cultural wisdom about self-control, how to deal with external temptation, and how to deal with weakness in one's character that makes one prone to be weak where and when one wishes not to be.

sense that it causes disharmony for the person who is the alcoholic and for the other people and other institutions he interacts with. Whether alcoholism is a disease or not is a great distraction. It is much ado about nothing. The facts are these: No one chooses to become alcoholic. Becoming alcoholic is unintentional. But many voluntary actions are required for someone to become alcoholic. Furthermore, many voluntary actions are required for someone who is alcoholic, who suffers from alcohol dependence, to stop drinking and stay stopped. Sometimes it takes a village. A.A. is one such village. It works. But this doesn't mean that it deserves—or, for that matter, even that it seeks or should seek—the phenomenal authority it has about the nature and causes of alcoholism.

REFERENCES

AA Comes of Age: A Brief History of Alcoholics Anonymous. 1957. New York: A.A. World Services.

Ainslie, George. 2001. *Breakdown of Will.* Cambridge: Cambridge University Press.

Bayne, Tim, and Neil Levy. 2006. "The Feeling of Doing: Deconstructing the Phenomenology of Agency." In N. Sebanz and W. Prinz (eds.), *Disorders of Volition.* Cambridge, MA: MIT Press.

The Big Book of Alcoholics Anonymous. 2001 (4th ed.; 1939, 1955, 1976). A.A. General Services Approved Literature. New York: A.A. World Services.

Frequently Asked Questions About A.A 1952. A.A. General Services Approved Literature. New York: A.A. World Services.

Elster, Jon. 1991. *Strong Feelings.* Cambridge, MA: MIT Press.

Fingarette, Herbert. 1988. *Heavy Drinking: The Myth of Alcoholism as a Disease.* Berkeley: University of California.

Flanagan, Owen. 1992. *Consciousness Reconsidered* Cambridge, MA: MIT Press.

Flanagan, Owen. 2007. *The Really Hard Problem: Meaning in a Material World.* Cambridge, MA: MIT Press.

Flanagan, Owen. 2009. "Can Do Attitudes." Reply to R.T McKay and D.C. Dennett "The Evolution of Misbelief." Behavioral and Brain Sciences, Vol. 32, Issue 06, December 2009, pp. 493–510.

Flanagan, Owen. 2011. "What It Is Like to Be an Addict." In J. Poland and G. Graham (eds.), *Addiction and Responsibility* Cambridge, MA: MIT Press, pp. 269–292.

Flanagan, O. in press. "Identity and Addiction: What Alcoholic Memoirs Teach." In *The Oxford Handbook of Philosophy and Psychiatry.* Edited by KWM Fulford, Martin Davies, Richard Gipps, George Graham, John Sadler, Giovanni Stanghellini and Tim Thornton.

Foucault, Michel. 1966 (French). 1970/1994. *The Order of Things. An Archaeology of the Human Sciences.* New York: Vintage.

Graham, George. 2010. *The Disordered Mind: An Introduction to Philosophy of Mind and Mental Illness.* New York: Routledge.

Holton, Richard. 2009. *Willing, Wanting, Waiting.* Oxford: Oxford University Press.

Heyman, Gene. M. 2009. *Addiction: A Disorder of Choice* Cambridge, MA: Harvard University Press.

Jellinek, E. M. 1946. "Phases in the Drinking History of Alcoholics: Analysis of a Survey Conducted by the Official Organ of Alcoholics Anonymous." *Quarterly Journal of Studies on Alcohol*, Vol. 7, pp. 1–88.

Jellinek, E. M. 1960. *The Disease Concept of Alcoholism*. New Haven, CT: Hillhouse.

James, William. 1902. *Varieties of Religious Experience.* New York: Random House.

Kurtz, Ernest. 1991 (2nd ed., orig. 1979). *Not God: A History of Alcoholics Anonymous.* Center City, MN: Hazelden.

Liedtke, W. B., McKinley, M. J., Walker, L. L., Zhang, H., Pfenning, A. R., Drago, J., Hochendoner, S. J., Hilton, D. L., Lawrence, A. J., and Denton, D. A.. 2011 "Relation of addiction genes to hypothalamic gene changes subserving genesis and gratification of a classic instinct, sodium appetite." *Proceedings of the National Academy of Science USA*, Vol. 108, Issue 30, pp. 12509–12514.

Loewenstein, George. 1996. "Out of Control: Visceral Influences on Behavior." *Organizational Behavior and Human Decision Processes*, Vol. 65, pp. 272–292.

McKellar, J. D., Stewart, E., and Humphreys, K. 2003. "Alcoholics Anonymous involvement and positive alcohol-related outcomes: Cause, consequence, or just a correlation? A prospective 2-year study of 2,319 alcohol-dependent men. "*Journal of Consulting and Clinical Psychology*", Vol. 71, Issue 2,:pp. 302–308.

Okrent, D. 2010. *Last Call: The Rise and Fall of Prohibition*. New York: Scribner.

Vaillant, George. E. 1995. *The Natural History of Alcoholism Revisited*. Cambridge, MA: Harvard University Press.

Wallace, R. J. 1999. "Addiction as Defect of the Will: Some Philosophical Reflections." *Law and Philosophy*, Vol. 18, No. 6, Addiction and Responsibility: Part I (November), pp. 621–654.

Watson, Gary. 1999. "Disordered Appetites." In Jon Elster (ed.), *Addiction: Entries and Exits*. New York: Russell Sage Foundation.

Yaffe, Gideon. 2001. "Recent Work on Addiction and Responsible Agency." *Philosophy & Public Affairs*, Vol. 30, No. 2 (Spring), pp. 178–221.

6

Varieties of Valuation in the Normal and Addicted Brain

Legal and Policy Implications from a Neuroscience Perspective

MARK E. WALTON AND NICHOLAS A. NASRALLAH

INTRODUCTION

Every day we face decisions between superficially attractive options and alternatives with greater long-term benefits. Such choices shape our existence and, in some cases, determine our survival. How we are able to exercise appropriate self-control and resist detrimental temptations in such situations, and why this might go awry in neuropsychiatric disorders, is of central importance to the behavioral sciences.

One prominent example is that addiction research is increasingly described as an instance of pathological decision making, where the potential incentives of drugs of abuse come to dominate and control behavior irrespective of associated costs, negative future consequences, or societal rules and norms (Bechara, 2005; Bernheim & Rangel, 2004; Herrnstein & Prelec, 1992; Heyman, 2009; Rahman, Sahakian, Cardinal, Rogers, & Robbins, 2001; Redish, Jensen, & Johnson, 2008; Robinson & Berridge, 2000). In chronic substance abuse patients, for instance, there would appear to be a faulty trade-off between the short-term payoffs of taking a drug and the potential long-term costs to health, finances, and family life. Indeed, several theories of addiction have emphasized the impulsive nature of the choices made by addicts in spite of the later costs (Ainslie, 2001; Dalley, Everitt, & Robbins, 2011), and there are influential models of addiction that treat drugs partly as an economic commodity no different from any other type of good that we might wish to obtain (Becker & Murphy, 1988; Bernheim & Rangel, 2004; Gruber & Koszegi, 2001).

Although there is an extensive history of neuroscientific research into self-control over our choices, most of the first studies focused on conditional situations (red light = stop, green light = go), and for a long time there was a surprising neglect of what may be seen as a more commonplace scenario, where decisions are based on how worthwhile a course of action might be. Over the past 15 years, however, this situation has reversed and there is now a flourishing field investigating how simple value-guided decisions are computed in the brain, aided by an integration of formal models and techniques from disciplines such as machine learning (Dayan & Niv, 2008; Sutton & Barto, 1998), behavioral ecology (Stephens & Krebs, 1986), and economics (Camerer, 2008) with experimental psychology and neuroscience.

Importantly, this research demonstrates what seems to be substantial overlap between the neural systems involved in reinforcement learning and value-based decision making and those activated and/or altered in addiction. For instance, dopamine transmission, which is affected by virtually all drugs of abuse, is required to motivate animals to pursue rewards (Berridge, 2007; Salamone, Correa, Farrar, & Mingote, 2007; Wise, 2004), and the activity of dopamine neurons and dopamine transmission in the ventral striatum (VStr) to reward-predicting stimuli correlates with several fundamental economic attributes, such as outcome magnitude, uncertainty, and delay (Fiorillo, Tobler, & Schultz, 2003; Gan, Walton, & Phillips, 2010; Roesch, Calu, & Schoenbaum, 2007; Tobler, Fiorillo, & Schultz, 2005). Many models of the loss of behavioral control that is central to addiction point to dysfunction in the same frontal-striatal-monoaminergic circuits that are implicated in guiding decision making (Dalley et al., 2011; Rangel, Camerer, & Montague, 2008). In other words, addiction could lead to a breakdown in control simply by hijacking the neural systems normally used for deciding what is worth doing.

However, while such simple descriptions of the conceptual and neuroanatomical overlap between normal value-guided decision making and addiction are compelling, there is also a danger that this coincidence may make it easy to overlook complexities of how decisions are made and changed in the brain. Neurophysiological studies demonstrate that outcome value influences processing in almost all areas of the brain—not only in those circuits traditionally implicated in reinforcement, motivation, and decision making, but also in the primary sensory and motor cortex (Kapogiannis, Campion, Grafman, & Wassermann, 2008; Kennerley & Walton, 2011; Serences, 2008). Therefore, a statement that addiction "results from a reconfiguration of the circuitry of the reward and decision-making systems" (Eagleman, Correro, & Singh, 2010, pp. 8–9), while undoubtedly true, might at one level simply be rephrased as "addiction is a neurological problem."[1]

There is now wide consensus that decision making and self-control involves multiple interacting neural systems encoding different aspects of value, only some of which need to be under our conscious control. Moreover, the brain regions involved in *learning* these different components of value can also be separate from those involved in *using* these values to make choices (e.g., Noonan et al., 2010). Strikingly, many of these distinctions at the neuroanatomical level have direct functional correlates. Such distinctions are of real importance when trying to relate addiction to neural dysfunction as apparently identical behavioral manifestations of failed self-control might arise after disruption to entirely separate decision processes. Conversely, this increased complexity also brings promise from the other direction. Disentangling the multiple valuation systems in the normal brain in tandem with a finer-grained understanding of addiction might provide clues to explain the different ways in which aberrant patterns of choice behavior may arise in this and other neuropsychiatric disorders.

Our main aim for this chapter is therefore to explore how our increasing understanding of the fractionation of the *normal* processes of valuation, self-control, and value- and rule-guided decision making in the brain may influence how we should think of addiction as a neurological disorder.[2] Accordingly, we will not provide an overarching review of the literature on how dysfunctions in neural circuitry may underlie different facets of addictive behavior or vulnerabilities to become addicted in the first place.[3] Nor will we attempt to define what types of maladaptive decision making might be categorized as an addictive behavior or whether there might be clear neurobiological markers for when something is addictive compared to a comparatively healthy obsession (a gourmet's gluttony versus an obese person's uncontrolled food intake, for instance). Instead, we will discuss the separate roles different brain systems might play in choice behavior, motivational drive, self-control, and aspects of addiction. In particular, we will focus on (1) areas in the frontal lobe such as the orbitofrontal cortex (OFC) and anterior cingulate cortex (ACC), and (2) the mesolimbic dopamine system projecting to the VStr (see Figure 6.1), contrasting the role

1. In fact, Eagleman and colleagues (2010) and others (e.g., Volkow & Li, 2004) are trying to make a broader point here that, as a neurological problem, drug addiction should be tackled from a medical standpoint and that drug policies should therefore emphasize treatment over punishment.

2. As the vast majority of research into the neuroscience of addiction has focused on the effects on the brain of drugs of abuse, our discussion will necessarily also concentrate on these specific disorders.

3 For excellent articles, see, for example, Redish et al. (2008), Robinson and Berridge (2008), Koob and Volkow (2010), and Everitt et al. (2008).

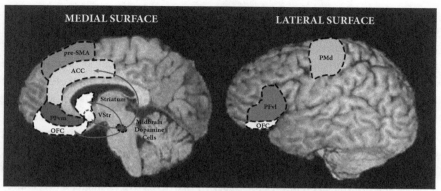

Figure 6.1 Selected frontal lobe and striatal brain areas superimposed on a medial (left-hand panel) and lateral (right-hand panel) image of a human brain. Arrows represent simplified representation of the major dopamine pathways originating from the midbrain dopamine cells terminating in the striatum and frontal lobe. ACC = anterior cingulate cortex; NAcc / VStr = nucleus accumbens / ventral striatum; OFC = orbitofrontal cortex; PFvm = ventromedial prefrontal cortex; PFvl = ventrolateral prefrontal cortex; PMd = dorsal premotor cortex; pre-SMA = presupplementary motor area.

of these regions in value-guided decisions with brain regions involved in externally determined, rule-guided choices. Finally, we will discuss ways in which these insights might shape law and policy dealing with addictive behaviors.

ACTIONS, HABITS, AND SELF-CONTROL

The past decade has seen growing interest in probing the neurobiology of value-guided decisions, where choices are based on our current needs, the opportunities that are available to us, and the likely costs and benefits that will ensue by choosing particular options.[4] Appropriate voluntary choice behavior in such contexts requires the integrity of regions in the frontal lobe on the ventral and medial portions of this structure such as the OFC and ACC (Rushworth & Behrens, 2008) (see Figure 6.1). Components of value-guided decisions also depend on parts of the striatum and structures in the medial part of the temporal lobe such as the amygdala. These substrates are sensitive to modulation by ascending neurochemical systems, including dopamine (Doya, 2008; Floresco, Onge, Ghods-Sharifi, & Winstanley, 2008; Rangel et al., 2008). As will be discussed in later sections, these circuits are largely distinct from those involved with appropriate rule-based action selection, which indicates a potential competition for control if the response option associated with the highest potential

4. This is a gross simplification of the factors that guide voluntary decisions. However, it serves here to distinguish this line of research from that into the neural basis of rule-guided behavior.

value is in conflict with what would be an appropriate action as determined by conditional rules.

The neural circuits involved in value-guided decisions do, however, overlap closely with those brain regions and neurochemicals that are known to be affected by drugs of abuse and are corrupted in addiction (Dalley et al., 2011; Koob & Volkow, 2011; Volkow, Fowler, Wang, & Swanson, 2004). Such correspondence has prompted a number of neurobiological theories of addiction to co-opt the language and models of value-guided decision making in describing core vulnerabilities and observed deficits (Bechara, 2005; Kalivas & Volkow, 2005; Redish et al., 2008; Volkow, Wang, Fowler, Tomasi, & Telang, 2011), with a particular emphasis on failure to resist impulsive desires (Ainslie, 2001; Dalley et al., 2011), overvaluing reward (Kalivas & Volkow, 2005), and disruptions in motivational drive (Robinson & Berridge, 2008).

However, as we will discuss in the following sections, value is not a unitary entity and no single brain region or even interconnected neural network encodes all aspects of value. If the maladaptive behaviors symptomatic of addiction are to be described within a decision-making framework centered on the neurobiology of value-guided decision making, it is imperative to understand the multiplicity of competing and separate systems that allow value to be constructed.

Competition between Goals, Habits, and Instincts in the Normal Brain

In an article published in 1961, two behaviorists, Keller and Marian Breland, documented a series of attempts to teach a variety of animals seemingly complex behaviors through simple conditioning (Breland & Breland, 1961). In spite of claiming success with over 6,000 individual animals ranging from reindeer to whales, the focus of their paper was their unexpected failure in a series of cases to control animal behavior. For instance, while pigs could seemingly be initially trained to pick up wooden coins and move to place them in a "piggy bank," the authors found with continued training that they became increasingly slow, often deliberately dropping the coins and spending time rooting for them on the ground. The authors' conclusion was that the animals' instincts were getting in the way of the reinforced behaviors (see Dayan, Niv, Seymour, & Daw, 2006 for further examples). Such innate behavioral repertoires in response to environmental stimuli that predict biologically valuable events, such as approaching cues that predict the delivery of reward, are often referred to as Pavlovian responses. As is evident from the examples above, these can be in direct opposition with other systems driven by the expected value of a selected action (Balleine et al., 2008; Rescorla & Solomon, 1967). Maladaptive competition between different valuation systems is not something limited to nonprimates; even chimpanzees struggle to exercise self-control in a task where selecting the smaller of two displayed amounts of food results in them receiving the larger amount of food (Boysen, Bernston, Hannan, & Cacioppo, 1996).

One notable effect reported by Breland and Breland was that animals' innate responses seemed paradoxically to take over as the amount of training the animals received increased. When in a new situation, actions are usually initially chosen in order to satisfy a current motivational goal based directly on the specific consequences of making that response. These choices have been termed "goal-directed" (Dickinson & Balleine, 1993). In the example of Breland and Breland, this would be the hungry pig wanting to obtain food and therefore choosing to pick up the coins and transport them to the piggy bank to cause this to happen. This is seen as a time-consuming and cognitively expensive strategy since the possible set of future consequences for each alternative course of action needs to be considered and compared before a decision can be made.[5] But goal-directed decisions do have substantial advantages: they provide a strong degree of control and flexibility as choices can be evaluated based on whether the eventual outcome satisfies current and long-term needs.

After repeated training in a sufficiently stable environment, actions instead can come to be elicited directly by a stimulus in the environment based on their learned value (for instance, reacting to the sight of the coins for the pigs or involuntarily moving to flip a light switch for us) without recourse to the specific outcome. This form of automatic action selection is known as a "habit" (Dickinson & Balleine, 1993).[6] This is a much more rapid system of action selection as it does not require forward planning but instead can rely on past experience that has endowed the stimulus-response association (coins = pick up and transport; light switch = press) with an abstract stored value (food to a hungry pig was good; light in a dark room was beneficial).

One problem with such a shortcut is that habitual actions are, by definition, somewhat rigid—this system makes it difficult to change behavior if, for

5. Outside of the constrained laboratory setting, it would obviously be impractical always to consider the potential consequences of each possible alternative far into the future. Instead, humans and animals may just consider whether a particular option is better than some average payoff likely within a particular environment ("satisficing": Simon, 1957) or, if currently engaged with a course of action, whether it still remains sufficiently worthwhile given the likelihood of there being any better alternative (formalized by Marginal Value Theorem in behavioral ecology: Charnov, 1976).

6. Note that the term "habit" here has a very specific definition that only partially overlaps with everyday usage. A habitual action is one that is performed without regard to the specific motivational consequences of outcome or to the causal relationship between the action and these consequences (Dickinson & Balleine, 1993). However, it need not imply uncontrolled compulsion to do something.

instance, something in the environment changes or the context requires a new type of response (consider the number of times one has unthinkingly turned on a light switch when leaving a darkened room). More importantly for the present discussion, habits are also more susceptible to Pavlovian influences from environmental cues than goal-directed decisions (Holland, 2004). In the case of Breland and Breland's pigs, as the process of taking the coins to the piggy bank became more automatic, this paradoxically allowed the animals' nearsighted innate tendencies to root for food, elicited by the association between the coins and reinforcement, to take over their behavior.

The processes that allow Pavlovian associations to be acquired and Pavlovian responses to be elicited rely on some of the brain structures implicated in value-guided decisions such as the amygdala and the VStr (Parkinson, Willoughby, Robbins, & Everitt, 2000) (Figure 6.1). However, these incentive processes and their neural systems required to learn about and express Pavlovian responses are largely separate from those required to learn to determine which actions to choose to obtain an expected outcome. Decisions based on goal-directed values depend on parts of the cortex such as the OFC and adjacent ventromedial prefrontal cortex along with dorsal parts of the striatum (Balleine et al., 2008; Rushworth & Behrens, 2008). By contrast, more lateral, motoric parts of the striatum, such as the putamen, are implicated in habitual action selection (Balleine et al., 2008). Dopamine in all of these regions is hypothesized to play a strong role both in the initial learning of both Pavlovian and instrumental values and in energizing responses to motivate animals to engage and persist with a particular response (Balleine et al., 2008; Berridge, 2007; Walton, Gan, & Phillips, 2011).

Importantly, these action selection circuits do not operate serially, but instead compete for control of action selection based on several factors, including the predictability of the environment and immediate task context (Daw, Niv, & Dayan, 2005; Dayan et al., 2006). This dissociation in neuroanatomy and function between Pavlovian, habitual, and goal-directed systems has potentially important implications for theories of maladaptive decision making, such as addiction.

Competition between Goals, Habits, and Instincts in the Addicted Brain

A number of theories of addiction have suggested that a key underlying cause of the disorder is a dualistic imbalance between a "deliberative," "executive," "goal-directed" action selection system and an "impulsive," "affective," "habit-based" system (Bechara, 2005; Everitt et al., 1999; McClure, Laibson, Loewenstein, & Cohen, 2004). Here, we have already described *three* distinct adaptive motivational mechanisms—goal directed, habitual, and Pavlovian—which can separately, or in tandem, guide how actions are normally chosen; in the subsequent sections, we will describe additional, fine-grained value representations within goal-directed systems. Just like Breland and Breland's pigs, biased competition between these systems can potentially cause irrational behavioral patterns that ensure short-term gains outweigh the long-term consequences. In vulnerable individuals, potentially addictive behaviors rapidly become both overvalued and habitual. Through the consequent loss of outcome-driven goal-directed control, these behaviors in turn become increasingly susceptible to influence by basic Pavlovian incentive processes elicited by stimuli in the environment, which, for those associated with the addiction, may in turn serve to drive an addict to pursue detrimental behaviors.

In several of these models of addiction, this transition from having voluntary control over a behavior to automatic, habitual responding is hypothesized to be driven by a change from a cortical, frontal lobe–based system to a subcortical, striatal-based one (Everitt & Robbins, 2005). Two frontal regions that are frequently included as critical nodes in neural models of addiction, value-guided decision making, and self-control are the OFC and ACC (Bechara, 2005; Everitt & Robbins, 2005; Goldstein et al., 2009; Kalivas & Volkow, 2005; Volkow et al., 2004; Volkow, Fowler, Wang, Swanson, & Telang, 2007; Winstanley, 2007). People with focal brain damage, caused by stroke or surgery, affecting these regions are often profoundly impaired in their ability to make appropriate decisions in their daily lives, in spite of the fact that their cognitive capacities and intelligence are left largely unaffected (Bechara, Damasio, Damasio, & Anderson, 1994; Fellows, 2007). In a direct comparison between such brain-damaged patients and chronic drug users, it was found that both displayed similar patterns of suboptimal decision making on a computerized decision-making task (Rogers et al., 1999).

Nonetheless, the precise contribution of frontal-striatal-dopaminergic circuits in the loss of control and compulsive behavior in addiction remains a matter of pressing concern. While some theories emphasize the importance of these networks in inhibiting inappropriate or impulsive actions (Eagleman et al., 2010; Everitt et al., 2008; Koob & Volkow, 2010; Winstanley, 2007), others focus on a role for them in representing motivational value or attentional salience, which may be important in underpinning a craving for drugs (Robinson & Berridge, 2008; Volkow et al., 2011). In part, we would argue that this lack of clarity arises as there remain many unanswered questions over the role of these networks in normal value-guided decision making. In the following sections we will highlight recent advances in this field, which have begun to demonstrate precise and dissociable contributions of different frontal lobe regions to these valuation and self-control. This may, in turn, influence our understanding of the contribution of these regions to addiction in humans.

VARIETIES OF VALUATION AND SELF-CONTROL

Value Representations in the Frontal Lobe

Preclinical studies of the ACC and OFC have consistently emphasized that both regions are involved in guiding appropriate goal-directed choice behavior, particularly when there is a requirement to modify behavior in response to a change in the environment (Rangel et al., 2008; Rushworth & Behrens, 2008; Walton et al., 2007; Walton, Rudebeck, Behrens, & Rushworth, 2011). To date, the cardinal test of flexible, reward-guided decision making is called reversal learning. Typically in such tasks, animals or people choose between a limited number of options, only one of which is initially associated with a positive outcome (for instance, a nutritious foodstuff to a hungry animal or a small amount of money for an undergraduate student). Once the participant has learned to consistently choose the beneficial option, the outcome contingencies are unexpectedly reversed, meaning that participants must now select one of the previously unrewarded options in order to continue to gain the reward.

Neither the ACC nor the OFC is required to make appropriate decisions in situations where a change in choice is prompted by an external instruction or a rule (Rushworth, Hadland, Gaffan, & Passingham, 2003; Shima & Tanji, 1998). This implies that these regions are not simply required to exercise self-control under any circumstances where the response contingencies change.

In fact, the precise contribution of these regions differs depending on what features guide a choice and how much control participants have over the responses they make (Rudebeck et al., 2008). For instance, activation of the ACC has been shown to be greater when participants had to evaluate the consequences of a voluntary choice when needing to change behavior than in situations when the experimenter told them what to do at this point. By contrast, the OFC was only involved when monitoring the outcome of a response they were instructed to make and not when freely able to make a decision (Walton, Devlin, & Rushworth, 2004). Therefore, the neural representation, and potentially the interpretation, of the consequences of a decision depends critically on the degree of volition people believed they had over its cause. In cases of addiction where there is hypoactivity of the ACC (e.g., Childress et al., 1999; Franklin et al., 2002), events may consequently be construed as falling out of the addict's own control. Once more, these findings highlight that our decisions are influenced by multiple distinct valuation signals, which cannot be compartmentalized within a simple dichotomy between deliberative versus affective systems.

Up to this point, we have tended to treat the term "value" in value-guided decision making as being synonymous with the benefits to be received from achieving a goal. It is self-evident, however, that our motivation to act depends not just on the eventual rewards, but also on the costs needed to be overcome in order to attain the goal (Walton, Rudebeck, Bannerman, & Rushworth, 2007). Both the ACC and OFC are implicated in facilitating choices of costly but ultimately beneficial options, and dysfunction in either region can cause failures to resist temptation in the face of easily and rapidly obtained alternative rewards. Nonetheless, again, these regions do not play a unitary role but instead are separately involved in processing different response costs, with decisions about whether to persist and overcome effort relying critically on the ACC, whereas delay-based choices depend more on OFC-centered networks (McClure, Ericson, Laibson, Loewenstein, & Cohen, 2007; Prevost, Pessiglione, Metereau, Clery-Melin, & Dreher, 2010; Rudebeck, Walton, Smyth, Bannerman, & Rushworth, 2006).

It is therefore evident that dysfunction of either the ACC or OFC causes a particular loss of self-control, characterized by either an inability to persist with the appropriate response in a changeable and uncertain environment or a failure to take on decision costs to achieve greater benefits. Such deficits might appear on the surface to mimic exactly the types of difficulties faced by addicts (for instance, lack of foresight, impulsivity, and an ability to correctly process the likely costs of a course of action), and have undoubtedly contributed to fine-grained theories of what roles these regions play in the loss of self-control in addiction.

However, to be able to translate between our understanding of how normal brain function underlies value-guided decision making and how dysfunction in these systems might give rise to aberrant choice behavior and loss of control in addiction, it is important to understand the subtle and separate contributions that these regions might play in these processes. As we shall go on to demonstrate in the next section, a detailed analysis of the patterns of decision making in these and other experiments demonstrate, first, that a seemingly identical aberrant behavior (for instance, a failure to stick with an appropriate action plan) can have quite different underlying causes, and second, that dysfunction within a single system can sometimes underpin a wide range of different deficits.

Multiple Routes to Impulsivity Following Frontal Lobe Damage

Decisions can be impulsive and deleterious if there is a direct problem with the way that choices are made. However, the same effect can also be brought about if a fully functioning decision-making system is receiving inaccurate information. While it may often be conceptualized that a loss in self-control reflects a malfunction in decision making, the weight of evidence suggests that it is the latter issue that drives many of the behavioral changes observed following damage to the ACC and OFC, and arguably in cases of addiction as well.

In order to work out what to do in a given situation, it is important to know how much weight to give to a single piece of evidence and therefore the degree to which it is possible to guide current choices based on past experience. Several lines of evidence suggest that the ACC mediates how much influence a particular outcome might have in guiding learning and future behavior, and therefore whether it is worth switching away from a current course of action (Behrens, Woolrich, Walton, & Rushworth, 2007; Rushworth & Behrens, 2008). Most strikingly, damage to this area causes a myopia about past outcomes, with only the most recent event, rather than the recent history of reward, exerting influence over the current decision (Kennerley, Walton, Behrens, Buckley, & Rushworth, 2006). Such a deficit can have profoundly different behavioral effects depending on the immediate context. An inability to utilize the integrated history of reinforcement to guide choices in a changeable environment, such as the reversal learning tasks discussed in the previous section, increases the tendency for impulsive, inappropriate changes in behavior and a failure to persevere with the correct action (Kennerley et al., 2006). Yet conversely, in more stable situations, precisely the opposite pattern of deficit can also been observed. Here, ACC disruption causes maladaptive increased persistence with a less beneficial option when it is, by chance, initially selected (Amiez, Joseph, & Procyk, 2006).

While similar inappropriate and changeable patterns of choices are also seen following disruption of the OFC, these appear to have a different underlying cause. In order to be able to learn the consequences of a decision, it is essential to be able to ascertain what past event might have caused a particular outcome to occur. While this is generally straightforward in many laboratory tasks where there is little spatial or temporal distance between a choice and its consequent outcome, in more realistic situations it can be much more problematic as there are innumerable options to choose between at any moment, and the consequences of a decision may only be felt days, weeks, or even years after the event, possibly in very different circumstances (take, for instance, the connection between smoking and lung cancer as an extreme example).

The ability to determine the precise association between a choice being made and the ensuing outcome is known as credit assignment, and disruption to the lateral part of the OFC impairs this form of learning (Walton, Behrens, Buckley, Rudebeck, & Rushworth, 2010). When fully functioning, such a fast learning system facilitates the ability to respond rapidly to changes in the environment and to learn how valuable a particular choice is likely to be, even when outcomes are distant from the decision point. However, when such a system is unavailable, such as following OFC disruption, the consequences of a choice can only be estimated based on the success of recent similar actions. Therefore, depending again on the precise context, such as how changeable the environment is, the loss of such a fast OFC-centered learning system can either cause patterns of inappropriate changes in behavior or result in maladaptive perseverance with a suboptimal strategy.

A role for the OFC in learning about and representing the specific consequences of a choice not only would be essential to appropriately adapt behavior in a changeable environment but also would make this region important for to enable decisions to resist immediate gratification in order to receive greater future rewards. While it is common to consider impulsivity as a failure to balance appropriately the cost of waiting against the eventual benefit of receiving the reward, and to assume that impulsive behavior in addiction is primarily caused by increased rates of delayed discounting of future rewards (e.g., Bickel & Marsch, 2001), such maladaptive decision making can also emerge through impairments in associative learning (Kacelnik, 2003). This comes about as people will only continue to choose a large delayed reward if they can assign the credit for that positive event to the earlier decision.

This implies that OFC dysfunction will *only* cause increases in choices of an immediate small reward over a delayed larger one in contexts where associative representations are taxed. Indeed, in a recent experiment, rats with lesions of the OFC showed no tendencies toward impulsive decisions if there was a salient visual cue (for instance, black-and-white stripes on the walls of the maze) that bridged the choice point, the section where the animal had to wait until the delay had elapsed, and the area where it finally received the food reward (Mariano et al., 2009). However, when such lesioned animals were run on an identical maze without these bridging cues, they were profoundly delay averse (Rudebeck, Walton, et al., 2006). Thus, the OFC is not required simply to inhibit the temptation of immediate rewards and to exert control to allow people to tolerate waiting for rewards, but is instead key to allow us to represent and update the causal connection between choices and their specific consequences across time and space. Such an ability is critical to facilitate far-sighted choices.

Therefore, while both the ACC and OFC can be said to be key components in deliberative, goal-direction decision-making systems for preventing detrimental impulsive choices in changeable environments, both do so through separate systems and through subtle contributions in value processing. While dysfunction in either region through brain damage or addiction can precipitate poor decision making, neither arises from a fundamental breakdown in the way in which self-control is exercised, as has been implied, but instead from a key change in the way the events and actions in the world are learned about and represented. Such findings may have important implications for our understanding of the difficulties addicts face in resisting the temptation of an immediate reward given that the negative consequences of an addiction may only be apparent at a point further in the future. We shall consider this in more detail in the final section.

Dopamine, Valuation, and Decision Making

There is wide agreement that dopamine transmission contributes to both addiction and value-guided decision making (Berridge, 2007; Doya, 2008; Everitt et al., 2008; Goldstein et al., 2009; Rogers, 2011). A related question to that discussed in the previous section therefore concerns what aspects of value are encoded by striatal dopamine and how changes in dopamine transmission might influence control over choice behavior. While dopamine projects widely throughout the brain, including dense innervation to the parts of the frontal cortex discussed above, we will here focus mainly on the mesolimbic dopamine projection to the VStr, which is a key substrate for the development and expression of drug addiction (Kalivas & McFarland, 2003; Wise & Bozarth, 1987). The VStr receives projections from parts of the OFC and ACC (Ferry, Ongur, An, & Price, 2000; Heidbreder & Groenewegen, 2003; Kunishio & Haber, 1994), and interactions between these regions are believed to be critical for several aspects of valuation and decision making.

There has been a rich history of association between dopamine and reward, which was often interpreted in both scientific circles and popular culture as implying that dopamine was the neural substrate of hedonic value (Wise, 1980). Indeed, several brain imaging studies have reported a correlation between dopamine levels measured in the VStr and the intensity of euphoria associated with a drug (Goldstein et al., 2009). However, the weight of evidence indicates that dopamine is not required to encode how much a reward is enjoyed or to form immediate subjective preferences between different outcomes (Berridge, 2007; Phillips et al., 2007; Salamone et al., 2007). Instead, mesolimbic dopamine plays an important role in motivating learning about what rewards are available in the environment and signaling other fundamental attributes of an outcome that may play an important role in biasing decision making, such as how likely it is that a particular amount of reward will occur at a particular time (Morris, Nevet, Arkadir, Vaadia, & Bergman, 2006; Roesch et al., 2007; Schultz, 2007). Such parameters of value may therefore be particularly vulnerable to addictive substances that affect the dopamine system.

As discussed in earlier sections, the value of a course of action is not simply determined by the anticipated benefits of the outcome, but also by the response costs that need to be overcome to obtain that goal. Disrupting VStr dopamine has a similar effect on effort-based decision making as ACC dysfunction: both cause a selective bias away from choices requiring a large amount of effort expenditure to obtain a high value reward when there is an alternative smaller gain to be had with much less work (Salamone, Cousins, & Bucher, 1994).

However, as was also highlighted in previous sections, there are many reasons that disruption of a system may result in a particular pattern of behavior, and therefore it is critical to determine what exact parameters of a decision VStr dopamine encodes. To this end, research has demonstrated that the magnitude of dopamine transmission in the VStr reliably scales with the anticipated benefits of a pending reward in a decision-making task (Gan et al., 2010). Nonetheless, dopamine does *not* encode the net value of an effortful response cost in a similar manner, even when the utility of the cost was equated to that of the benefit (Gan et al., 2010). This implies that an unwillingness to overcome response costs following reductions in VSt dopamine might not be a fundamental failure of motivation, but instead be the result of a functional decision-making system misvaluing the likely benefits of putting in effort. Such selective encoding could also lead to maladaptive patterns of behavior in situations where VStr dopamine transmission is enhanced, such as by certain drugs of abuse, as there would be a preferential augmentation of the predicted benefits of a course of action without a concomitant alteration in perception of the cost.

These studies describe situations where all the value parameters are known and fixed. However, a characteristic of many addictive behaviors is a drive toward options that carry with them some novelty, uncertainty, and risk, and such behaviors are partly controlled by dopamine.[7] For example, a widely reported side effect of several types of drugs that modulate the dopamine system is that they can cause an increase in risk-seeking tendencies, which may even result in pathological gambling behavior in a subset of patients (Voon et al., 2011). Recent work has shown that chronic adolescent drug exposure, which causes a maladaptive preference for risky decisions (Nasrallah, Yang, & Bernstein, 2009), is characterized by a relative increase in VStr dopamine transmission for those risky options over safe ones (Nasrallah et al., 2011).

It is still currently unknown what precise contribution VStr dopamine transmission plays in guiding cost-benefit decisions. However, as with the OFC and ACC, it is possible that perturbations of mesolimbic dopamine do not directly affect mechanisms for controlling choices, but instead alter how the value functions associated with the benefits of future rewards are learned about and represented. Under this scheme, uncertainty-driven dopamine activity might

7. We shall here refer to "risk" to describe options where there is a probability of a potential negative as well as a positive outcome and a "risky decision" as one where that option is chosen over an alternative that has a safe, if lesser, benefit. This terminology diverges from the way risk is often described in economics and neuroscience, where it refers to the standard deviation or entropy of a distribution of possible outcomes such that a 50% probability has the maximum risk.

augment positive prediction errors—the discrepancy between a predicted and experienced outcome when the latter is better than the former, which are also coded by dopamine neuronal responses (Schultz, 2011). In normal brains, such a system would promote behaviors that help reduce uncertainty and gain benefits, even when doing this requires costs to be overcome. However, in situations where the dopamine system fails to be appropriately regulated, such as in addiction, this could motivate a loss of control over behavior, with risky choices becoming favored in spite of the negative consequences of pursuing such courses of action. Indeed, a recent study showed that chronic adolescent drug exposure results in selectively increased learning rates for better-than-expected outcomes (Clark et al., 2011), which alone could explain the maladaptive risk seeking in this group later in life.

RULES, VALUES, AND SELF-CONTROL

While many of our choices are based on our current needs, the opportunities that are available to us, and the likely costs and benefits that will ensue by choosing to take particular options, there are also many circumstances where our behavior is constrained by prescribed rules and the surrounding context that determine what response to make in a given situation. There are many levels of abstraction of such rule-guided, conditional behavior, ranging from simple stimulus-response associations—pressing the brake in response to a red light, for instance—to more abstract rules, such as legal prohibitions against exceeding specified speed limits on roads. Self-control in these circumstances is usually considered in terms of the difficulties of learning to execute the correct response. Unlike in value-guided decision making, however, the options are usually externally determined to be categorically correct or incorrect in a particular context.

Studies using techniques that either measure or disrupt brain activity have again converged on a general picture that parts of the frontal lobe and striatum are required to respond appropriately in these types of tasks (Murray, Bussey, & Wise, 2000; Rushworth, Croxson, Buckley, & Walton, 2008; Wallis, 2008). Strikingly, however, these neural circuits are largely anatomically separated from those underlying value-guided decision making.

For instance, research has demonstrated that the ventrolateral part of the prefrontal cortex (PFvl: Figure 6.1) is required to rapidly acquire conditional rules that allow instructing stimuli to be linked with particular actions in a particular context (Boussaoud & Wise, 1993; Bussey, Wise, & Murray, 2001; Rushworth et al., 2005; Toni, Schluter, Josephs, Friston, & Passingham, 1999; Wallis & Miller, 2003). While several different brain regions, such as the dorsal premotor cortex, the presupplementary motor cortex (pre-SMA), and parts of the basal ganglia including the dorsal striatum and subthalamic nucleus (Figure 6.1), are involved in learning and implementing conditional rules and inhibiting responses, what marks out PFvl is its importance when there are multiple features in the world, some of which may be separated in space or time from the response, that could be guiding action selection (Petrides, 2002; Rushworth et al., 2005).

The regions underpinning rule-guided behavior not only are distinct from those commonly implicated as mediating value-guided decisions but also are seldom directly implicated with aspects of addiction. While there have been a few studies showing altered patterns of activation in the PFvl and pre-SMA in chronic drug users that correlate with difficulties, respectively, in resisting distraction by drug cues or in inhibiting responses (e.g., Kaufman, Ross, Stein, & Garavan, 2003; Nestor, McCabe, Jones, Clancy, & Garavan, 2011; Tabibnia et al., 2011), other experiments have found *improved* inhibitory control following acute cocaine use that correlated with increases in signals in the PFvl (Garavan, Kaufman, & Hester, 2008). This might suggest that addiction cannot be caused by a simple failure to control behavior according to prescribed rules, but instead that these rule-based circuits for some reason become superseded during action selection by value representations based on distorted needs and motivation.

A key question, therefore, is how these rule-guided networks interact with value-guided circuits, especially when rules and desires are in competition, and how these interactions are affected by addiction. Some clues to the former come from recent studies about how people make choices concerning what food to eat (Hare, Camerer, & Rangel, 2009; Hare, Malmaud, & Rangel, 2011). As has been shown on many occasions, parts of the frontal lobe implicated in making value-guided decisions—such as the mOFC—represent the overall value of a food item, incorporating not only taste but also potentially its anticipated health impact. When active dieters were given choices about whether to accept or spurn offers of food that were unhealthy but palatable (a chocolate bar, for instance), those who were more likely to successfully exercise self-control showed increased activity in parts of the rule-guided network—the lateral prefrontal cortex, including the PFvl. Importantly, these signals were also then correlated with the degree to which their value signal in the mOFC was weighted toward how healthy the foodstuff was. By contrast, in those dieters who were unable to resist their temptation, the signal in the PFvl was diminished and consequently value-related activation in the mOFC now only reflected the anticipated taste ratings and not its health impact.

In other words, the way our brains represent value is dynamic and malleable, and self-control can result in direct modification of the features and outcomes considered subjectively beneficial in value-guided decision networks. This suggests that failures in self-control in some forms of addiction may arise not simply from specific dysfunction within value- or rule-based neural networks, but instead from impaired interaction between the systems, such that imposed rules and guidance become less able to influence how addicts value courses of action and ultimately how decisions are made. In such cases, it may therefore be possible to help addicts overcome their compulsions if strategies can be found to allow them to focus on long-term benefits of abstaining from an addictive behavior. In the following section, we will consider what such policies might be in the light of neuroscientific findings.

NEUROSCIENTIFIC PERSPECTIVES ON CRIMINAL JUSTICE AND DRUG POLICY

In the preceding sections, we have set out the way in which normal value-guided decision making involves competition and cooperation between different neural systems encoding value and have suggested how dysfunction within these systems may cause the pathological loss of self-control characteristic of addiction. In this section, we will use these ideas as a springboard to suggest ways that law and public policy could be shaped to deal with addiction.

Tacit in our article is a belief that addiction is a brain disorder and, as such, should be treated as one. Addiction is undoubtedly complex and consists of many phases and components for which the precise neural underpinnings are far from fully understood. Different facets of different addictions in different people will likely turn out to involve at least partially separate neural dysfunction and behavioral sequelae (Redish et al., 2008). Nonetheless, drugs of abuse, at least, have been shown to hijack and demonstrably alter neural signaling involved in the normal processes of valuation and decision making. At some point in their lives, the majority of people take potentially addictive substances or engage in potentially addictive activities, yet only a consistently small percentage progress to addiction. A pressing area for further research is determining whether there are identifiable neural endophenotypes associated with particular vulnerabilities (Dalley et al., 2011; Kalivas & Volkow, 2005), which could be used, in advance, to identify and help those at risk, and may also be useful to help inform treatment strategies.[8]

8. While our perspective here is a neuroscientific one, we do not wish to downplay the importance of social and environmental factors in the development and maintenance of addiction. In fact, there may be interesting interplay between the two levels of description. Recent studies have shown that chronic stress causes both adaptations in frontostriatal networks and dopamine (Dias-Ferreira et al., 2009; Ungless, Argilli, & Bonci, 2010) and maladaptive decision making. Moreover, stress can cause relapse into drug taking (Shaham, Shalev, Lu, De Wit, & Stewart, 2003; Ungless et al., 2010).

While we do not wish here to discuss the complex question of the degree of moral responsibility of an addict—or indeed, of any person whose behavior could be described as a dysfunction in decision making—who has identifiable alterations in defined neural systems, we do believe that consideration of the neuroscience may be beneficial in terms of implementing drug policy. In particular, we want to highlight the ways that legal rules predicated primarily on a deterrence theory of criminal justice may have a diminished effect on addicts' ability to control their long-term choices. Deterrence, along with retributivist goals, plays a primary role in shaping criminal law. The deterrence theory of criminal justice views criminal penalties (incarceration, for example) as a cost designed to neutralize the seeming benefit to the perpetrator of a criminal course of action.[9] In this view, one goal of our justice system is to make use of our understanding of decision making to influence the behavior of individuals in a society. Our subsequent argument, that changes in decision processes underlying addiction may affect the ability of the law to appropriately deter particular behaviors, can potentially be interpreted to suggest that addiction undermines punishment as well.[10] But our discussion here will focus specifically on some possible ways that the findings described in this chapter come to bear on criminal justice and drug policy.

First, as we have described, one of the key components altered in addiction—dopamine in the VStr—plays only a limited role in representing the costs or negative consequences of a course of action, but instead signals, in isolation, the potential benefits to be gained from a choice (Gan et al., 2010). Therefore, while making addictive behavior harder to accomplish or prohibited by law may have *short-term* effects on reducing such activities, in isolation it is likely to have comparatively little influence on the long-term patterns of choices that are made, since this will not do much to counteract against the maladaptive coding of the potential benefits of a risky option or to alter how that drive for a particular reinforcer is represented by dopamine.

Indeed, taken to an extreme, one could controversially hypothesize that punitive costs might become altogether less salient to a drug abuser. Dopamine primarily encodes events that are surprisingly better than expected, but it plays a limited role when they are worse. Moreover, recent research has

9. It should be noted that here we will be using deterrence in the context of special deterrence. Special deterrence of individuals applies to a particular group or groups, such as addicts, and is distinct from general deterrence, which would address the issue of deterring all individuals who might become addicts if they are not threatened with punishment.

10. Not only is it possible that addicts will come to be perceived as less responsible for their actions and thus less deserving of punishment, but also it may come to be shown that addicts are insensitive to punishment. This potential, however, is certainly speculative and necessitates additional research into how addicts acutely perceive punitive costs.

demonstrated specific reduction in cost sensitivity resulting from chronic drug exposure that is expressed both behaviorally, in terms of maladaptive pursuit of uncertain large rewards, and through alterations in VStr dopamine transmission (Nasrallah et al., 2011). If such an addiction-induced effect generalized across types of costs (risk, time, effort, and monetary, for example) to include criminal-imposed costs (such as incarceration), this could reduce the deterrence effect of criminal law.[11] Future work confirming this potential insensitivity may lead to several, competing policy solutions. For instance, if addiction simply causes a change in the weighting of potential costs and benefits of a course of action without disrupting the decision-making mechanism itself, one may argue that a greater punishment is needed for this population in order to achieve the intended level of deterrence. Alternatively, if addicts are biologically impaired in making *the appropriate* decision, they may be deemed to exhibit the impaired volition requisite for reduced culpability.

A related factor is that the separation between brain systems that encode how to respond when behavior is guided by externally determined rules and when behavior is guided by internally generated values, and the potential breakdown in the influence of the former over the latter in addiction, makes it unlikely that simply imposing rules will have much influence over an addict's decisions without further help to allow the rule-based system to win out over the pathological desire to engage with a particular behavior. However, the lack of obvious dysfunction within rule-based neural networks in at least some cases of addiction also implies that control could be regained if policies could be devised to allow addicts to alter the focus of their attention and to allow their behavior to be guided by externally determined principles rather than internal drives.

As discussed in the preceding section, there is limited experimental neuroscientific research to date in this area, and it is not immediately clear what strategies could be put in place as an alternative to punishment to help facilitate self-control. Nevertheless, some recent brain imaging and physiological studies investigating the regulation of emotion and how that affects valuation and decision-making networks may provide some clues. For instance, the use of relaxation techniques can cause a bias away from risky decisions and a reduction in risk signals in the VStr (Martin & Delgado, 2011). Such relaxation protocols also result in reduced activation in the VStr to a stimulus associated with an immediate monetary reward, an effect that is coupled with increases in signals in prefrontal cortex including the PFvl (Delgado, Gillis, & Phelps, 2008).

---

11. Though see Heyman (2009) or Pickard and Pearce's chapter in this volume for an alternative perspective.

The studies by Hare and colleagues also suggest that people can be helped both by internally determined strategies and by external cues to modulate their desires for tasty but unhealthy foodstuffs (Hare et al., 2009; Hare et al., 2011).

Importantly, we have described how maladaptive patterns of choices that arise with OFC or ACC dysfunction, and at least partially from increased dopamine transmission, may not simply be examples of unfettered impulsivity caused by a malfunctioning decision-making system, but may instead reflect appropriate choices based on inaccurate information. If the latter holds true for at least some cases of addiction, then such findings hold out the potential that there may be cognitive treatments that could be utilized to help train addicts make advantageous decisions in the face of temptation. Such cognitive treatments could be required as part of mandatory rehabilitation sentences imposed for drug-related offences. This type of criminal law policy would also lack a deterrence effect, but could potentially reduce recidivism rates among drug-abusing populations. Moreover, it may eventually be possible to determine neural signatures indicating the likelihood that addicts will be able to exercise rule-based self-control or even to develop targeted brain stimulation protocols to boost activity in regions required for appropriate self-control (Goldman et al., 2011).

Extrapolating from the behavioral work in animals, which demonstrated that they were more likely to be influenced by maladaptive Pavlovian associations when habitually engaging with a behavior than when they were making goal-directed choices, it will be valuable to determine ways to encourage addicts to think directly about the consequences of their actions to allow them to gain control over their lives. A related strategy might be put in place on the basis of the findings that OFC dysfunction only causes maladaptive impulsive decisions if there is no explicit cue to bridge between the choice point and the outcome (Mariano et al., 2009; Rudebeck, Walton, et al., 2006). For those addicts in whom there are changes in OFC function, it might be possible to bias them toward farsighted choices if there can be some cue that allows them explicitly to associate the advantages to be gained from refraining from an addictive behavior or similarly that enables the negative consequences from an addictive choice to be connected with the decision to select that option. Accordingly, cue and countercue policies may be used to influence the behavior of addicts before an illegal course of action is pursued (see Bernheim & Rangel, 2004). Putting images depicting the harmful consequences of smoking on a cigarette packet, for instance, might remove the need for the OFC to represent the causal connection between the choice to smoke and the potential for future lung disease.

Finally, regardless of how successful such behavioral and cognitive interventions might be, it is important to remember that value-based decisions do not involve deterministic selections based precisely on the expected values of the options, but are instead driven by stochastic processes. This means that, on occasion, suboptimal alternatives will be selected. If placed in situations where addictive choices are available, even an addict with strong self-control may select that deleterious option. It is therefore important for the addict to find strategies to avoid contexts where such options present themselves (for instance, an alcoholic in a bar), and potentially for policies to be developed that limit the cues in the environment associated with the addictive behavior to prevent addicts being unconsciously drawn toward such environments (alcohol advertising at sports matches, for instance). From a legal perspective, it may also be necessary to build in some tolerance to failures to comply with laws against certain addictive activities such as drug taking.

CONCLUSION

In this chapter, we have argued that (1) value-guided decision making is a multifaceted process and cannot be reduced to a simple dichotomous division between a deliberative, reflective system and an affective, impulsive one; (2) addiction involves a corruption of normal neural circuits involved in value-guided, but not rule-based, decision making; and (3) advances in our understanding of the role of separate brain areas and chemicals in decisions may give clues as to why addicts persist with engaging in harmful behavior and may suggest strategies to try to prevent this occurring. While we believe the logic between these three strands is strong, we acknowledge that a large amount of the evidence is still indirect. There has been little research to date that has directly investigated the influence of drugs of abuse on value-guided decision making (Ostlund & Balleine, 2008; Schoenbaum & Shaham, 2008). Indeed, several decades of research into the neuroscience of addiction has yet to lead to many tangible treatments.[12] Moreover, it is likely that the precise neuropathology will depend on the particular addictive behavior being investigated.[13] Nonetheless, as our understanding of both the neural basis of value-guided decision making and the different forms of addiction advances, there should be great scope to use neuroscience to help shape law, public policy, and treatment strategies for addicts, with the ultimate goal of helping them regain control over their behavior.

12. This might partly relate to the fact that the animal model of choice for addiction is the rodent, which probably lacks homologs of the lateral prefrontal regions in humans that are implicated as being a critical component for determining self-control.

13. For example, while impulsive tendencies can predict the likelihood of abusing stimulants, such traits do not correlate with escalation of intake of opiate drugs (Dalley et al., 2007; McNamara, Dalley, Robbins, Everitt, & Belin, 2010).

ACKNOWLEDGMENTS

MEW is funded by a Wellcome Trust Research Career Development Fellowship. We would like to thank Carinne Piekema for helpful comments on this manuscript.

REFERENCES

Ainslie, G. (2001). *Breakdown of Will*. Cambridge: Cambridge University Press.

Amiez, C., Joseph, J. P., & Procyk, E. (2006). Reward encoding in the monkey anterior cingulate cortex. *Cereb Cortex*, 16(7), 1040–1055.

Balleine, B. W., Daw, N. D., & O'Doherty, J. P. (2008). Multiple forms of value learning and the function of dopamine. In P. W. Glimcher, C. F. Camerer, E. Fehr, & R. A. Poldrack (Eds.), *Neuroeconomics: Decision Making and the Brain* (pp. 367–387). London, UK: Academic Press.

Bechara, A. (2005). Decision making, impulse control and loss of willpower to resist drugs: a neurocognitive perspective. *Nat Neurosci*, 8(11), 1458–1463.

Bechara, A., Damasio, A. R., Damasio, H., & Anderson, S. W. (1994). Insensitivity to future consequences following damage to human prefrontal cortex. *Cognition*, 50(1–3), 7–15.

Becker, G. S., & Murphy, K. M. (1988). A theory of rational addiction. *Journal of Political Economy*, 96(4), 675–700.

Behrens, T. E., Woolrich, M. W., Walton, M. E., & Rushworth, M. F. (2007). Learning the value of information in an uncertain world. *Nat Neurosci*, 10(9), 1214–1221.

Bernheim, B. D., & Rangel, A. (2004). Addiction and cue-triggered decision processes. *Am Econ Rev*, 94(5), 1558–1590.

Berridge, K. C. (2007). The debate over dopamine's role in reward: the case for incentive salience. *Psychopharmacology (Berl)*, 191(3), 391–431.

Bickel, W. K., & Marsch, L. A. (2001). Toward a behavioral economic understanding of drug dependence: delay discounting processes. *Addiction*, 96(1), 73–86.

Boussaoud, D., & Wise, S. P. (1993). Primate frontal cortex: neuronal activity following attentional versus intentional cues. *Exp Brain Res*, 95(1), 15–27.

Boysen, S. T., Bernston, G. G., Hannan, M. B., & Cacioppo, J. T. (1996). Quantity-based interference and symbolic representations in chimpanzees (Pan troglodytes). *J Exp Psychol Anim Behav Process*, 22(1), 76–86.

Breland, K., & Breland, M. (1961). The misbehavior of organisms. *American Psychologist*, 16(11), 681–684.

Bussey, T. J., Wise, S. P., & Murray, E. A. (2001). The role of ventral and orbital prefrontal cortex in conditional visuomotor learning and strategy use in rhesus monkeys (Macaca mulatta). *Behav Neurosci*, 115(5), 971–982.

Camerer, C. F. (2008). Neuroeconomics: opening the gray box. *Neuron*, 60(3), 416–419.

Charnov, E. L. (1976). Optimal foraging: the marginal value theorem. *Theor Pop Biol*, 9, 129–136.

Childress, A. R., Mozley, P. D., McElgin, W., Fitzgerald, J., Reivich, M., & O'Brien, C. P. (1999). Limbic activation during cue-induced cocaine craving. *Am J Psychiatry*, 156(1), 11–18.

Clark, J. J., Nasrallah, N. A., Hart, A. S., Collins, A. L., Bernstein, I. L., & Phillips, P. E. (2011). Altered risk-based decision making following adolescent alcohol use results from an imbalance in reinforcement learning in rats. *PLoS One*, 7(5), e37357.

Dalley, J. W., Everitt, B. J., & Robbins, T. W. (2011). Impulsivity, compulsivity, and top-down cognitive control. *Neuron*, 69(4), 680–694.

Daw, N. D., Niv, Y., & Dayan, P. (2005). Uncertainty-based competition between prefrontal and dorsolateral striatal systems for behavioral control. *Nat Neurosci*, 8(12), 1704–1711.

Dayan, P., & Niv, Y. (2008). Reinforcement learning: the good, the bad and the ugly. *Curr Opin Neurobiol*, 18(2), 185–196.

Dayan, P., Niv, Y., Seymour, B., & Daw, N. D. (2006). The misbehavior of value and the discipline of the will. *Neural Netw*, 19(8), 1153–1160.

Delgado, M. R., Gillis, M. M., & Phelps, E. A. (2008). Regulating the expectation of reward via cognitive strategies. *Nat Neurosci*, 11(8), 880–881.

Dias-Ferreira, E., Sousa, J. C., Melo, I., Morgado, P., Mesquita, A. R., Cerqueira, J. J., Costa, R. M., & Sousa, N. (2009). Chronic stress causes frontostriatal reorganization and affects decision-making. *Science*, 325(5940), 621–625.

Dickinson, A., & Balleine, B. W. (1993). Actions and responses: the dual psychology of behaviour. In N. Eilan, R. A. McCarthy, B. Brewer (Eds.), *Spatial representation: Problems in philosophy and psychology* (pp. 277–293). Malden: Blackwell Publishing, xi, 409 pp.

Doya, K. (2008). Modulators of decision making. *Nat Neurosci*, 11(4), 410–416.

Eagleman, D. M., Correro, M. A., & Singh, J. (2010). Why neuroscience matters for a rational drug policy. *Minnesota J Law Sci Technol*, 11(1), 7–26.

Everitt, B. J., Belin, D., Economidou, D., Pelloux, Y., Dalley, J. W., & Robbins, T. W. (2008). Neural mechanisms underlying the vulnerability to develop compulsive drug-seeking habits and addiction. *Philos Trans R Soc Lond B Biol Sci*, 363(1507), 3125–3135.

Everitt, B. J., Parkinson, J. A., Olmstead, M. C., Arroyo, M., Robledo, P., & Robbins, T. W. (1999). Associative processes in addiction and reward. The role of amygdala-ventral striatal subsystems. *Ann N Y Acad Sci*, 877, 412–438.

Everitt, B. J., & Robbins, T. W. (2005). Neural systems of reinforcement for drug addiction: from actions to habits to compulsion. *Nat Neurosci*, 8(11), 1481–1489.

Fellows, L. K. (2007). The role of orbitofrontal cortex in decision making: a component process account. *Ann N Y Acad Sci*, 1121, 421–430.

Ferry, A. T., Ongur, D., An, X., & Price, J. L. (2000). Prefrontal cortical projections to the striatum in macaque monkeys: evidence for an organization related to prefrontal networks. *J Comp Neurol*, 425(3), 447–470.

Fiorillo, C. D., Tobler, P. N., & Schultz, W. (2003). Discrete coding of reward probability and uncertainty by dopamine neurons. *Science*, 299(5614), 1898–1902.

Floresco, S. B., Onge, J. R., Ghods-Sharifi, S., & Winstanley, C. A. (2008). Cortico-limbic-striatal circuits subserving different forms of cost-benefit decision making. *Cogn Affect Behav Neurosci*, 8(4), 375–389.

Franklin, T. R., Acton, P. D., Maldjian, J. A., Gray, J. D., Croft, J. R., Dackis, C. A., O'Brien, C. P., & Childress, A. R. (2002). Decreased gray matter concentration in the insular, orbitofrontal, cingulate, and temporal cortices of cocaine patients. *Biol Psychiatry*, 51(2), 134–142.

Gan, J. O., Walton, M. E., & Phillips, P. E. (2010). Dissociable cost and benefit encoding of future rewards by mesolimbic dopamine. *Nat Neurosci*, 13(1), 25–27.

Garavan, H., Kaufman, J. N., & Hester, R. (2008). Acute effects of cocaine on the neurobiology of cognitive control. *Philos Trans R Soc Lond B Biol Sci*, 363(1507), 3267–3276.

Goldman, R. L., Borckardt, J. J., Frohman, H. A., O'Neil, P. M., Madan, A., Campbell, L. K., Budak, A., & George, M. S. (2011). Prefrontal cortex transcranial direct current stimulation (tDCS) temporarily reduces food cravings and increases the self-reported ability to resist food in adults with frequent food craving. *Appetite*, 56(3), 741–746.

Goldstein, R. Z., Craig, A. D., Bechara, A., Garavan, H., Childress, A. R., Paulus, M. P., & Volkow, N. D. (2009). The neurocircuitry of impaired insight in drug addiction. *Trends Cogn Sci*, 13(9), 372–380.

Gruber, J., & Koszegi, B. (2001). Is addiction "rational"? Theory and evidence. *Quarterly Journal of Economics*, 116(4), 1261–1303.

Hare, T. A., Camerer, C. F., & Rangel, A. (2009). Self-control in decision-making involves modulation of the vmPFC valuation system. *Science*, 324(5927), 646–648.

Hare, T. A., Malmaud, J., & Rangel, A. (2011). Focusing attention on the health aspects of foods changes value signals in vmPFC and improves dietary choice. *J Neurosci*, 31(30), 11077–11087.

Heidbreder, C. A., & Groenewegen, H. J. (2003). The medial prefrontal cortex in the rat: evidence for a dorso-ventral distinction based upon functional and anatomical characteristics. *Neurosci Biobehav Rev*, 27(6), 555–579.

Herrnstein, R. J., & Prelec, D. (1992). A theory of addiction. In G. Loewenstein & J. Elster (Eds.), *Choice Over Time* (pp. 331–360). New York: Russell Sage Foundation.

Heyman, G. M. (2009). *Addiction: A Disorder of Choice*. Cambridge, MA: Harvard University Press.

Holland, P. C. (2004). Relations between Pavlovian-instrumental transfer and reinforcer devaluation. *J Exp Psychol Anim Behav Process*, 30(2), 104–117.

Kacelnik, A. (2003). The evolution of patience. In G. Loewenstein, D. Read, & R. Baumeister (Eds.), *Time and Decision: Economic and Psychological Perspectives on Intertemporal Choice* (pp. 115–138). New York: Russell Sage Foundation.

Kalivas, P. W., & McFarland, K. (2003). Brain circuitry and the reinstatement of cocaine-seeking behavior. *Psychopharmacology (Berl)*, 168(1–2), 44–56.

Kalivas, P. W., & Volkow, N. D. (2005). The neural basis of addiction: a pathology of motivation and choice. *Am J Psychiatry*, 162(8), 1403–1413.

Kapogiannis, D., Campion, P., Grafman, J., & Wassermann, E. M. (2008). Reward-related activity in the human motor cortex. *Eur J Neurosci*, 27(7), 1836–1842.

Kaufman, J. N., Ross, T. J., Stein, E. A., & Garavan, H. (2003). Cingulate hypoactivity in cocaine users during a GO-NOGO task as revealed by event-related functional magnetic resonance imaging. *J Neurosci*, 23(21), 7839–7843.

Kennerley, S. W., & Walton, M. E. (2011). Decision making and reward in frontal cortex: complementary evidence from neurophysiological and neuropsychological studies. *Behav Neurosci*, 125(3), 297–317.

Kennerley, S. W., Walton, M. E., Behrens, T. E., Buckley, M. J., & Rushworth, M. F. (2006). Optimal decision making and the anterior cingulate cortex. *Nat Neurosci*, 9(7), 940–947.

Koob, G. F., & Volkow, N. D. (2010). Neurocircuitry of addiction. *Neuropsychopharmacology*, 35(1), 217–238.

Koob, G. F., & Volkow, N. D. (2011). Neurocircuitry of addiction. *Neuropsychopharmacology*, 35(1), 217–238.

Kunishio, K., & Haber, S. N. (1994). Primate cingulostriatal projection: limbic striatal versus sensorimotor striatal input. *J Comp Neurol*, 350(3), 337–356.

Mariano, T. Y., Bannerman, D. M., McHugh, S. B., Preston, T. J., Rudebeck, P. H., Rudebeck, S. R., Rawlins, J. N., Walton, M. E., Rushworth, M. F., Baxter, M. G., & Campbell, T. G. (2009). Impulsive choice in hippocampal but not orbitofrontal cortex-lesioned rats on a nonspatial decision-making maze task. *Eur J Neurosci*, 30(3), 472–484.

Martin, L. N., & Delgado, M. R. (2011). The influence of emotion regulation on decision making under risk. *J Cogn Neurosci*, 23(9), 2569–2581.

McClure, S. M., Ericson, K. M., Laibson, D. I., Loewenstein, G., & Cohen, J. D. (2007). Time discounting for primary rewards. *J Neurosci*, 27(21), 5796–5804.

McClure, S. M., Laibson, D. I., Loewenstein, G., & Cohen, J. D. (2004). Separate neural systems value immediate and delayed monetary rewards. *Science*, 306(5695), 503–507.

McNamara, R., Dalley, J. W., Robbins, T. W., Everitt, B. J., & Belin, D. (2010). Trait-like impulsivity does not predict escalation of heroin self-administration in the rat. *Psychopharmacology (Berl)*, 212(4), 453–464.

Morris, G., Nevet, A., Arkadir, D., Vaadia, E., & Bergman, H. (2006). Midbrain dopamine neurons encode decisions for future action. *Nat Neurosci*, 9(8), 1057–1063.

Murray, E. A., Bussey, T. J., & Wise, S. P. (2000). Role of prefrontal cortex in a network for arbitrary visuomotor mapping. *Exp Brain Res*, 133(1), 114–129.

Nasrallah, N. A., Clark, J. J., Collins, A. L., Akers, C. A., Phillips, P. E., & Bernstein, I. L. (2011). Risk preference following adolescent alcohol use is associated with corrupted encoding of costs but not rewards by mesolimbic dopamine. *Proc Natl Acad Sci U S A*, 108(13), 5466–5471.

Nasrallah, N. A., Yang, T. W., & Bernstein, I. L. (2009). Long-term risk preference and suboptimal decision making following adolescent alcohol use. *Proc Natl Acad Sci U S A*, 106(41), 17600–17604.

Nestor, L., McCabe, E., Jones, J., Clancy, L., & Garavan, H. (2011). Differences in "bottom-up" and "top-down" neural activity in current and former cigarette smokers: evidence for neural substrates which may promote nicotine abstinence through increased cognitive control. *Neuroimage*, 56(4), 2258–2275.

Noonan, M. P., Walton, M. E., Behrens, T. E., Sallet, J., Buckley, M. J., & Rushworth, M. F. (2010). Separate value comparison and learning mechanisms in macaque medial and lateral orbitofrontal cortex. *Proc Natl Acad Sci U S A*, 107(47), 20547–20552.

Ostlund, S. B., & Balleine, B. W. (2008). On habits and addiction: an associative analysis of compulsive drug seeking. *Drug Discov Today Dis Models*, 5(4), 235–245.

Parkinson, J. A., Willoughby, P. J., Robbins, T. W., & Everitt, B. J. (2000). Disconnection of the anterior cingulate cortex and nucleus accumbens core impairs Pavlovian approach behavior: further evidence for limbic cortical-ventral striatopallidal systems. *Behav Neurosci*, 114(1), 42–63.

Petrides, M. (2002). The mid-ventrolateral prefrontal cortex and active mnemonic retrieval. *Neurobiol Learn Mem*, 78(3), 528–538.

Phillips, P. E., Walton, M. E., & Jhou, T. C. (2007). Calculating utility: preclinical evidence for cost-benefit analysis by mesolimbic dopamine. *Psychopharmacology (Berl)*, 191(3), 483–495.

Prevost, C., Pessiglione, M., Metereau, E., Clery-Melin, M. L., & Dreher, J. C. (2010). Separate valuation subsystems for delay and effort decision costs. *J Neurosci*, 30(42), 14080–14090.

Rahman, S. J., Sahakian, B. J., Cardinal, R. N., Rogers, R. D., & Robbins, T. W. (2001). Decision making and neuropsychiatry. *Trends Cogn Sci*, 5(6), 271–277.

Rangel, A., Camerer, C., & Montague, P. R. (2008). A framework for studying the neurobiology of value-based decision making. *Nat Rev Neurosci*, 9(7), 545–556.

Redish, A. D., Jensen, S., & Johnson, A. (2008). A unified framework for addiction: vulnerabilities in the decision process. *Behav Brain Sci*, 31(4), 415–437; discussion 437–487.

Rescorla, R. A., & Solomon, R. L. (1967). Two-process learning theory: relationships between Pavlovian conditioning and instrumental learning. *Psychol Rev*, 74(3), 151–182.

Robinson, T. E., & Berridge, K. C. (2000). The psychology and neurobiology of addiction: an incentive-sensitization view. *Addiction*, 95 *Suppl 2*, S91–117.

Robinson, T. E., & Berridge, K. C. (2008). Review. The incentive sensitization theory of addiction: some current issues. *Philos Trans R Soc Lond B Biol Sci*, 363(1507), 3137–3146.

Roesch, M. R., Calu, D. J., & Schoenbaum, G. (2007). Dopamine neurons encode the better option in rats deciding between differently delayed or sized rewards. *Nat Neurosci*, 10(12), 1615–1624.

Rogers, R. D. (2011). The roles of dopamine and serotonin in decision making: evidence from pharmacological experiments in humans. *Neuropsychopharmacology*, 36(1), 114–132.

Rogers, R. D., Everitt, B. J., Baldacchino, A., Blackshaw, A. J., Swainson, R., Wynne, K., Baker, N. B., Hunter, J., Carthy, T., Booker, E., London, M., Deakin, J. F., Sahakian, B. J., & Robbins, T. W. (1999). Dissociable deficits in the decision-making cognition of chronic amphetamine abusers, opiate abusers, patients with focal damage to prefrontal cortex, and tryptophan-depleted normal volunteers: evidence for monoaminergic mechanisms. *Neuropsychopharmacology*, 20(4), 322–339.

Rudebeck, P. H., Behrens, T. E., Kennerley, S. W., Baxter, M. G., Buckley, M. J., Walton, M. E., & Rushworth, M. F. (2008). Frontal cortex subregions play distinct roles in choices between actions and stimuli. *J Neurosci*, 28(51), 13775–13785.

Rudebeck, P. H., Walton, M. E., Smyth, A. N., Bannerman, D. M., & Rushworth, M. F. (2006). Separate neural pathways process different decision costs. *Nat Neurosci*, 9(9), 1161–1168.

Rushworth, M. F., & Behrens, T. E. (2008). Choice, uncertainty and value in prefrontal and cingulate cortex. *Nat Neurosci*, 11(4), 389–397.

Rushworth, M. F., Buckley, M. J., Gough, P. M., Alexander, I. H., Kyriazis, D., McDonald, K. R., & Passingham, R. E. (2005). Attentional selection and action selection in the ventral and orbital prefrontal cortex. *J Neurosci*, 25(50), 11628–11636.

Rushworth, M. F., Croxson, P. L., Buckley, M. J., & Walton, M. E. (2008). Ventrolateral and medial frontal contributions to decision-making and action selection. In S. A. Bunge & J. D. Wallis (Eds.), *Neuroscience of Rule-Guided Behavior* (pp. 129–158). New York: Oxford University Press.

Rushworth, M. F., Hadland, K. A., Gaffan, D., & Passingham, R. E. (2003). The effect of cingulate cortex lesions on task switching and working memory. *J Cogn Neurosci*, 15(3), 338–353.

Salamone, J. D., Correa, M., Farrar, A., & Mingote, S. M. (2007). Effort-related functions of nucleus accumbens dopamine and associated forebrain circuits. *Psychopharmacology (Berl)*, 191(3), 461–482.

Salamone, J. D., Cousins, M. S., & Bucher, S. (1994). Anhedonia or anergia? Effects of haloperidol and nucleus accumbens dopamine depletion on instrumental response selection in a T-maze cost/benefit procedure. *Behav Brain Res*, 65(2), 221–229.

Schoenbaum, G., & Shaham, Y. (2008). The role of orbitofrontal cortex in drug addiction: a review of preclinical studies. *Biol Psychiatry*, 63(3), 256–262.

Schultz, W. (2007). Multiple dopamine functions at different time courses. *Annu Rev Neurosci*, 30, 259–288.

Schultz, W. (2011). Potential vulnerabilities of neuronal reward, risk, and decision mechanisms to addictive drugs. *Neuron*, 69(4), 603–617.

Serences, J. T. (2008). Value-based modulations in human visual cortex. *Neuron*, 60(6), 1169–1181.

Shaham, Y., Shalev, U., Lu, L., De Wit, H., & Stewart, J. (2003). The reinstatement model of drug relapse: history, methodology and major findings. *Psychopharmacology (Berl)*, 168(1–2), 3–20.

Shima, K., & Tanji, J. (1998). Role for cingulate motor area cells in voluntary movement selection based on reward. *Science*, 282(5392), 1335–1338.

Simon, H. A. (1957). *Models of Man*. New York: Wiley.

Stephens, D. W., & Krebs, J. R. (1986). *Foraging Theory*. Princeton, NJ: Princeton University Press.

Sutton, R. S., & Barto, A. C. (1998). *Reinforcement Learning: An Introduction*. London: MIT Press.

Tabibnia, G., Monterosso, J. R., Baicy, K., Aron, A. R., Poldrack, R. A., Chakrapani, S., Lee, B., & London, E. D. (2011). Different forms of self-control share a neurocognitive substrate. *J Neurosci*, 31(13), 4805–4810.

Tobler, P. N., Fiorillo, C. D., & Schultz, W. (2005). Adaptive coding of reward value by dopamine neurons. *Science*, 307(5715), 1642–1645.

Toni, I., Schluter, N. D., Josephs, O., Friston, K., & Passingham, R. E. (1999). Signal-, set- and movement-related activity in the human brain: an event-related fMRI study. *Cereb Cortex*, 9(1), 35–49.

Ungless, M. A., Argilli, E., & Bonci, A. (2010). Effects of stress and aversion on dopamine neurons: implications for addiction. *Neurosci Biobehav Rev*, 35(2), 151–156.

Volkow, N. D., Fowler, J. S., Wang, G. J., & Swanson, J. M. (2004). Dopamine in drug abuse and addiction: results from imaging studies and treatment implications. *Mol Psychiatry*, 9(6), 557–569.

Volkow, N. D., Fowler, J. S., Wang, G. J., Swanson, J. M., & Telang, F. (2007). Dopamine in drug abuse and addiction: results of imaging studies and treatment implications. *Arch Neurol*, 64(11), 1575–1579.

Volkow, N. D., & Li, T. K. (2004). Drug addiction: the neurobiology of behaviour gone awry. *Nat Rev Neurosci*, 5(12), 963–970.

Volkow, N. D., Wang, G. J., Fowler, J. S., Tomasi, D., & Telang, F. (2011). Addiction: beyond dopamine reward circuitry. *Proc Natl Acad Sci USA*, 108(37), 15037–15042.

Voon, V., Gao, J., Brezing, C., Symmonds, M., Ekanayake, V., Fernandez, H., Dolan, R. J., & Hallett, M. (2011). Dopamine agonists and risk: impulse control disorders in Parkinson's disease. *Brain*, 134(Pt 5), 1438–1446.

Wallis, J. D. (2008). Single neuron activity underlying behavior-guiding rules. In S. A. Bunge & J. D. Wallis (Eds.), *Neuroscience of Rule-Guided behavior* (pp. 23–44). New York: Oxford University Press.

Wallis, J. D., & Miller, E. K. (2003). Neuronal activity in primate dorsolateral and orbital prefrontal cortex during performance of a reward preference task. *Eur J Neurosci*, 18(7), 2069–2081.

Walton, M. E., Behrens, T. E., Buckley, M. J., Rudebeck, P. H., & Rushworth, M. F. (2010). Separable learning systems in the macaque brain and the role of orbitofrontal cortex in contingent learning. *Neuron*, 65(6), 927–939.

Walton, M. E., Devlin, J. T., & Rushworth, M. F. (2004). Interactions between decision making and performance monitoring within prefrontal cortex. *Nat Neurosci*, 7(11), 1259–1265.

Walton, M. E., Gan, J. O., & Phillips, P. E. (2011). The influence of dopamine in generating action from motivation. In R. B. Mars, J. Sallet, M. F. Rushworth, & N. Yeung (Eds.), *Neural Basis of Motivational and Cognitive Control* (pp. 163–187). Cambridge, MA: MIT Press.

Walton, M. E., Rudebeck, P. H., Bannerman, D. M., & Rushworth, M. F. (2007). Calculating the cost of acting in frontal cortex. *Ann N Y Acad Sci*, 1104, 340–356.

Walton, M. E., Rudebeck, P. H., Behrens, T. E., & Rushworth, M. F. (2011). Cingulate and orbitofrontal contributions to valuing knowns and unknowns in a changeable world. In M. R. Delgado, E. A. Phelps, & T. W. Robbins (Eds.), *Decision Making, Affect, and Learning* (pp. 235–261). Oxford: Oxford University Press.

Winstanley, C. A. (2007). The orbitofrontal cortex, impulsivity, and addiction: probing orbitofrontal dysfunction at the neural, neurochemical, and molecular level. *Ann N Y Acad Sci*, 1121, 639–655.

Wise, R. A. (1980). Action of drugs of abuse on brain reward systems. *Pharmacol Biochem Behav*, 13 Suppl 1, 213–223.

Wise, R. A. (2004). Dopamine, learning and motivation. *Nat Rev Neurosci*, 5(6), 483–494.

Wise, R. A. (2009). Roles for nigrostriatal—not just mesocorticolimbic—dopamine in reward and addiction. *Trends Neurosci*, 32(10), 517–524.

Wise, R. A., & Bozarth, M. A. (1987). A psychomotor stimulant theory of addiction. *Psychol Rev*, 94(4), 469–492.

7

Are Addicts Responsible?

WALTER SINNOTT-ARMSTRONG

My title asks the wrong question. That is what I will try to show eventually. But first we need to ask:

WHY ASK?

Many of us use addictive substances. Many of us know people who are addicted to various substances. So addiction affects many of us in personal ways. Addiction is also a societal issue. It tears apart families, leaves children needy, and fills prisons, which reduces everyone's security and pocketbooks. Experts estimate that drug addiction costs over $250 billion per year in the United States alone. That makes it worthwhile to study addiction.

But why ask whether addicts are responsible? One reason is that addiction raises profound puzzles and illustrates general points that can be useful for theories of responsibility. More practically, whether people view addicts as responsible seems to affect how they are treated by courts, by psychiatrists, and by their friends.

Finally, why ask these questions now? One reason is that recently science has discovered a lot of cool stuff about brains and genes as well as minds and societies that greatly enhances our understanding of addiction (e.g., Robbins et al. 2010). We know more today about how addiction begins and progresses, how it compares with normal motivation, and how to treat it.

ONE CASE STUDY

Let's start by listening to a self-described addict, the poet William Burroughs:

> I lived in a room in the Native Quarter of Tangier. I had not taken a bath
> in a year nor changed my clothes or removed them except to stick a needle

every hour into the fibrous grey wood flesh of terminal addiction....I could look at the end of my shoe for eight hours. I was only roused to action when the hourglass of junk ran out. If a friend came to visit—and they rarely did since who or what was left to visit—I sat there not caring that they had entered my field of vision—a grey screen always blanker and fainter—and not caring when he walked out of it. If he had died on the spot, I would have sat there looking at my shoe waiting to go through his pockets. Wouldn't you?...A dope fiend is a man in total need of dope. Beyond a certain frequency, need knows absolutely no limit or control. In the words of total need: "*Wouldn't you?*" Yes, you would. You would lie, cheat, inform on your friends, do *anything* to satisfy total need. Because you would be in a state of total sickness, total possession, and not in a position to act in any other way. Dope fiends are sick people who cannot act other than they do. A rabid dog cannot choose but to bite. (Burroughs 1959, xli, xxxix; quoted in Heyman 2009, 51)

Burroughs' personal vision of addiction raises several issues.

First, he says, "A rabid dog cannot choose but to bite." He does not deny that a rabid dog does choose to bite. Indeed, he seems to admit that he himself chooses and acts, despite his professed inability to choose or act other than he does. Neither a rabid dog nor an addict is like a river that does not choose to flow. That is important if responsibility requires choice (except possibly in cases of negligence), as some claim.

Second, Burroughs explains his choice in terms of "not caring" about anything other than dope (and his shoe). We normally blame people when they misbehave because they do not care about other people, so lack of caring also seems important to responsibility. However, we also normally assume that people are capable of caring, even if they do not actually care. That assumption might not apply to everyone. If we choose to care about something, such as a person, that choice will not automatically make us start caring. Compare patients with severe depression who cannot bring themselves to care about anything. If such depressives are not responsible, as many assume, then how could addicts be responsible for not caring about anything other than their dope?

Third, Burroughs asks, "Wouldn't you?" He answers, "Yes, you would." This affirmative answer presumably means that, if you yourself somehow got as hooked on heroin as he was, then you would choose and fail to care as he did. This counterfactual suggests that his problem is not due to anything special—or especially bad—about him or his character. His problem results from our shared human nature mixed with drugs in certain circumstances. If this is correct (though many deny it), then it seems inappropriate to blame him as a person—at least in the way that we blame people for burglary when most of us would not burgle even if we badly needed money.

Fourth, Burroughs describes his condition without qualification: "total need... absolutely no limit or control... total sickness, total possession." Perhaps this is just poetic license. He is a poet, after all. In any case, these claims are exaggerations. If he really had "absolutely no limit or control," then he would have overdosed quickly. And it is not hard to understand why he exaggerates. He wants us to excuse him, and perhaps he also wants to excuse himself. Our question is whether he deserves to be excused.

Fascinating as Burroughs is, he is just one example and probably not a typical one. We should not generalize too quickly from his case—or from any one case—to addiction in general. Here's why.

VARIETY

Addiction comes in many forms. It varies widely and wildly with respect to who is addicted, what they are addicted to, and whether they want to be addicted.

What are addicts addicted to? The paradigms of addictive substances are illegal drugs, including heroin, cocaine, morphine, barbiturates, amphetamines, and so on. People can also become addicted to legal drugs, including alcohol, nicotine, and caffeine. Some experts believe that people can also be addicted to behaviors, including gambling, sex, work, shopping, and the Internet (Ross 2008). It is controversial whether behavioral "addictions" are really addictions at all, but they are worth comparing to substance addictions, which are the main topic here (though most of what I say also applies to supposed behavioral addictions).

Potentially addictive substances differ in the percentage of users who become addicted and how quickly users become addicted, with much individual and group variation. These substances also differ in the health effects of heavy use: from lung cancer and sclerosis of the liver to risk of mental illness and "fibrous grey wood flesh." Withdrawal symptoms also vary. John Lennon sings that "cold turkey" is horrible. Others, however, claim it is no worse than a bad flu (Pickard & Pearce, this volume). Still, if you have a bad flu and know that your suffering can be relieved by taking a medication that is right in front of you, then it would be hard not to take the medicine, even if it had certain risks. In contrast, cocaine withdrawal is reported to be more like depression, with loss of energy and interest, but cocaine withdrawal is reportedly not painful in the same way as heroin withdrawal. Alcohol withdrawal is supposed to be the most severe, sometimes leading to hallucinations, delirium tremens, and even death. These variations in withdrawal symptoms are relevant to responsibility if high costs of quitting make an addict less responsible for not quitting.

Next, who gets addicted? All levels of socioeconomic status (SES), intelligence (IQ), and education include some addicts, but rates of addiction are positively correlated with low SES, low IQ, young age, childhood abuse, stress, personality disorders, and religion. Unsurprisingly, Mormons don't get addicted as often as other people. Though correlation does not establish causation, these correlations seem to suggest that people are not responsible for some factors that make them more susceptible to addiction. Genetics can teach the same lesson insofar as genes can make some individuals unknowingly more susceptible to addiction than others.

In addition, people have many different motivations for using drugs, including pleasure, stimulation, acceptance, escape, and even insight (for fans of Timothy Leary). People do take drugs for pleasure or fun, but they also often use drugs to avoid pain: either physical pain (such as morphine after surgery) or mental pain (perhaps from stress, anxiety, sadness, anger, frustration, hopelessness, or just boredom). Peer pressure is another motivation for those who crave acceptance by peers, as many do. Some people take drugs to improve their functioning, such as when workaholics take speed. After becoming addicted, people sometimes take drugs just to maintain normal functioning, as when former heroin addicts take up methadone maintenance, but also when cocaine addicts take just enough to feel normal. These motivations can affect responsibility if motivation reveals an agent's character or true self, and if agents are more responsible for acts that reflect their true characters or selves.

Addicts also differ in their attitudes toward their drug use and their addiction. They can be willing or unwilling addicts (Frankfurt 1971). Unwilling addicts have a second-order desire not to desire to take the substances to which they are addicted (along with, presumably, also a desire not to take them, a desire to desire not to take them, a desire not to be addicted to them, no desire to desire to take them, and so on). In contrast, a willing addict desires to desire to take drugs or to be addicted (and, presumably, does not also desire not to desire to take drugs or to be addicted and does not desire to desire not to take drugs or to be addicted), and a wanton neither desires to desire them nor desires not to desire them (and might either consider or not consider that second-order issue). The parentheses show additional possibilities (if you can keep the negations straight), and there can be variation within each group. Some willing addicts are doctors who have ready access to drugs, take them for pleasure or maintenance, and never suffer serious harms or take much risk. Other "willing" addicts are what Kennett (this volume) calls "resigned" addicts.

A long-time homeless addict might have no realistic option other than life on the streets with drugs and life on the streets without drugs. The latter might be the lesser of two evils, since life on the street without drugs is so horrible. Faced with only these options, then, it might be reasonable to desire to desire to take drugs (and not to desire to desire not to take drugs and maybe even to desire to desire to be addicted). These second-order desires are mentioned here, because they are crucial to responsibility according to Frankfurt (1971) and others (see Woolfolk et al. 2006).

These distinctions show only part of the variety among addicts, but they suffice to issue a challenge: How can anyone say anything intelligent about responsibility that will cover all addicts? In order to answer the question of whether addicts in general are responsible, we need to specify what is common to all real addicts that reduces or removes responsibility.

CONTROL

To understand what makes addicts less responsible, we first need to specify: Less responsible than what? We need a comparison class. The natural comparison is with heavy users who are not addicted, since this group is presumably responsible.

What is the difference between heavy use and addiction? The answer lies in control. Burroughs says that "dope fiends" are "not in a position to act in any other way" and "cannot act other than they do" (1959, xli). In contrast, I am a heavy user of ice cream and golf, but I can stop eating ice cream when I go on a diet, and I can stop playing golf when a nongolfing friend visits. I do not ignore my friends and just stare at my shoe in the way that Burroughs said he would. Of course, Burroughs was extreme. Some addicts go out of control when they have just taken drugs or when they are on a binge, but not all addicts stare at their shoes all the time. Many greet their friends and engage in complex activities. Some addicts lead otherwise normal lives. Still, they seem to be missing some kind of ability to stop taking drugs, and that is what makes them addicts instead of mere heavy users.

What exactly does it mean to say that addicts lack *control* or the *ability* to stop or that they *cannot* stop taking drugs? Hard determinists often claim that nobody can act in any way other than they do. Here "cannot" means something like "prevented by some cause" regardless of whether the cause is a choice or a seizure, a desire or a push. This use of "can" does not violate any semantic rules. The problem is only that this use is useless here. This use of "cannot" cannot distinguish anyone from anyone else, since addicts are no more or less determined than nonaddicts, so it cannot be used to distinguish addicts from heavy users.

We also say things like, "I can't watch a movie tonight, because I have to work." This justification for not watching a movie does not deny that I have the physical and psychological ability to watch the movie. All it denies is that I have good enough reason. The point is that it would be irrational or irresponsible for me to watch a movie, at least given my values. However, when Burroughs says that he cannot stop taking drugs, his point is not that it would be irrational or irresponsible for him to stop taking drugs. Some methods of quitting (such as killing himself) might be irrational, but that is clearly not what Burroughs means.

What does he mean? Burroughs seems to claim that he lacks control over his drug use in a way that I do have control over my golf and ice cream consumption and in a way that heavy drug users who are not addicted have control over whether they abstain. As I said, Burroughs exaggerates when he claims that he cannot act in "any other way," but there is a grain of truth beneath his exaggeration.

That grain of truth is hidden not only by exaggerations but also by a heap of inspecificities and varieties (see Fischer & Ravizza 1998 and Pettit 2001 on kinds of control). Addicts do not lack control in the extreme way that people during seizures or with muscular or nerve disorders cannot control their limbs, but many other factors can reduce control in various ways.

One way to control something uses external aids. Do you control whether a certain weight touches the floor? An indirect way to prevent the weight from touching the floor is to put the weight on a stand that separates the weight from the floor. This indirect kind of control is analogous to an addict controlling drug use by moving to an island where there are no drugs or, less dramatically, by hanging out only with Mormons. Such moves have high costs, to be sure, but they can work.

Other methods of control are more direct. You might try to hold the weight up by yourself. Then you lack control over whether the weight touches the floor if the weight is too heavy for you to hold up. Analogously, addicts lack control over their drug use if their desires for drugs are so strong that nobody could resist or if they personally cannot resist, even if some others with unusually strong willpower could resist. Weakness is another way to lack control. People who normally could lift 100 pounds might be too sick or tired to lift 100 pounds. Analogously, drug addicts' desires for drugs might be too strong for them to resist when their willpower has been weakened by addiction, though not when they are healthy. A third way to lack control involves persistence. Many people can lift and hold up a 20-pound weight easily for a minute but not for a day. Before the day is up, they get bored, lose hope, or forget what they are doing, and the weight goes down every time they try, even if they are not too tired to keep it up longer at that moment, and even if they had strong incentives to keep it up. This case is analogous to drug addicts who eventually give in to persistent desires for drugs even though they have enough willpower to resist their desires at the moment. Persistence is central to recent discussions of resolutions (Holton 2011; Holton & Berridge, this volume). This third way to fail is more common than is recognized, but the other models of failure of control fit other addicts on other occasions. There is too much variety among addicts to expect them all to fail in the same way.

Another way to lack control is more cognitive. Instead of desires and choices, addicts can also lack control over attention and beliefs (Garavan & Hester 2007). Drug cues can make it very difficult for addicts to pay attention to other things that they value, and attention can then affect desires and decisions. When they face constant drug cues, intrusive thoughts about drugs can resemble obsessions, so many addicts eventually relent or relapse, even if they would not have used drugs in the absence of drug cues. In addition to attention, addicts can also lose control over beliefs, especially their evaluative beliefs. Addicts regularly seem to overestimate benefits of using drugs (including expected pleasure or relief), overestimate costs of not using (including the likelihood and intensity of cravings and withdrawal pains), underestimate harms of using (including health effects), and underestimate benefits of not using (including the value of other activities as well as friends). They also seem to discount the future in extreme ways: hyperbolically (see Ainslie, this volume). And some addicts fail to take in or use information about fictive losses that is relevant to rational choice (Chiu et al. 2008, on smokers). These mistakes involve addicts' beliefs, but they can still make addicts lose control if addicts cannot correct their mistakes (see Bernheim & Rangel 2005, 21, 25–27).

Yet another way to lack control resembles coercion or duress. When a robber convincingly threatens, "Your money or your life," you lack control over your money. When a storm will sink a ship if its captain does not throw goods overboard (Aristotle 1941, 1110a), the captain lacks control over whether he will toss the goods. Analogously, some addicts lack control over taking drugs because they will suffer serious losses if they stop taking drugs. These losses might include severe withdrawal pains that it would be unreasonable to expect or require anyone to undergo in order to conform to drug laws (though it might not be unreasonable to expect people to undergo these pains in order to avoid stealing or killing in order to get money to buy drugs). Other losses might include isolation from friends or family or reduced performance for some time in one's job. Such costs of quitting can sometimes justify postponing quitting until tomorrow and the next day and so on for a long time. Then addicts cannot quit in the same sense in which I have not been able to play golf for a month because I have been under constant pressure to meet a deadline.

To accommodate this variety, we need a broad account of control. There are at least four common accounts of control.

One account focuses on wants or desires and claims that an agent has control over a type of action if and only if the following conditionals are true:

  (i) If the agent desires overall to perform that type of action, then usually he does it; and
  (ii) If the agent desires overall not to perform that type of action, then usually he doesn't do it.

On this account, golfers have control over playing golf if and only if they usually play golf when they desire overall to play golf and usually do not play golf when they desire overall not to play golf. The qualification "usually" is necessary because they might fail to play golf when they want to because the only golf course is closed or their car breaks down or they miss their starting time. Similarly, the qualification "overall" is necessary because desires can conflict. If a golfer decides not to play, even though he has some desire to play, because he has a stronger desire to go swimming, then the golfer still has control over whether he golfs or swims.

A second account refers not to desires but instead to reasons. On this kind of account, an agent has control over a type of action if and only if the following conditionals are true:

  (i') If the agent has a strong overall reason to perform that type of action, then usually he does it; and
  (ii') If the agent has a strong overall reason not to perform that type of action, then usually he doesn't do it.

On this account, golfers have control over playing golf if and only if they usually play golf when they have strong overall reason to play golf and usually do not play golf when they have strong overall reason not to play golf.

These want-tracking and reason-tracking accounts might seem very close, especially to internalists who assume that all reasons are based on desires. However, these accounts come apart in some cases that are relevant to addiction. In particular, if agents have no reason to fulfill some desires, then those agents can act on their desires without tracking their reasons. For example, some heavy users claim that they want drugs in the sense of having a strong desire even though they no longer like drugs or get any pleasure from them (and also would not suffer withdrawal if they quit) (see Holton & Berridge, this volume). If so, these users might have control over their drug use on the desire-tracking account because they take drugs when they want to and cease when they want not to. However, such users would lack control on the reason-tracking account if they continue to use drugs because of their strong desires even when they know that they have little or no reason to use drugs and strong reason not to use drugs.

A third account refers not to the reasons that the agent has but instead to the reasons that the agent recognizes or believes in. On this kind of account, an agent has control over a type of action if and only if the following conditionals are true:

(i")   If the agent believes that he has a strong overall reason to perform that type of action, then usually he does it; and

(ii") If the agent believes that he has a strong overall reason not to perform that type of action, then usually he doesn't do it.

To distinguish this account from the preceding, we need to consider cases where the agent has reasons without recognizing them (or believes in reasons without having any). Imagine that a strong desire to take drugs causes a user to think only about drugs and then forget or not notice conflicting consider-ations, such as detrimental effects on self or loved ones. This user has reasons not to take drugs and also would want not to take drugs if he paid attention to the reasons not to take drugs, but his strong desires for drugs prevent him from becoming aware of those conflicting considerations (at least at the time when he takes drugs), so he does not actually want not to take drugs. In this case, it can be true that he takes drugs when he wants and does not take drugs when he wants not to take drugs, and then he has control on the desire-tracking account. In contrast, he lacks control on the reason-tracking account, because he does not act according to the reasons that he never notices or becomes aware of. Nonetheless, it still might be true that he would respond to reasons if he did notice them, and then he would have control on this third account.

Once this distinction is drawn, it seems natural to propose that control requires both that one's acts track one's beliefs about reasons and also that one's beliefs about reasons track the reasons one has. On this kind of account, an agent has control over a type of action if and only if all of these conditionals are true:

(i''')   If the agent has a strong overall reason to perform that type of action, then usually he believes that he has that reason;

(i'''') If the agent believes that he has a strong overall reason to perform that type of action, then usually he does it;

(ii''') If the agent has a strong overall reason not to perform that type of action, then usually he believes that he has that reason; and

(ii'''') If the agent believes that he has a strong overall reason not to per-form that type of action, then usually he does not it.

Something like this seems to be what is intended in most common reasons-responsiveness accounts of ability, freedom, or control (cf. Duggan & Gert 1979; Fischer & Ravizza 1998).

This reasons-responsiveness account elucidates the various ways to lose control that were mentioned above. If an addict has a desire that is too strong for anyone or for this addict to resist either in any circumstances or in the addict's current circumstances, then the addict will take drugs even when the addict has strong enough reason not to take drugs. His desires make him act against his reasons. If the addict cannot get his mind off of drugs, then the addict might forget about the reasons not to take drugs, and end up acting against those reasons; so loss of cognitive control (such as control over attention) can also lead to loss of control over action on this reasons-responsiveness account. And, just as a person who is threatened with "Your money or your life" loses the ability to act on strong reasons to keep the money, so an addict who faces severe withdrawal pains or loss of friends if he quits can lose the ability to act on strong reasons to quit.

This reasons-responsiveness account also illuminates control over willing as well as control over action. Consider unwilling addicts who try but fail to quit in response to strong reasons to quit. They do not control whether they use drugs, so they lack freedom of action. Nonetheless, they control whether they attempt and intend to quit. These choices to try to quit respond to their reasons, so they have free will to that extent at those times (when they try to quit). However, at other moments when they choose to use drugs, these other choices do not respond to their reasons, so they lack control over those choices at those times. In contrast, some other addicts (possibly including resigned addicts) might have even less control over their wills and intentions because they do not even try to quit when they have strong reason to try to quit. Thus, the reasons-responsiveness account of control can help to draw useful distinctions among addicts.

This reasons-responsiveness account of control can also be used to define addiction—to distinguish addicts from nonaddicts (see Sinnott-Armstrong & Pickard, 2013). Addiction can be understood as a strong appetite that significantly reduces control over drug use. On this definition, lack of control over drug use is not enough by itself for addiction. If an addict has no control over whether she takes drugs only because she has no way to get any drugs or only because she is forced to take drugs (or is pressured by her culture into taking drugs, perhaps during religious ceremonies), then that lack of control cannot make her an addict. What makes her an addict is that her internal condition—her strong appetite—is what significantly reduces her control. (Compare Gert et al. 2006 on the absence of a distinct sustaining cause.) This definition explains the difference between addiction and love of golf, because lovers of golf who are not addicted can recognize and act on reasons not to play golf.

OBJECTIONS

Some critics object that individuals who are called addicts do not really lack control. This challenge is sometimes expressed by saying that addicts do not have a compulsion (Pickard & Pearce, this volume) or that addiction is voluntary (Heyman 2009). Either way, the point is that addicts consciously choose to take drugs and that they retain at least some control, such as control over which drugs to take and when and how to take them. Drug use is not like having a seizure or a reflex; nor is it automatic or unconscious.

The problem with this objection is that conscious choice does not prove control. If a robber threatens, "Your money or your life," you choose to hand over your money. You do so willingly and happily, given your limited options. Nonetheless, you do not control what you do with your money. The robber controls that. Again, compulsive hand washers choose to wash their hands, even after their hands become raw and bleeding from too much washing. Their washings are not like seizures. They know what they are doing, intend to do it for a reason (to relieve tension or anxiety), and control how they do it within limits. Nonetheless, they do not control whether they wash their hands too often. Similarly, what we need to ask is not whether addicts choose, but whether they have control over whether they take drugs or gamble.

Lots of evidence speaks against control. First come self-reports by addicts. Recall Burroughs' poetic comparison to a rabid dog that cannot choose but to bite. Then Alcoholics Anonymous requires members to admit that they are powerless over alcohol, at least without help from a "higher power." And clinics report that many patients try hard but fail to quit. They often stop for a short period, but most relapse eventually and go back to using drugs or gambling. Some patients even take Antabuse (Disulfiram), which they know will make them extremely nauseous if they drink alcohol, but they drink anyway. Failure to abstain in the face of such high costs is evidence of lack of control, just as one's failure to lift 200 pounds to avoid a serious harm is evidence that one cannot lift that much weight.

Admittedly, none of the evidence against control is conclusive. There is also contrary evidence for control. Burroughs quit heroin with help from a clinic when his parents stopped sending him money (Heyman 2009, 63–64), and most veterans who used heroin heavily in Vietnam quit using when they returned to their homes in the United States (Heyman 2009, 75–76). The stories of failures to quit come from clinics, but that sample might be skewed, because the addicts who go to clinics might be an atypical subset who either cannot give up on their own or have mental illnesses that make them unable to quit (Heyman 2009, 82–85). Clinics that teach appropriate life skills have great success in helping addicts who use drugs escape their bad lives (Pickard & Pearce, this volume).

Alcoholics Anonymous reports high rates of recovery. Indeed, some programs reportedly work simply by offering vouchers to addicts when they test clean each week (Budney & Higgins 1998).

However, this evidence for control is also far from conclusive. Alcoholics Anonymous can report high recovery rates for addicts who finish the program partly because addicts leave the program if it is not working for them, and they complete the program only when they have quit. Any program will work for anyone who tries hard enough and sticks with it long enough, but that claim is empty, because anyone who fails obviously did not try hard enough or stick with it long enough—simply by definition of "enough."

Compare also Pickard and Pearce's program: "Before they can begin the 18-month program, we require them to stop, or adequately control, the use of alcohol, to stop the use of illicit drugs, and to stop taking certain kinds of prescribed medication, such as benzodiazepines, other sedatives, and hypnotics" (Pickard & Pearce, this volume, XXX). This entrance requirement makes perfect sense, given the therapeutic strategy: "these drugs impair the capacity to do the psychological work that the program involves: in particular, the capacity to explore painful and difficult memories and emotions, and to learn new, healthier ways of coping with them" (Pickard & Pearce, this volume, XXX). However, the high success rate of their treatment program might be explained at least partly by the entrance requirement if potential patients who fail the entrance requirement would not be able to stop abusing drugs and alcohol even if they did receive the prescribed therapy.

The program described by Pickard and Pearce can still do tremendous good for those who are allowed into it. Even then, however, their program might make the people able to do something they were not able to do before the program. If you want to run fast, this program works: get a coach to teach you better technique and build your leg muscles. Still, success does not show that you could run faster before the program. Instead, it shows that you gained new abilities during the program. Analogously, addicts might lack control before they enter a treatment program and then gain control as a result of the program. If so, then the program really cures them, for it changes them from an addict without control into a former addict with control. That is an important and impressive success, but it would not undermine the claim that addicts lacked control at times before treatment when they were addicts.

Other programs work without training. One program in Vermont simply gave vouchers worth less than $100 per week to every addict who tested clean. Their success rate was surprisingly high, even though many of their patients had spent over $100 per day on their drug habits. The fact that these so-called addicts could quit for such a small reward suggests that they did have significant control over their choices and actions before entering the program. However, another possibility is that the patients who succeeded in this program were not really addicts to begin with. They were only heavy users. Potential patients who refused to enter the program or who entered but then failed to show up clean might be the only ones who lacked control and were really addicted. Moreover, when the program stopped because funding ran out, many of those who had quit while receiving vouchers quickly went back to using drugs. This might suggest that money (and personal attention) temporarily gave them the ability to refrain from using drugs while the program existed. If so, then they still might lack the ability to refrain in other circumstances.

Recall also the Vietnam veterans who used heroin regularly in high quantities while in Vietnam. Only 12% continued to use heroin when they returned (Heyman 2009, 75–76). Still, if the dramatic change in circumstances (either stress, access, cues, peer pressure, or all of these) when they returned home explains their recovery, then these data do not show that they had control while they were in Vietnam or that any addict can quit without a dramatic change in circumstances. Also, of course, they did not all quit, so maybe some but not all of them lacked control and, hence, were real addicts.

Another kind of case is doctors who are caught using drugs and then threatened with losing their jobs if they do not quit immediately. Reportedly, a very high percentage quit with treatment, even though they do not change their circumstances as dramatically as veterans returning home from war. Still, being caught and threatened with losing one's job can be dramatic, they might not be able to control their use without treatment, and some of them still fail to quit. So, as before, these cases do not show that all heavy drug users have control over whether they continue to use drugs.

Other statistics apply to drug users more generally instead of special groups like veterans and doctors. Rates of drug use are highest in the late teens and twenties and most people "mature out" of drug use by age 35 (Heyman 2009, 70–71). Nonetheless, circumstances change as people mature. Moreover, the tendency to quit drugs by age 35 might result from the simple fact that older people have more control. After all, their brains change. They are also less susceptible to peer pressure. Also, older people probably tried more often, so there is more chance that one attempt to quit will have succeeded. As a result, what these data show is at most that many mature people are able to quit in their new circumstances. They don't show that these people were able to quit in other circumstances when they were younger. Maybe they became able to do what they were not able to do in their youth.

Another kind of evidence for control is that the level of drug use is affected by cohort, environment, income, and price. These factors affect drug use much more than they affect most other mental illnesses (Heyman 2009, 31–39). Heyman defines acts as voluntary when they "vary systematically as a function of their consequences" but as involuntary when they "are elicited by preceding stimuli (e.g. urges) and are influenced little or not at all by their consequences" (Heyman 2009, 104). Drug use by addicts is voluntary under this definition. However, this does not show that addicts have enough of the kind of control that is required for responsibility. After all, peers and inducements can also affect which small areas claustrophobes enter: Some claustrophobes will sometimes get into an elevator if they need to get to their daughter's wedding on the top floor in time or if their peers taunt them. But they are still not responsible for failing to enter an elevator in other situations. Thus, Heyman's definition of voluntary acts cannot determine whether addicts are responsible.

DEGREES

This leaves us in a mess: Do people who seem to be addicts really have control or not? No answer seems to fit all of the evidence on both sides.

The solution is to recognize that control comes in degrees. Addicts have *some* control over their choices and actions. Nonetheless, they do not have *full* control, and they have *less* control than nonaddicts, including some heavy drug users.

Indeed, control varies along several dimensions—including time, circumstance, and incentive. Individual addicts respond to some reasons in some circumstances, but they fail to respond to other reasons in other circumstances, including circumstances where their actions are irrational. Typically, addicts respond to fewer reasons and in a smaller range of circumstances than nonaddicts, which means that they have less control, at least in those circumstances.

The ways in which a particular person lacks control need not fit into a neat package that seems intuitive from the outside. A drug addict who is undeterred by a long jail sentence might be able to avoid drugs for a small reward in money or vouchers, at least for a while. One alcoholic might always drink in bars but never at home, whereas another alcoholic drinks at home but never in public. An addict might proudly abstain for months and then binge uncontrollably for no apparent reason. Even when the pattern among such factors makes no sense from the outside, the fact that an addict refrains in some circumstances does not show that the addict has complete or even much control in other circumstances.

This perspective might seem obvious and innocuous, but it undermines many traditional debates. Those who claim that addicts have control and deny that they have a compulsion require a lot for compulsion and only a little for control. Those who claim that addicts have a compulsion and lack control require a lot for control and only a little for compulsion. They are arguing about whether the glass is half empty or half full. The solution is to recognize that the glass is both half empty and half full. We don't have to choose between half truths either about water or about addiction.

Consider a doctor who happily takes drugs, has unhampered access to drugs, and would not quit if his wife threatened to leave him or if there were only a risk of being caught and fired; but then he is caught and threatened with losing his job if he does not enter therapy and quit. So he does. In this case, he has control over whether he tries to quit and also over whether he succeeds in quitting after he is caught. Nonetheless, he still might not have control over whether he quits at times when his only reasons to quit include risks or his family, even though he would honestly report that he values them more than drugs. At that earlier time, this doctor might control when, where, and what he takes but not whether he takes drugs within a week or a month. Overall, does he have or lack control? Yes—he both has and lacks control to some degree.

How much reduction in control makes someone an addict? How can we draw a line on the continuum of control between addicts and nonaddicts? Common language cannot help, because common language here, as elsewhere, is too flexible to determine a specific answer. Logic cannot help, because equally coherent views can draw the line at different places. It is hard to imagine a metaphysical or scientific basis for drawing the line one place rather than another. In the end, then, there is no way to justify drawing a line at one place rather than another except pragmatically. That means that where we should draw the line depends in part on what our specific goals are.

Compare vision. An optometrist can tell patients whether their eyesight is 20-20, 20-30, 20-40, or 20-400, as well as whether they are color blind, are nearsighted or farsighted, or have less than usual night vision (cf. Fingarette 1972, 38–39). However, it takes policy makers to determine how good an individual's vision must be in order to get a license to drive a car (or to drive a school bus or to pilot a plane) or to get disability benefits, serve in the military or the police, and so forth. The lines between adequate and inadequate vision are drawn at different places for different practical purposes, depending on the likelihood and harms of different kinds of mistakes in different circumstances.

The same goes for lines between addicts and nonaddicts. Courts might draw the line relatively high in order to count fewer people as addicts and thereby hold more people responsible, whereas private citizens might draw the line relatively low in order to count more of their friends as addicts so that they can express their understanding and sympathy and then help their friends conquer their drug and alcohol problems. Therapists might sometimes draw the line relatively low in order to count more potential patients as addicts for the purposes of eligibility for treatment, but then sometimes draw the line relatively high so as to count fewer patients as addicts when they think that telling patients that they are addicted will undermine successful treatment. And scientists might draw the line between addicts and nonaddicts at whatever level of control is most highly correlated with the factor that they are studying (such as neural structure or function or genetic or environmental factors).

These pragmatic considerations are crucial not only for applying the word "addict" but also for applying words like "control" and "can." A psychiatrist might encourage a patient by saying, "You can stop." This claim is fine if the patient has enough control to make encouragement useful. But then a friend might say, "You can't stop," and this apparently conflicting claim might also be fine if the person's control is reduced enough to deserve sympathy. Both sides might place the individual on the same place in the continua of control and ability, but they draw their lines between adequate and inadequate control, between what the agent can and cannot do, and between addiction and nonaddiction at different places for different practical purposes.

The point is not that any line is as good as any other. Given the purposes and normative constraints of a particular context, such as law, therapy, or science, it can be better to draw the line at some places rather than others. It can even be wrong to draw the line too low or too high when labeling someone as an addict. Still, the applicable purposes and norms can vary.

This variation in purposes can be confusing, especially when it is not explicit, but there is nothing illegitimate about drawing the line at different places for different purposes. That is what the law does for vision as well as many other concepts. We just need to keep in mind what we are doing and avoid overly simplistic questions like, "But is he really an addict?"

RESPONSIBLE

Addiction and control are not the only things that come in degrees. So does responsibility. To see this, we need to specify what responsibility is.

It is common to see blameworthiness as some function of responsibility and harm (or seriousness of wrong-doing). A person who causes a death is more blameworthy than a person who causes a bruise even if both were equally responsible. Since harm comes in degrees, so does blameworthiness. Similarly, praiseworthiness (or, more accurately, credit-worthiness) is also a function of responsibility and benefit (and maybe also difficulty and risk or sacrifice by the agent), so praiseworthiness also clearly comes in degrees. Still, even though blameworthiness and praiseworthiness come in degrees, and responsibility is crucial to both, this does not yet show that responsibility comes in degrees. The degrees in blameworthiness and praiseworthiness might be due only to the degrees of harm and benefit or factors other than responsibility.

To see that responsibility does come in degrees, consider children and adolescents. Suppose that otherwise typical 5-, 10-, 15-, and 20-year-old people each causes a death (or a bruise) intentionally with the same motive (such as jealousy or anger). Because different levels of understanding, impulsivity, susceptibility to peer pressure, and so on occur at their different ages, these children seem responsible to different degrees even though they caused the same harm. The US Supreme Court recently recognized this kind of variation in responsibility in the cases of *Roper v. Simmons* (2005) and *Graham v. Florida* (2010), but most people do not need the Supreme Court to tell them that responsibility increases in degrees as children mature.

Consider also provocation, which reduces murder to manslaughter and can excuse some assaults in many legal systems. Provocation comes in degrees, because some words are more provocative than others, provocative words can be repeated more or less often either in the person's face or from a distance, and the provoked person's emotions can rise to various levels. The law needs to decide how much provocation is sufficient to turn murder into manslaughter or to excuse a punch (or a failed attempt to punch), but the line might be drawn at different places for different harms or crimes, and the practical need to draw a line is compatible with recognizing that the underlying responsibility varies in degrees.

Degrees of duress also illustrate degrees of responsibility, if duress is seen as an excuse rather than a justification. Responsibility also varies with degree of mental illness (compulsion or delusion), even if the law needs to draw a line in particular cases. And if extreme emotional upset provides a whole or partial excuse, that emotion varies in degrees as well. There are, then, many reasons to admit degrees of responsibility, and these reasons apply to moral as well as legal responsibility.

Opponents sometimes reply that responsibility is a necessary minimal condition of any degree of blameworthiness and praiseworthiness. They are surely correct that people are not blameworthy or praiseworthy at all if they fail certain minimal conditions. An epileptic who causes death during a seizure that was unforeseeable is not at all blameworthy or responsible. However, such minimal conditions for any responsibility at all do not undermine the claim that responsibility varies in degrees after it passes that minimal threshold (just as the fact that some people are totally blind does not undermine the claim that visual acuity varies in other people).

Once we recognize that both control and responsibility vary in degrees, the next question is whether they covary or, in other words, whether degree of control matches or is correlated with degree of responsibility. Consider the cases of provocation and adolescence. The very same factors that reduce responsibility after provocation—number of repetitions "in your face" and the resulting level of emotional disturbance—also reduce responsiveness to reasons (the percentage of times that the provoked person will avoid striking out because he realizes that doing so is against his interest) and, hence, also reduces the degree to which the provoked person controls the actions. Similarly, the factors that reduce the degree of responsibility in children of different ages—reduced understanding and increased impulsivity and susceptibility to peer pressure—also reduce adolescents' awareness of or responsiveness to reasons and, hence, the degree to which adolescents control their actions, according to the above account. This covariation might be explained by some third factor that independently affects both control and responsibility, but that reduced degree of control still at least seems to be what explains reduced degree of responsibility in provocation and adolescence (other things being equal).

This conclusion then applies to addiction. Drug users are more addicted when they have less control and then they also have less responsibility. We cannot ask whether addicts are responsible, because addiction is too varied and comes in degrees, as does responsibility, but there can still be an important relation between degree of addiction and degree of responsibility that is mediated by degree of control.

TRANSFERENCE

Some critics object that, even if addicts have very little control, they are still responsible for what they do now, because they were responsible in the past for becoming addicted in the first place. After all, they were not yet addicted when they first began to use drugs. Their responsibility for their first dubious act transfers to responsibility for later acts of the same sort that result from their first dubious act.

Of course, people are not responsible for all effects of their actions, because some effects are unforeseeable. However, critics seem to assume that people do or should know the risks when they first use drugs. This assumption is questionable in many cases, especially because many people begin using drugs when they are adolescents, and there are reasons to discount the foresight of adolescents. Still, the transfer principle behind the objection can be formulated conditionally like this:

(T) If a person, P, is responsible for doing an act, A, and if P does or ought to know that doing A will create a risk that P will later cause an effect, E, then P is responsible for E. (Cf. Vargas 2005.)

According to this principle, if Percy is responsible for taking drugs the first time, and if at that time Percy does or ought to know that taking drugs the first time creates a risk that Percy will later become addicted and cause harm, then Percy is responsible for that later harm. This consequent is supposed to be true even if at the later time Percy has too little control to count as responsible without some transfer principle like (T).

Notice, first, that this transfer principle is about responsibility rather than blameworthiness. Imagine that Percy drinks alcohol for the first time on his 21st birthday. It is both legal and common to drink alcohol at this age, so there seems to be nothing legally or morally wrong with these acts at this age. Hence, Percy is not blameworthy for doing these first acts. That means that a transfer principle would not apply to Percy if its antecedent required the agent to be blameworthy for the earlier act. However, the formulation of (T) above requires only that the agent was responsible for the earlier act. Percy is responsible for taking that fateful first drink. Hence, if Percy did know or ought to have known that his first drink would create a risk of addiction, loss of control, and harm, then Percy is responsible for that later addiction, loss of control, and harm, according to (T).

The focus on responsibility rather than blame also comes out when we consider responsibility for good effects, which can be called credit. Imagine that I train myself so that I will be unable to stop myself from helping people in need, and then I help someone in need. Transfer principle (T) implies that I am responsible for fulfilling that person's needs even though I was out of control when I helped him. Thus, what transfers is responsibility, not necessarily blame, even though the principle is more often used to transfer blame.

Notice also that this transfer principle is limited in scope. In particular, it does not apply to addicts who became addicted through no fault of their own. Some surgery patients become addicted to painkillers, such as morphine, that they needed for their surgeries. A different kind of case is a 12-year-old who is forced by a drug dealer to use drugs. Perhaps the drug dealer credibly threatened to kill him or his family if he did not serve the dealer as a drug mule, and then the dealer forced him to become addicted as a way of ensuring his loyalty and silence. In cases like these, where a person is not responsible (or has very little responsibility) for becoming addicted, there is little or no initial responsibility to transfer to later acts after control is lost or diminished. My conclusion—that drug users are less responsible when they have less control and are more addicted—applies to these cases, even if responsibility does transfer as the objection claims.

Transfer principle (T) also does not apply unless the person does or ought to know that taking drugs will create a risk of later becoming addicted and causing harm. It might seem that everyone ought to know this. But consider an adolescent who tries cocaine once and has been told by a trusted authority that no user ever becomes addicted the first time. Unfortunately, it turns out that a few users do become addicted the first time, and this adolescent is one of the unlucky few. It seems unfair to say that this adolescent ought to have known the risk of becoming addicted with only one use. Without this antecedent, transfer principle (T) will not apply to cases like this.

Moreover, transfer principle (T) has exceptions. Consider Paula, who is paralyzed while bungee jumping or driving drunk. Paula is responsible for her earlier act and knew or ought to have known that her act would create a risk of paralysis that, in turn, would create a risk of not being able to help someone in need. Now add that Paula's son falls into a river and drowns, and Paula could have jumped in and saved her son if she had not been paralyzed. Transfer principle (T) implies that Paula is responsible for her son's drowning. That seems incorrect. To avoid this absurd implication, transfer principle (T) must be either given up or qualified in some way (cf. Vargas 2005). But then it is not clear whether a properly qualified transfer principle will still apply to most cases of addiction.

Anyway, the transfer principle is at least not obvious. But then that principle cannot be used to establish that severe addicts with little or no control are responsible for their current drug use, simply because they were responsible when they first began using drugs many years ago. Perhaps their acts prior to addiction add some responsibility to their acts after becoming addicted, but long ago acts still might not make addicts fully or even very responsible.

CONCLUSION

All of this shows that we should not ask the question in my title: Are addicts responsible? Instead, we should ask how responsible individual addicts are or how much responsibility they have. That will depend on how much control they have left or how badly addicted they are and possibly also on how they became addicted and on other factors that I have neglected here, such as whether they sought help and tried to quit. All of these factors complicate the question and its answers.

No matter how difficult, we need to reconceptualize this whole issue in terms of degrees. We already do that when we think about friends and family or even strangers on the street. We recognize that some people have a lot more control than others, even if they are all addicted to some degree. We adjust our attitudes toward them in light of those degrees of control. Some people do draw a single line between sick people and bad people. However, there is no need to draw such a simple line in our personal lives, and doing so creates a variety of problems and puzzles.

Psychiatry is recognizing the need to introduce degrees. The Diagnostic and Statistical Manual of Mental Disorders, Fifth Edition (DSM-5) includes specifiers of whether substance use disorders are mild, moderate, or severe, though these degrees are measured by the number of symptoms and sometimes the frequency of use rather than by degrees of control. These specifiers create practical difficulties and aren't always used by clinicians, but they make the diagnosis somewhat more faithful to the actual phenomena of control and addiction.

This recognition should also come to law because it would be a useful lesson for the courts. It explains why we need drug courts. The law can say that these addicts retain some responsibility, and that is what justifies us in forcing them to go into treatment. Still, their responsibility is reduced, and that's why we aren't warranted in punishing them, at least not for mere possession. If addicts start stealing cars and killing people to get their money, then that is a different matter. But for many types of crimes reduced punishment would be justified because of their reduced control and their reduced responsibility.

Many details remain to be worked out. The main point here is only that we need to remember that control and responsibility come in degrees. We also need to rethink traditional issues in that light. That approach will be more fruitful than continuing to debate simply whether addicts are or are not responsible. So now I should go back and retitle this chapter.

REFERENCES

Aristotle. 1941. *Nicomachean Ethics*, translated by W. D. Ross, in *The Basic Works of Aristotle*, ed. R. McKeon. New York: Random House.

Bernheim, B. D., & Rangel, A. 2005. From Neuroscience to Public Policy: A New Economic View of Addiction. *Swedish Economic Policy Review* 12: 11–56.

Budney, A. J., & Higgins, S. T. 1998. *National Institute on Drug Abuse Therapy Manuals for Drug Addiction, Manual 2. A Community Reinforcement plus Vouchers Approach: Treating Cocaine Addiction*. Rockville, MD. National Institute on Drug Abuse, National Institute of Health Publication 98–4309.

Burroughs, W. S. 1959. *Naked Lunch*. New York: Grove Weidenfeld.

Chiu, P. H., Lohrenz, T. M., & Montague, P. R. 2008. Smokers' Brains Compute, but Ignore, a Fictive Error Signal in a Sequential Investment Task. *Nature Neuroscience* 11(4): 514–520.

Duggan, T., & Gert, B. 1979. Free Will as the Ability to Will. *Nous* 13: 197–217.

Fingarette, H. 1972. *The Meaning of Criminal Insanity*. Berkeley: University of California Press.

Fischer, J. M., & Ravizza, M. 1998. *Responsibility and Control: A Theory of Moral Responsibility*. Cambridge: Cambridge University Press.

Frankfurt, H. 1971. Freedom of the Will and the Concept of a Person. *Journal of Philosophy* 68: 5–20.

Garavan, H., & Hester, R. 2007. The Role of Cognitive Control in Cocaine Dependence. *Neuropsychology Review* 17: 337–345.

Gert, B., Culver, C., & Clouser H. D. 2006. *Bioethics: A Systematic Approach*. New York: Oxford University Press.

Heyman, G. 2009. *Addiction: A Disorder of Choice*. Cambridge, MA: Harvard University Press.

Holton, R. 2011. *Willing, Wanting, Waiting*. New York: Oxford University Press.

Pettit, P. 2001. *A Theory of Freedom: From the Psychology to the Politics of Agency.* Cambridge: Polity Press.

Robbins, T. W., Everitt, B. J., & Nutt, D. J. 2010. *The Neurobiology of Addiction: New Vistas.* Oxford: Oxford University Press.

Ross, D., Sharp, C., Vuchinich, R. E., & Spurrett, D. 2008. *Midbrain Mutiny: The Picoeconomics and Neuroeconomics of Disordered Gambling.* Cambridge, MA: MIT Press.

Sinnott-Armstrong, W., & Pickard, H. 2013. What Is Addiction? In *The Oxford Handbook of Philosophy and Psychiatry*, ed. K. W. M. Fulford, M. Davies, R. Gipps, G. Graham, J. Sadler, G. Stanghellini, & T. Thornton, 851–864. Oxford: Oxford University Press.

Vargas, M. 2005. The Trouble with Tracing. *Midwest Studies in Philosophy* 29(1): 269–291.

Woolfolk, R. L., Doris, J. M., & Darley, J. M. 2006. Identification, Situational Constraint, and Social Cognition: Studies in the Attribution of Moral Responsibility. *Cognition* 100: 283–301.

8

Just Say No?

Addiction and the Elements of Self-Control

JEANETTE KENNETT

INTRODUCTION

According to a standard view, both in philosophy and common sense, self-control is called for in the face of temptation, which inclines you toward something you judge it better not to do. When we think of temptations we usually think in terms of appetitive desires or urges—for junk food or alcohol and so forth. We exert self-control when we resist that extra slice of chocolate cake because we value health or slimness, say, or leave a party early to prepare for an important talk for the next day, or restrain an urge to punch someone who has angered us. Occasional failures of self-control are tolerable and probably inevitable, but a person who persistently fails to exercise control over his appetites and impulses in key areas of life, and so to live up to his values, tends to attract condemnation.

While some philosophers have been skeptical of this standard picture,[1] it can provide a useful starting point for investigating self-control in the context of addiction. Substance dependence or addiction is usually characterized in terms of a loss of control over the substance use, and as a consequence over other important areas of life such as employment and relationships: the cycle of craving and withdrawal experienced by the addict are an ever present threat

---

1. For example, Bigelow, Dodds, and Pargetter (1990) and Frank Jackson (1984) deny that strength or weakness of will depend in any interesting way on evaluative judgment. According to Jackson, one can exercise strength of will in acting *against* one's better judgment. See Kennett (2001, 54–71), for a discussion of their views.

to self-control, and addiction itself is often seen as the outcome of a series of previous failures of will.

Neil Levy (2011) has recently suggested, in line with the influential dual-processing model of cognition, that the relevant resource for success-ful self-control is controlled cognitive processing capacity. He argues that the folk-psychological notion of weakness of will invoked above is an instance of a broader phenomenon of the switch from rational controlled processing to a more intuitive mode of processing. Levy's suggestion appears to be borne out by recent work in the neuroscience of addiction. This work seems to provide evidence that the addicted person's drug-related judgments and decisions are indeed often driven by automatic processes, which operate outside of conscious control.

I argue that though this model is a very useful one, the picture it provides of self-control and its loss in addiction (and elsewhere) is incomplete. There *is* a normative aspect to self-control, implicit in the common-sense account, that is not captured by the purely procedural account to be drawn from dual-process theories of cognition—and which we only uncover when we consider what self-control is *for* and why it is valuable. In this chapter I examine the variety of ways in which self-control may be exercised and threatened in order to more fully understand what is going wrong in the lives of addicts. I conclude that self-control is not just a matter (and not always a matter) of having sufficient, available, controlled processing capacity. For at least a significant subgroup of addicts the main problem may not be a lack or depletion of the cognitive resources relevant to self-control.[2] Rather, it may be that they have little con-fidence in their ability to exert control over their external circumstances and shape the lives they would value having and the people they would value being.

REASON VERSUS DESIRE: CASHING OUT THE METAPHOR

On the standard view, the paradigmatic loss of self-control involves succumb-ing to strong desires that run contrary to judgment. The metaphor is of a battle between reason and desire, or between values and mere desires. This battle is exemplified in Frankfurt's picture of the unwilling addict. The unwilling addict fails to have the will she wants to have. She is violated by and alienated from her own desires. Perhaps the unwilling addict can sometimes resist the lure of

---

2. Levy has elsewhere (2006) defended an extended mind thesis and thus would agree that our capacities for self-control are partly dependent upon external scaffolding. But it is not clear to me that he would regard some of the cases described later in this chapter as cases where a person's cognitive resources and ability to deploy system 2 reasoning are impaired. If not, it would appear that he is committed to saying there is no loss of self-control in such cases and this would be a key point of disagreement between us.

drugs. But the persistence of drug-related cravings wears down her resistance and eventually she gives in. Perhaps sometimes she gives in while continuing to believe that using is a bad idea. Perhaps she experiences judgment shift under the press of her desires and comes to judge, temporarily, that using just this time is justified.[3]

This kind of picture of the addict's resistance as being worn down by her desires has in recent times found support from psychology. For example, it has been suggested that self-control depends on a resource that operates like strength or energy, and depletion of this resource makes self-control less effective (e.g., Baumeister, Bratslavsky, Muraven & Tice 1998; Muraven, Tice & Baumeister 1998; Baumeister 2002). Baumeister and colleagues have conducted a series of studies described by Levy, which have variously shown that subjects who have already completed a self-control task (e.g., regulating emotional response while watching a movie, choosing radishes over freshly baked cookies, or suppressing forbidden thoughts) do worse than controls on subsequent self-control tasks requiring perseverance or resisting of temptation, including tasks such as resisting forbidden foods that tapped into a subject's pre-existing personal commitments.

On Baumeister's view willpower is rather like muscle power. Muscles may become tired through overexertion—there is clearly a limit on how long one can hold up a heavy weight, for example—and as that limit is approached one might either realize that "I *can't* hold this up any longer" or, in light of the discomfort one is experiencing, decide that "I don't *want* to hold it up any longer. It would be *better* to put it down." Muscle power can also, as we know, be conserved, strengthened, and renewed. So, too, one's capacity for self-control may be conserved by avoiding situations of temptation, strengthened by learning

3. Many philosophers resist the notion of clear-headed weakness of will or akrasia. Some like Levy (2011) and Holton (1999) follow the Socratic view in understanding weakness of will in terms of judgment shift and distinguish it from akrasia. While an addict, for example, ordinarily judges that she should not use drugs, when the craving hits she temporarily judges that using this time is best. This is consistent with Gene Heyman's claim (2009) that addicts adopt a local rather than a global perspective on choice. Perhaps when not craving drugs, the person is capable of judging from a global perspective, which takes account of her long-term interests. But when craving hits, her focus narrows and she chooses the immediate good. While doubtless true of many addicts, this doesn't undermine descriptions of the unwilling addict as one who does not value taking the drug—at least on plausible accounts of valuing, such as that offered by Gary Watson, who argues that a person's values are "that set of considerations which he—in a cool and non-deceptive moment—articulates as definitive of the good, fulfilling and defensible life" (Watson 1982, p. 105). Levy's focus is on the judgment shift model, but akrasia also involves a loss of self-control. If some drug use is akratic rather than weak-willed—as I shall suggest—and if akrasia cannot be accounted for under a dual-process model, then it would strengthen my claim that the dual-process model cannot fully explain loss of control in addiction.

and regular practice of various techniques of self-control such as narrowing or altering the focus of one's attention or forming a negative ideation of the temptation (Kennett & Smith 1996; Kennett 2001), or renewed by rest or, according to Baumeister and colleagues (Gailliot et al. 2007), something as simple as glucose.

While Baumeister's work seems to confirm our intuitive understanding and ordinary experience of self-control and the challenges to it, we seem to have exchanged one metaphor for another. It is helpful to think of self-control as dependent upon a depletable resource. But what is the resource that is depleted when self-control is lost? How should we understand weakness and strength of will?

Levy (2011) draws upon the influential dual-processing model of cognition to argue that the relevant resource for self-control is controlled cognitive processing capacity. This is what fails in weakness of will. Dual-process models of cognition contrast automatic processes (also referred to as implicit, reflexive, impulsive, or system 1 processes) with controlled (or explicit, reflective, deliberative, or system 2) processes.

Automatic processes can be understood as "control of one's internal psychological processes by external stimuli and events in one's immediate environment, often without knowledge or awareness of such control" (Bargh & Williams 2006, p. 1). By contrast, prototypical controlled processes are characterized as slow and effortful and are intentionally or consciously deployed. As Sherman et al. (2008) have pointed out, a central tenet of dual-process models is that controlled processes represent resource-dependent self-regulatory processes that control the effects of automatically activated implicit processes, which may conflict with consciously held beliefs or goals. The exertion of self-regulatory resources enables judgments and behaviors that are more in keeping with the individual's consciously endorsed values.

However, system 2 resources are limited and cognitively expensive. When we are under cognitive load (i.e., distracted by other tasks) or our attentional resources are depleted due to fatigue, stress, and so forth, system 1 dominates and our judgments and behavior will be more strongly influenced by our automatic, affect-driven attitudes. There is evidence, for example, that when we are tired or distracted we are more likely to judge and be influenced in our behavior in accordance with ingrained stereotypes than, say, with our explicit egalitarian principles (Kennett & Fine 2009; Fine 2006).[4] Levy (2011) notes that the effects of cognitive load resemble the effects of ego depletion and concludes that "[s]elf-control is a system 2 process and its loss switches us to system 1" (p. 145).

---

4. But see Dijksterhuis & Van Olden (2006) for an opposing view.

Given that synchronic self-control—that is, self-control exercised under conditions of temptation—is heavily dependent on the attentional techniques mentioned above, Levy's analysis has considerable plausibility. Cravings may force themselves upon and come to dominate our attention. Controlling the focus of our attention requires cognitive effort, and this may wear out when we are trying to combat repeated intrusive appetitively driven thoughts. Levy (2011) suggests the following mechanism for judgment shift under conditions of temptation:

> In response to temptation, subjects spontaneously generate or retrieve from memory arguments in favour of weak-willed action. Since they lack the cognitive resources to reject these arguments, they experience judgment-shift. They come to judge that the benefits of succumbing to temptation are higher, or the costs of giving in lower, or both, and act accordingly. (p. 143)

This model of self-control and its loss initially suggests two possibilities for explaining the loss of control characteristic of addiction. First, it might not be that addicts are worse at self-control than nonaddicts. They just have more constant and intense calls on their willpower. Resisting addictive cravings depletes the addicted person's (normal) effortful controlled processing capacity and eventually she gives in.[5] Second, addicts may have reduced controlled processing capacities, and this would leave their judgments and choices especially vulnerable to the influence of the automatic system.

Both of these scenarios for the loss of self-control in addiction find additional significant empirical support from addiction neuroscience. Antoine Bechara proposes that "willpower emerges from the dynamic interaction of two separate but interacting neural systems: an impulsive system in which the amygdala is a critical neural structure involved in triggering the affective/emotional signals of immediate outcomes and a reflective system in which the VMPC is the critical neural structure involved in triggering the affective/emotional signals of long term outcomes" (2005, p. 1459).

Bechara cites evidence that supports the first hypothesis of increased calls upon the substance user's willpower. He notes that drugs "acquire powerful affective and emotional properties" and identifies a subgroup of addicts who display an exaggerated autonomic response to drug-related cues, suggesting that their amygdala is overresponsive to reward (p. 1461). He suggests that hyperactivity in the impulsive system weakens the control of the reflective system. The hypersalience of drug-related cues and the intensity of cue reactivity

5. Compare with Feinberg's claim that though no desire is literally irresistible "they must be resisting it always." This might constitute an unfair burden

(as measured on functional magnetic resonance imaging) have been found to correlate with the likelihood of relapse to drug use and are combined with hyporesponsiveness to natural rewards (pp. 1461–1462). He concludes consistently with the dual-processing model that "substance related cues trigger bottom up mechanisms in substance abusers, influencing top-down mechanisms such as impulse and attentional control." They have the capacity to "hijack the top down goal-driven cognitive resources needed for the normal operation of the reflective system and exercising the willpower to resist drugs" (Bechara 2005, p. 1461). Addiction neuroscience, then, provides evidence for the view that addicts do at times lack the capacity to resist *at that time* due to the persistent, strong, and intrusive nature of drug cravings.

Support for the notion that addicts have reduced controlled processing capacities is also found in a range of studies cited by Bechara (2005) or conducted by him and his colleagues (Verdejo-Garcia et al. 2006). Substance abusers show impairments across a variety of decision-making and control tasks, including the Iowa Gambling Task, response inhibition tasks, and cognitive flexibility tasks, and in the ability to resist the intrusion of unwanted thoughts and memories, consistent with corresponding damage or diminished neural activity in regions of the prefrontal cortex. Their executive function is impaired (perhaps as a result of neuroadaptations caused by drug use, as suggested by Volkow & Li 2005), and their judgments and decisions are thus more likely to be driven from below. A significant subgroup of drug users appear insensitive to future consequences, both positive and negative. This group resembles so-called acquired sociopathy patients with ventromedial prefrontal cortex (VMPC) damage—who display significant decision-making deficits and failure to learn from previous mistakes.

Bechara's work suggests that some addicts may thus face the double disadvantage of antecedently weak controlled processing capacity *and* more constant calls upon that capacity to resist addictive cravings. The hypersalience of drug-related cues and the intensity of pleasure response to drugs, combined with a lowered response to natural pleasures and impaired executive function, make it almost inevitable that their unaided efforts to resist drugs will fail.

Bechara also draws attention to a third subgroup of addicts who do not show behavioral or physiological signs of decision-making deficits (Bechara 2005, p. 1462). These individuals tend to be better functioning than other users but may still not count, or may not count themselves, as making autonomous choices with respect to their drug use or as living up to their values. Are these addicts accounted for by a dual-process model? Levy, at least, is not committed to the claim that loss of control in addiction must turn upon the decision-making deficits noted above. Addiction in this group could simply involve the kinds of resource depletion seen in everyday failures of will. While addicts in the first two groups may be closer on the spectrum of failures of control to compulsion, this group may suffer from garden variety weakness of will—and so may be thought to be more culpable for their failure to exercise self-control.

The neuroscience and the psychology together appear to provide a neat way of cashing out both ordinary and philosophical talk of self-control, strength and weakness of will, and compulsion, in ways amenable to empirical investigation. Should we, then, rest content with a dual-process account of self-control and its application to the case of addiction? I want to suggest that while addicted people are (usually but not always) impaired in self-control in the ways described, the controlled resource depletion theory provides an incomplete picture of the losses of control suffered by addicts. Controlled processing capacity is an important resource, but it is not the only resource required for successful self-control. Moreover, loss of self-control is not always a result of being mugged by our appetites. We need to look more closely at the variety of ways in which our control may be threatened in order to more fully understand what is going on in the lives of addicts.

I'm going to begin by looking at control over single actions and the ways in which they can go wrong and then expand the story to encompass control over broader aspects of one's life.

INTENTIONAL SELF-CONTROL

Let's begin with *intentional* self-control, that is, the control I exercise over my actions in order to do what I intend. When I perform familiar or habitual actions I am in control of what I do, but this may not require any or much explicit effort on my part. Making tea, brushing my teeth, checking the mail, typing these words—these are all things I do intentionally, but much of the control or regulation of the actions is delegated to the automatic system. I think about what to say but not about where to place my fingers on the keyboard. The rhythm of making tea is so familiar that my mind is free to wander while I set out the cups, attending only lightly as I pour the freshly boiled water over the leaves. If an action is novel, more in the way of conscious attention and effort is required for success. But it would appear that my successful intentional actions usually and properly count as being under my control whether or not they are directly under the guidance of the reflective system.

Perhaps we should understand my self-controlled actions as counterfactually dependent on the availability of system 2 resources. I must be in a position to take explicit control of the action if needed. If attentional resources are not available, I should not count as being in control. Or perhaps we should think of self-control as control over my impulses, emotions, and intentions themselves, and only derivatively of my actions.

To make progress with these questions, we need to examine more closely what happens when we lose control and fail to do as we intend. Are all such losses able to be characterized in terms of failures of attention, impulse control, deliberative capacity, and the like?

A range of factors, both internal and external to the agent, can interfere with successful intentional action. The key internal factor that is focused on in discussions of loss of self-control in addiction is craving. The user's desires to abstain from drug use are simply not causally strong enough to carry the day. But while very strong desires may impede the successful carrying out of an intention, other internal factors are equally or more important in addiction and elsewhere. As I've argued elsewhere,[6] sometimes we fail to do what we intend, not because we don't want strongly enough to do so but because our decisions and desires are defeated by other psychological factors. Shyness, anxiety, fear, anger, grief, or lack of confidence may all interfere with the capacity to perform some intended action, here and now.

I break down while giving the eulogy at the funeral of a loved one and am unable to complete the tribute I so wanted to make. I want to ask Arnie out for dinner but I'm overcome by shyness as I look into his ice-blue eyes and I blush and stammer incoherently. I fail to suppress a sneer that betrays my contempt for the executive to whom I'm making an important presentation. I tense up and botch the dive that would have earned me Olympic selection. In all these cases I lose control of my action and fail to do what I intended, and indeed what I most wanted, to do.

External circumstances may also threaten my capacity to do what I intend. Sometimes our actions misfire. The dollar plunges when I'm trying to make my fortune buying foreign currency. The wind blows as I'm trying to hit the target. A loud mobile phone ring spoils the telling of a witty anecdote in my lecture. What I end up doing is not what I intended to do: make a fortune, hit the target, amuse the audience. In these cases, too, I lose control of what I'm doing. Control with respect to the external environment is as important to successful action as control over my internal environment.[7]

Regaining control of what I'm doing requires that I regulate or adjust for my *internal* states—for example, deep breathing to relax myself before attempting the dive, or emailing the object of my desire instead of asking him out face to

---

6. Kennett (2001).

7. Levy has argued elsewhere (2007) that agents' *capacities* can depend on features of their environment and that the way to respond to addiction is to change the environment in which they choose. We are in agreement on this point. Social support, nurture, training, and so forth support and strengthen the capacity for self-control in addiction. Constant presentation of drug-related stimuli undermines it. My claim is that some environmental features may block the *exercise* of self-control without necessarily reducing the agent's controlled processing capacity or switching the agent from system 2 to system 1. I count this as a loss of self-control. Levy disagrees—though of course he doesn't deny that it's a loss of sorts.

face. And often it requires also that I regulate the *external* conditions I face or that I adjust for those conditions—I can't prevent the wind from blowing but I can make allowances for it as I take the shot. I can ask audiences to switch off their mobile phones so the lecture isn't interrupted.

In the case of resisting the urge to use drugs, successful self-control requires addressing both the internal and external circumstances the person confronts. So the addict might try to regulate her internal states by, for example, learning techniques of detached observance of the craving or by learning to direct her attention away from the drug-related stimulus. She may also attempt to regulate or change the external circumstances that might interfere with control, such as not going to places where she knows she'll be tempted to indulge, discarding all her drug-related paraphernalia, and so forth. These well-established methods of self-control seem to be consistent with dual-processing theory and addiction neuroscience—they seem to affirm that successful self-control involves either exercising or conserving system 2 capacity.

Nevertheless, I argue that there is more to understanding and addressing loss of control in addiction than this. Considering the ways in which intentional control is exercised and how it may fail is instructive. It suggests that the dual-process account cannot cover all of the cases in which we count as self-controlled or all of the cases in which we fail.

First, while the internal impediments to successful action outlined above may be driven from below in line with the dual-processing account (with the important exception of lack of confidence), it is not clear that the cure for them rests on the availability and exercise of controlled processing capacity. Exercising synchronic control over *internal* states such as nerves is not always a matter of deploying available controlled processing capacity. Sometimes thinking too much about the elements of an action undermines performance. If I'm merging into fast-moving traffic, hesitation can spell disaster. If I explicitly call to mind each of the elements required for success as I stand on the end of the 10-meter board, I'll lose confidence. I surely do better to let muscle memory guide my dive.

Moreover, since controlled processing is a limited resource, the self-controlled *person* is, plausibly and contra the suggestion above, the person who doesn't need to draw on this resource too often in order to act as she desires, values, or intends. She has a *well-schooled* automatic system that preserves self-control even when attentional resources are depleted. This suggests a diachronic aspect to self-control that goes beyond the muscle-building/strength metaphor. The drug user will be better protected against relapse, and more capable of sustaining her intention not to use, if she can exercise preconscious control over her impulses.[8]

8. See in this regard interesting work reported by Wiers et al. (2010), where heavy drinkers were trained to push away pictures of alcohol using a joystick and drank half as much as other heavy drinkers in a subsequent taste test. In a subsequent clinical study patients given repeated

Second, it should be obvious that we can't always control for *external* circumstances by making allowances or restructuring our environment. Control over my actions isn't always up to me. Sometimes circumstances may be such that I give up. If the wind is very gusty and strong, my attempts at target shooting may be pointless and I become discouraged. We often need the world to cooperate with our endeavors if we are to have any realistic prospect of success. Hostile physical and social environments undermine agent control. This is a point we will take up in more detail in the next section with respect to addiction.

Third, while loss of self-control is taken to be central to addiction, it is clear that intentional control, that is, control over the particular actions one is performing, may be exercised by a hopeless heroin addict or alcoholic (absent effects of intoxication) as efficiently as by a model of temperance.[9] Indeed, it is evidence of their capacity for intentional control that persuades many people that drug users *can* say no to drugs and so should be held fully responsible for the harmful consequences arising from their drug use. After all, they do not use drugs unintentionally and may devote considerable attentional and planning resources to activities surrounding the acquisition and administration of their drug of choice.

But the mere fact that one acts intentionally in securing and administering a desired substance isn't sufficient for us to conclude that the drug user is capable of what I will call *normative self-control*. Mere intentional self-control may be exercised in accordance with the individual's values or may be exercised in the service of an action the individual does not, all things considered, think is a good thing to do and maybe something that runs counter to what she thinks she ought to do. The kind of control addicts display may be what Mele has called *errant self-control* (Mele 1990). As he notes, considerable self-control may be required to perform an action that runs counter to one's own or wider social values. A teenager may have to steel himself to throw a rock through a window to impress the gang or to repress feelings of sympathy for the victim of a gang beating. Similarly, drug users may have to steel themselves to perform otherwise disvalued actions connected with their drug use, such as stealing from family and friends. They may need to overcome nerves, feelings of revulsion, and other affective obstacles. Drug use itself may at times be a triumph of controlled processing, as this first-person account suggests.

Addiction is often conceived of as a failure of will. . . . But in fact, and not necessarily incompatibly, addicts often suffer from an excess of will. Ask

retraining of alcohol action tendencies showed automatic alcohol avoidance tendencies and reduced cravings compared with controls (Wiers 2010).

9. This is consistent with addicts persistently underestimating the rewards of future goods (applying a steep discount rate). They may thus fail to institute strategies of diachronic self-control that would enable future control of actions in line with longer-term goals or values.

yourself what it takes to do that, say, every day. I tell you what it takes : it takes will-power. You have absolutely got to stop listening to your body; you have to overcome a thousand bodily recalcitrances and make yourself keep pouring. Ask yourself what it takes to keep doing this even while everyone around you is telling you that you need to stop, and so on. It takes a masterful will. (Sartwell, n.d., "Addiction and Authorship")

Whatever it is that drives Sartwell to drink, it doesn't seem to be a case of impulse or the anticipation of pleasure overwhelming his resolve, and it doesn't seem to be explained by depletion of controlled processing capacity. While I cannot presume to diagnose what has gone wrong in Sartwell's case, I suggest it shows that we need to look beyond the dual-process model and beyond a focus on the individual's capacity to control particular actions surrounding drug use, to reach a full understanding of the losses of control characteristic of addiction. In doing so we will consider more directly why self-control is valuable.

NORMATIVE SELF-CONTROL AND THE GOOD LIFE

The kind of self-control that those in the grip of addiction most notably appear to lack is *normative* control. The capacity for self-control, in this sense—which I take to be a very familiar sense—is the capacity to govern oneself in accordance with one's values and the (usually diachronic) reasons one generates. While the capacity for intentional control over one's actions is required in order for one to count as an agent at all, normative control constitutes us as autonomous, self-governed individuals. It is control over the self and not just over particular actions that a self might perform. These two forms of control are at different points on a spectrum of agent control, and it should be obvious that one may have the first without the second.[10] It is all too easy to imagine the drug user who asks, "What have I become?" as she takes a deep breath and approaches her intended mugging victim and as she later surveys the wreck of her relationships, career, and all that she once held dear.

The weak-willed or akratic person and the compelled person fail to govern themselves in accordance with their values. It is in this respect we say that they have lost control. Their actions are not responsive to the reasons that flow from their *values*—even though they may be appropriately responsive to various local contingencies, such as the price of the drugs, the presence of the police, and so forth. When we say of an addict that her life is running out of her control, we don't mean that she is incapable of responding to such contingencies and initiating successful intentional action. We mean that her life (and her particular

10. I have defended this view elsewhere. See Kennett (2001).

actions) is no longer governed by her values, and so lacks the shape and coherence that this brings.[11]

This brings us to the normative question of what self-control is for and why it is valuable. Let me now sketch what I hope is a relatively uncontroversial account of the elements of a valuable life and of the agential capacities that support it and then consider how and why substance-dependent individuals are impaired in their ability to enjoy these goods.[12]

The value of a life might be registered merely in terms of the aggregation of the well-being a person experiences moment by moment through her life, but such an approach, though it might be adequate for (say) a cat, would fail to properly account for those goods that are most central to a distinctively human life. Compare a life composed of a series of short-term, but on the whole pleasant, experiences and sensations, such as might arise from eating or bathing or being massaged or listening to nice music, with a life in which the person, say, developed enduring and happy relationships, was a hardworking and much appreciated committee member for the local hospital, wrote a well-received biography, and pursued a passion for growing orchids. Suppose this second life also contained significant early hardship and illness (to which the later charitable work was in part a response) such that it is clear that the aggregate of momentary well-being or *synchronic* well-being in the first life was greater than in the second life. Nevertheless, the second person might look back on her life with greater satisfaction. It is plausible to suppose that hers is the more valuable life.

Flourishing lives, it seems, are marked by such things as relationships that stand the test of time. They are marked by challenges and by the rewards that accrue to a person who has stuck at a task and completed it. Anyone who has successfully parented a child, or managed an organization over an extended period, or completed a degree, or undertaken elite sports knows that these achievements involve difficult, boring, and sometimes painful experiences. Nevertheless, as we often say, "It was worth it." We should say, then, that though good lives may come in many different forms, they all have significant *diachronic value.*[13]

Diachronic goods include a range of moral and social goods that accrue to persons who successfully engage in *projects* and occupy certain *roles*. While

11. I don't deny, of course, that some addicts are acting in accordance with their values and that some addicts may not have values: that is, some addicts may not think in terms of what is valuable and what there is most reason to do in the light of those values. These possibilities are explored below.

12. The sketch that follows is taken from Kennett and Matthews (2006).

13. This discussion of synchronic and diachronic welfare draws on David Velleman's paper "Wellbeing and Time." (Velleman 1991)

some of our projects are quite short term—shopping for and cooking dinner, for example—our diachronic well-being depends on the success of what Bernard Williams has called "ground projects." According to Williams (1981, p. 5), we each have "a set of desires, concerns or...projects...which help to constitute a *character*." A person's ground projects are the force "which propel...him into the future, and give...him a reason for living." While any desire, even the simple desire for a glass of water, propels us some way into the future, the cluster of projects and concerns that give our lives meaning and distinctively agential value are longer term. Through taking on these projects we provide ourselves with reasons that extend into the future and shape the actions and decisions we will take then. In adopting, pursuing, juggling, modifying, and completing our various projects, we extend our agency across time and, to a significant extent, become authors of our own unique life stories.

Ground projects typically include such things as learning a skill, playing a sport, studying, pursuing a career, raising a family, maintaining a friendship, or working for a political or moral cause. The loss or failure of these projects (or most of them) would, suggests Williams, remove the meaning from the person's life. We can see why by focusing on our various roles. Seeing through our projects depends on the capacity to occupy and sustain certain roles over extended periods of time. Roles, in this sense, are close cousins of projects. So, for example, it is in the role of parent that one takes on the project of raising children; it is in the role of fiction writer that one takes on the project of writing a novel; and so on. The roles we occupy are critical to our identity, to how we see ourselves and how we are seen. Writer's block is frightening, not just because it threatens the completion of the novel but because it threatens my conception of myself as a writer. The so-called empty nest syndrome is not simply about a mother missing her children when they leave home. She mourns the loss of her role even while she acknowledges the success of her project.

The completion of ground projects, the successful fulfilment of important social roles, and the enjoyment of the values these provide clearly require self-control. Consider the example of a person studying for a degree. Unless that person is able to be governed over time by the set of reasons—to attend classes, to study, and so forth—generated by this project, the project will fail. Individuals must have the capacity to plan, sustain, and regulate their activities over lengthy periods of time. Self-control is a necessary condition of access to a variety of goods that help constitute a life as meaningful, as flourishing, and, importantly, as one's own.

Possession of the diachronic goods also reinforces normative self-control. One's diachronic plans, projects, and commitments provide a structure that obviates the need for constant decision making and choice. Important decisions are already made and do not need to be revisited unless circumstances change. Diachronic goods such as loving relationships, absorbing work, and interesting hobbies protect one against passing temptations and provide motivational resources for the exercise of self-control. The person with a rich array of interests, relationships, and commitments can remind herself of all she has to lose by giving in to temptations that threaten those goods. The person who lacks those goods is not so protected.

We exercise normative self-control, then, when we act so as to regulate our lives and activities in accordance with our values. If we are unable to do so, we do in an important sense lack control over ourselves. So understood, normative self-control, like intentional self-control, is to some degree hostage to fortune. Both internal and external circumstances may undermine it.

What is notable about substance-dependent individuals is that for the most part their grip on the kinds of projects, relationships, and commitments that mark good and flourishing lives is tenuous. They often do not occupy the kinds of social roles that confer meaning, structure, and social recognition. Whether or not they are impaired in the exercise of intentional control, their day-to-day lives often do not appear to be guided or regulated by a conception of what would constitute a good life or by a conception of their diachronic welfare. They lack normative control of their lives. There are two related possibilities to be considered for this lack.

First, some drug users may lack a plausible conception of the good life. This may be the result of drug use itself or of other life circumstances. Drug use over time may lead to corruption or corrosion of the drug users' values.[14] Perhaps they used to value family and friends but now take a wholly instrumental view of other people. Perhaps they have forgotten the pleasures they used to enjoy. Gene Heyman (2009) argues that a distinguishing feature of addictive substances is that they undermine competing rewards, including social goods of the kind outlined above. He says that "A substance is behaviorally toxic when it poisons the field making everything else relatively worse" (p. 145). Such corruption of the addict's preference structure is, however, only partly explicable by dual-process theory. Another possibility is that deprived life circumstances have resulted in an impoverished conception of the good life—some users simply cannot conceive of the value to be found in dedication to long-term projects related to education, or work, or sport—with a resulting focus on immediate goods. In such cases, too, a dual-process model cannot account for the lack of normative control.

Second, it is possible that the user has a conception of the good life as centrally involving the kinds of diachronic goods and roles outlined above, but

---

14. The impact of addiction on the values of drug users has not been systematically investigated. An Australian Research Council–funded project led by the author is currently addressing drug users' perceptions of self-control and value in the context of addiction.

it doesn't inform the way he lives. If the second of these is correct, it may be that the impotence of his conception of the good life is due to the executive failures and impairments already described and can be fully accounted for by a dual-process model. In many cases, though I suspect this is too simplistic a diagnosis of the problem. I think it more likely that in these cases the person does not see the life he would value having as being available to him. What gets obscured by the use of dual-processing models to analyze loss of control in addiction is the fact that normative reflection and choice is undertaken in an autobiographical context. It usually engages our sense of self and our capacity to see ourselves diachronically. To the extent that we cannot, in reflection or imagination, realistically project ourselves into a particular future, it is not a practical guide for our current choices. Bechara, to be sure, has characterized a subgroup of addicts as displaying "myopia for the future," but this is not what I am talking about here. I am suggesting that some addicts (e.g., Sartwell) are perfectly capable of affectively appreciating the future consequences of their actions. They are not at all impaired in their capacities for mental time travel. And they do not fail to appreciate what is genuinely valuable or irrationally discount the value of future goods. But internal and external circumstances combine to make these values and the actions required to secure them seem an improbable continuation of their life story. They lack the full array of resources required for normative self-control.

A TAXONOMY OF ADDICTION

Not all addicts are alike. They do not form a single kind. To sum up the discussion thus far, it is useful to present a (no doubt somewhat artificial) taxonomy of addiction, based on the one offered by Harry Frankfurt (1971), and of the kinds of failures or impairment associated with each subtype.

The Willing Addict

Willing addicts probably don't exist as Frankfurt describes them, since addiction as a state doesn't seem like something that could be valued for its own sake, but there is a subgroup of addicts for whom drug use and the experiences derived from it are seen as part of a good and flourishing life. Drug use may be an important and ritualistic constituent of their social or intimate relations or religious experiences, and drug dependence may be seen as the price to be paid for them. The effects of certain drugs may be to provide artistic inspiration and experiences and may be seen as providing valuable insights into oneself and others. Drug experiences can be considered an irreplaceable source of meaning and of pleasure and as such form part of one's identity. For such individuals the health consequences of heavy use are no doubt seen as unfortunate but are outweighed by the benefits. Perhaps some willing addicts are self-deceived, but it is unlikely that all are. Since a significant proportion of the adverse health and social impacts of drugs are a consequence of their illegality, and since in principle safer recreational drugs could be developed that would avoid the health impacts of current legal drugs such as alcohol, there is no case to conclude that drug use and even drug dependence are in principle inconsistent with normative self-control.

The Unwilling Addict

The unwilling addict, as Frankfurt describes him, hates his addiction and fights against it. The unwilling addict lacks autonomy because he does not have the will he wants to have. He does not value taking the drug but he is unable to conform his first-order desires to his values. While the unwilling addict as Frankfurt describes him clear-headedly detests and rejects the desires on which he acts, even as he succumbs, it is sufficient for my purposes that he tries but fails to live in accordance with values that are antithetical to his drug use. So in my view an unwilling addict could experience the reversals of judgment that Levy describes so long as they are temporary and he at least intermittently tries, but fails, to stay clean, keep commitments, and so forth. The unwilling addict may have an enhanced response to the pleasures of drug use, reduced capacity to exert executive control over his actions, or both. But he is not an unwilling addict if he does not over time judge that some other way of life would be better for him and devote some of his voluntary cognitive resources to resisting drug use. The unwilling addict most clearly fits the dual-process account of self-control and its loss as applied to addiction.

The Wanton Addict

The wanton, as Frankfurt conceives of him, does not care which of his desires moves him, he never stands back from his desires and assesses the ends they incline him to pursue, and so he is moved indifferently by whichever desire is currently strongest. The wanton addict may suffer "myopia for the future" in common with acquired sociopathy patients (Bechara, Damasio & Damasio 2000). It is not necessarily the case, however, that the wanton cannot articulate the likely outcomes of his actions; it is just that having no overarching values to provide unity and purpose to his life, he does not identify with or care about his future. It is not merely that his future concerns are trumped by his current desires in deliberation; these concerns do not figure in deliberation at all. They are not seen by him to be reason providing. Wanton addicts are not self-controlled agents, because they are not normative agents; they constitutively live in the moment, but this seems consistent with their possessing sufficient available semantic processing capacity to weigh their current options. In this respect they resemble certain amnesic patients, whose autonomic system and semantic processing and attentional capacities may be normal but whose incapacity to occupy a personal past and future leaves them grossly impaired. These agents surely lack self-control, but they are neither weak-willed, nor akratic, nor coerced by their desires. In characterizing the lack of self-control displayed by the wanton addict, we need to go beyond dual-process theory.

The Resigned Addict

The resigned addict is one who has a conception of what is truly valuable and who may be acutely aware of the absence of diachronic value in his own life but who does not believe that such a life is open to him. The loss or unavailability of the diachronic goods leads him to focus on the available synchronic goods. For this group drug use offers temporary relief, or escape, or the simulacrum of social connectedness, and they are resigned to the fact that this is all that is open to them. They are not, like the unwilling addict, doing battle with their desires. But they do not, like the willing addict, endorse them or endow them with normative force either. They have given up. From their own point of view (as well as from a third-person perspective), it is true to say that their lives are in an important sense out of their control.

Can we understand this attitude of resignation from within the resources of a dual-processing framework and as exemplified in the neuroscience of addiction? I argue that we cannot.

Cheshire Calhoun has argued that:

> ...the standard view tempts us to imagine that the principal or sole internal threat to agency is from our own unruly impulses. I think this is false. Careful reflection on how our lives as agents may internally fail suggests there are an array of related psychological states that undermine agency not by supplying uncontrollable motivating forces but by depriving the individual of either interest in her own reasons or interest in deliberating on the basis of them. (Calhoun 2008, p. 194)

This picture fits, I suggest, a significant subgroup of addicts who clearly lack normative control over their lives. In their case internal threats to self-control may include fatigue, depression, self-loathing, apathy, and most importantly a lack of confidence in their capacity to attain a life they would value having. In these cases the psychological states leading to an attitude of resignation about one's drug use are causally connected to the external conditions of their life, which may, objectively, make a flourishing life a fairly remote possibility.

Sometimes, as we've noted, external conditions may be such that I must give up on an intention or a plan. If it is too windy target shooting is out of the question. But broader social or personal circumstances may also make it difficult or impossible for me to succeed at certain activities and in such cases, too, I may give up on forming certain kinds of intentions. Poverty, social exclusion, illness, oppression, abuse, and trauma may all restrict what I can successfully intend and do. They can restrict my agency—my control. As Calhoun says, "When exercising one's agency has ceased to be reliably connected to producing intended effects, deliberation may well seem pointless and the future hopeless" (2008, p. 205). In such circumstances agency contracts, and we stop trying to act in accordance with values that seem unachievable and may instead focus on the here and now.

> ...[F]irst and foremost is I'm extremely lonely...I'm totally unemployable. I'm over the hill, got no references, no appreciable skills, patchy work history at best, former alcoholic and addict, homeless...it's very depressing. I mean [participating in treatment] is not the answer to all my problems. Recovery is not going to make my problems go away. (Weinberg and Kogel 1995, p. 217)

Robinson (2003, p. 33) argues that among participants in her study of homeless mentally ill people, drug and alcohol use, overdosing, and other harmful behaviors should be "understood as 'symptoms' of forms of social exclusion as well as of...trauma and mental disorder." The use of drugs as a coping or even survival mechanism was clearly evident. Chris Middendorp (2009a) agrees, saying that "heroin addiction may be best understood as the consequence of profound social dislocation, rather than an individual's weakness. Children do not ask to be traumatised and they do what they can to survive the despair.

Middendorp describes in detail the case of Robbie, a homeless alcoholic:

> When his wife died of cancer and just months later his teenage son died in a car accident, the life Robbie knew vaporised. In his own words, "fate hollowed me out". He couldn't cope. He was unable to work and within a year was evicted from his house for rental arrears.
>
> Despite spending a week getting sober in a detox unit every year or two, Robbie felt there was not much merit in abstinence. "It's easier living in the park when you're sloshed," was Robbie's standard justification. (Middendorp 2009b)

For a long time Robbie fitted the mold of what I am calling the resigned addict. Such individuals may not lack the capacity for self-control if this is conceived of in the purely procedural terms of the dual-process model. There is no evidence that Robbie's problem was a lack or loss of controlled processing capacity. Nevertheless, people like Robbie and the homeless man quoted above often—perhaps justifiably—believe that they cannot, by their own efforts, control their lives in accordance with their conception of what a flourishing life would be. In these circumstances many give up on deliberating, planning, and acting on the basis of those values. This contraction of their agency is appropriately characterized in terms of a loss of control over the self.

CONCLUSION

Robbie's story has a happy ending. Assisted into good-quality housing with ongoing social support he was able to rebuild connections in the mainstream community. With a safe place to call home his need to drink was reduced, he rediscovered domestic and social skills, and six years later he was stable and happy. As Middendorp points out, Robbie's example shows us that we shouldn't underestimate anyone's capacity to rebuild his or her life. But as he says: "The key to accomplishing this—and here's the crucial point—is *having access to the resources that offer a life worth rebuilding.*"

What are the lessons to be learned, then, from this discussion of addiction and self-control? I suggest it shows that self-control is not just a matter of freeing up or boosting system 2 processing capacity and that we will miss much that is important to understanding addiction if we focus solely on cognitive models. Cognitive load and ego depletion don't fully explain the relapses to drug use cited above. Self-control requires also that the agent sees himself as having other, better, *achievable* options. In the absence of such options agents may understandably give up on self-government, in effect giving up on themselves, and focus on the synchronic goods provided by drug use. In sum, as the case of the resigned addict demonstrates, normative self-control turns out to be a complex, socially situated achievement. It is not just a matter of willpower, however this is conceived. People who are dependent on drugs need adequate resources, both psychological and social, to "just say no."

REFERENCES

Bargh, J. A., & Williams, E. L. (2006) The automaticity of social life. *Current Directions in Psychological Science* 15, 1–4.

Baumeister, R. F., Bratslavsky, E., Muraven, M., & Tice, D. M. (1998) Ego depletion: Is the active self a limited resource? *Journal of Personality and Social Psychology* 74 (5), 1252–1265.

Baumeister, R. F. (2002) Ego depletion and self-regulation failure: A resource model of self-control. *Alcoholism-Clinical and Experimental Research* 27 (2), 281–284.

Bechara, A. (2005) Decision making, impulse control and loss of willpower to resist drugs: A neurocognitive perspective. *Nature Neuroscience* 8 (11), 1458–1463.

Bechara, A., Damasio, H., & Damasio, A. R. (2000) Emotion, decision making and the orbitofrontal cortex. *Cerebral cortex* 10 (3), 295–307.

Bigelow, J., Dodds, S. M., & Pargetter, R. (1990) Temptation and the Will. *American Philosophical Quarterly* 27 (1), 39–49.

Calhoun, C. (2008) Losing one's self. In C. MacKenzie and K. Atkins (eds.), *Practical Identity and Narrative Agency*. New York & London: Routledge.

Dijksterhuis, A., & van Olden, Z. (2006) On the benefits of thinking unconsciously: Unconscious thought can increase post-choice satisfaction. *Journal of Experimental Social Psychology* 42, 627–631.

Fine, C. (2006) Is the emotional dog wagging its rational tail, or chasing it? *Philosophy Explorer* 9, 83–98.

Frankfurt, H. G. (1971) Freedom of the will and the concept of a person. *Journal of Philosophy* 68, 5–20.

Gailliot, M. T., Baumeister, R. F., DeWall, C. N., Maner, J. K., Plant, E. A., Tice, D. M., Brewer, L. E., & Schmeichel, B. J. (2007) Self-control relies on glucose as a limited energy source: willpower is more than a metaphor. *Journal of Personal and Social Psychology* 92(2), 325–336.

Heyman, G. M. (2009) *Addiction: A Disorder of Choice*. Cambridge, MA.: Harvard University Press.

Holton, R. (2009) *Willing, Wanting, Waiting*: Oxford University Press.

Jackson, F. (1984) Weakness of will. *Mind* 93, 1–18.

Kennett, J. (2001) Agency and responsibility : a common-sense moral psychology. Originally a thesis (PhD), Monash University, early 1990s, Clarendon Press: Oxford University Press, Oxford; New York.

Kennett, J., & Fine, C. (2009) Will the real moral judgment please stand up? *Ethical Theory and Moral Practice* 12(1), 77–96.

Kennett, J., & Matthews, S. (2006) The moral goal of treatment in cases of dual diagnosis. In J. Kleinig & S. Einstein (eds.), *Ethical Challenges for Intervening in Drug Use: Policy, Research and Treatment Issues*. Office of International Criminal Justice.

Kennett, J., & Smith, M. (1996) Frog and toad lose control. *Analysis* 56(2), 63–73.

Levy, N. (2006) Autonomy and addiction. *Canadian Journal of Philosophy* 36(3), 427–447.

Levy, N. (2007) The social: A missing term in the debate over addiction and voluntary control. *American Journal of Bioethics* 7(1), 35–36.

Levy, N. (2011) Resisting "Weakness of the Will." *Philosophy and Phenomenological Research* LXXXII(1), 134–155

Mele, A. R. (1990) Errant self-control and the self-controlled person. *Pacific Philosophical Quarterly* 71, 47–59.

Middendorp Chris (2009a) Heroin: A curse or a source of meaning. *The Age* June 22 2009   http://www.theage.com.au/opinion/heroin-a-curse-or-a-source-of-meaning-20090621-cshv.html (accessed 8/17/11)

Middendorp Chris (2009b) Being homeless does not mean being hopeless. *The Age* August 4 2009   http://www.theage.com.au/opinion/being-homeless-does-not-mean-being-hopeless-20090803-e77l.html#ixzz1VEdhSSxc (accessed 8/17/11)

Muraven, M., Tice, D. M., &Baumeister, R. F. (1998) Self-control as a limited resource: Regulatory depletion patterns. *Journal of Personality and Social Psychology* 74(3), 774–789.

Robinson, C. (2003) *Understanding Iterative Homelessness: The Case of People with Mental Disorders*. Melbourne: Australian Housing and Urban Research Institute.

Sartwell, C. (n.d.) Addiction and authorship http://www.crispinsartwell.com/addict2. htm (accessed 9/23/2011).

Sherman, J. W., Gawronsko, B., Gonsalkorale, K., Hugenberg, K., Allen, T. J., & Groom, C. J. (2008) The self-regulation of automatic associations and behavioral impulses. *Psychological Review* 115, 314–335.

Velleman, J. D. (1991) Well-being and time. *Pacific Philosophical Quarterly* 72(1), 48–77.

Verdejo-Garcia, A., Bechara, A., Recknor, E. C., & Perez-Garcia, M. (2006). Executive dysfunction in substance dependent individuals during drug use and abstinence: an examination of the behavioral, cognitive and emotional correlates of addiction. *Journal of the International Neuropsychological Society: JINS*, 12(3), 405–415.

Volkow, N., & Li, T. K. (2005) The neuroscience of addiction. *Nature Neuroscience* 8, 1429–1430.

Watson, G. (1982) *Free Will*. Oxford Oxfordshire; New York: Oxford University Press.

Weinberg, D., & Kogel, P. (1995) Impediments to recovery in treatment programs for dually diagnosed homeless adults: An ethnographic analysis. *Contemporary Drug Problems* 22(2), 193–236.

Wiers, R. W., Rinck, M., Kordts, R., Houben, K., & Strack, F. (2010) Retraining automatic action-tendencies to approach alcohol in hazardous drinkers. *Addiction* 105, 279–287.

Williams, B. (1981) *Moral Luck: Philosophical Papers, 1973–1980*. Cambridge Cambridgeshire; New York: Cambridge University Press.

9

Addiction in Context

Philosophical Lessons from a Personality Disorder Clinic

HANNA PICKARD AND STEVE PEARCE

There are exceptions to every rule in human psychology, but, on the whole, addicts do not lead flourishing lives. The *Diagnostic and Statistical Manual of Mental Disorders*, fourth edition, text revision (*DSM-IV-TR;* American Psychiatric Association 2000) defines substance dependence as a maladaptive pattern of use, leading to clinically significant impairment or distress, manifested by three or more of the following criteria occurring at any time in the same 12-month period:

  (i) tolerance
 (ii) withdrawal
(iii) the amount or length of use is greater than intended
 (iv) there is a persistent desire or unsuccessful efforts to control use
  (v) time spent obtaining, using, and recovering from the substance is substantial
 (vi) important social, occupational, or recreational activities are given up or reduced because of substance use
(vii) substance use is continued despite knowledge of the physical or psychological harm it causes

The picture painted is of a life that spirals out of control, as the person cannot find a way to resist their temptation to use: horizons narrow; harm to self and, no doubt, to significant others increases; and the good life fades from view. But, quite apart from their substance dependence, addicts do not tend to come from backgrounds that promote flourishing. Addiction is associated with physical or sexual abuse as a child (Widom et al. 1995: only in women); a propensity for antisocial traits, anxiety, depression, and impulsivity (Compton et al. 2007; Farrell et al. 2001; Heyman and Gibbs 2006; Kirby et al. 1999); lower social and emotional functioning (Compton et al. 2007); low self-esteem or self-worth (Gossop 1976); and, finally, poverty (for a comprehensive review of socioeconomic data, see Heyman 2009). Once again, there are exceptions. But on the whole, addicts come from a background of poor opportunity and experience a host of comorbid psychiatric problems (for a review of how socioeconomic status affects brain development, see Hackman et al. 2010).

These associated problems are essential to understanding chronic, as opposed to short-lived, addiction. Large-scale national survey data suggest that substance dependence peaks in adolescence and early adulthood but, in the majority of cases, has resolved permanently, without clinical intervention, by the late twenties or early thirties (for a comprehensive review of these findings, see Heyman 2009; cf. Foddy and Savulescu 2006). It appears that addicts who suffer from additional psychiatric disorders are the exception: those who seek clinical treatment are more than twice as likely to suffer from at least one other psychiatric disorder as those who do not engage with services (Regier et al. 1990); and, compared to what is predicted by the national survey data, they are also significantly more likely to relapse. The stereotype of addiction as a chronic disorder, with little hope of recovery, is not an accurate picture for the general population. It is an accurate picture for psychiatric patients.[1]

This suggests that chronic addiction is unlikely to be successfully understood, let alone treated, if the issue of psychiatric comorbidity is not addressed. This paper focuses on one particularly common dual diagnosis: substance dependence and personality disorder. We suggest that the successful treatment of addicts within specialist services for personality disorder sheds light on why addicts use alcohol and drugs despite the attendant negative consequences, and how treatment for dual-diagnosis patients might helpfully proceed. Put simply, addicts use substances to cope with the psychological distress associated with personality disorder and other psychiatric conditions, and will continue to do so unless they learn alternative coping strategies to manage negative emotions, address underlying issues, and gain

---

1. Pickard (2012) complements this paper and argues that these data challenge the common conception of addiction as a chronic, relapsing neurobiological disease. Note that these data also suggest an explanation for the otherwise puzzling finding that, out of the many Vietnam veterans who returned to the United States addicted to opiates, the few who sought clinical treatment were five times *more* likely to relapse than the many who stopped using opiates spontaneously (Robins 1993; Heyman 2009). The veterans who sought clinical treatment may have suffered from additional psychiatric disorders that complicated their recovery and increased the chance of relapse.

opportunities for a better life, containing positive, alternative goods. We further suggest that this explanation, although underpinned by neurobiological research, does not fundamentally depart from folk psychological explanations of action. In particular, we appeal to five rough-and-ready folk psychological factors to explain addictive drug use: (i) strength of desire and habit, (ii) willpower, (iii) motivation, (iv) functional role, and (v) decision and resolve.

The paper divides into six parts. First, we describe the comorbidity between substance dependence and personality disorder, and sketch the nature of recent, evidence-based specialist treatment for personality disorder. On the whole, the interventions employed are not recherché or particularly medical: they are common-sense methods for developing the capacity for choice and control. The effectiveness of such methods tells against popular depictions of addiction as a form of compulsion. Thus, second, we canvass and reject the three standard reasons offered in support of this picture. Third, we delineate the five rough-and-ready folk psychological factors that we suggest explain addiction and describe how they are targeted in treatment. Fourth, we suggest that reflection on the trajectory from addiction to recovery shows how we can develop a common but opaque thought, namely, that agency, understood as the capacity for choice and control, comes in degrees. Addicts are agents: their behavior is voluntary. But their agency is often limited: their choices are few, and their control is meager. Part of the clinical aim is to augment it. Fifth, we suggest one repercussion of our discussion for the criminal law surrounding addiction: punishment and treatment may be more complementary than they can initially appear. We conclude with a brief, general summary of the argument presented.

SUBSTANCE DEPENDENCE AND PERSONALITY DISORDER

Comorbidity between substance dependence and personality disorder is high. The prevalence of personality disorder in the UK general population is estimated at 4.4% (Coid et al. 2006). In inpatient treatment for addiction, 78% of drug users and 91% of alcoholics suffer from at least one personality disorder (DeJong 1993). In outpatient treatment, 37% of drug users and 53% of alcoholics suffer from at least one personality disorder (Weaver et al. 2003). Fifty percent of people referred for personality disorder treatment have suffered from a substance misuse disorder in their lifetime (Skodol et al. 1999). Finally, within the general population, the median prevalence of personality disorder within substance dependence across 25 studies is 61% (Thomas et al. 1999).

High comorbidity between substance dependence and personality is, in fact, predictable a priori by comparison of the criteria for diagnosis. Apart from tolerance and withdrawal, the criteria for substance dependence point toward psychological traits such as impulsivity and low tolerance for frustration (criteria [iii] and [iv]) as well as self-harm (criterion [vii]). These traits are core symptoms of borderline and antisocial personality disorder.[2]

Personality disorder was long considered impossible to treat. But this has started to change. In 2003 the UK Department of Health launched a new initiative *Personality Disorder: No Longer a Diagnosis of Exclusion* (2003) to combat stigma and improve quality and access to services. A wave of new treatments and evidence-based research began, both in the United Kingdom and in the United States. Alongside the appropriate prescription of medication, there is now growing evidence for a variety of effective psychological treatments. These include:

(i) Varieties of cognitive-behavioral therapy, such as dialectical behavior therapy (Linehan and Dimeff 2001), STEPPS (Blum et al. 2008), and "stop and think" training, to help manage self-harm and other counterproductive behaviors

(ii) Motivational interviewing techniques, to engage service users and foster the desire to change (Rollnick and Miller 1995)

(iii) Emotional intelligence to develop the knowledge and ability to identify triggers, understand emotions, and manage behavior (Goleman 1998)

(iv) Mentalization-based therapy to develop self- and other-understanding and empathy (Fonagy and Bateman 2006)

(v) Therapeutic Communities, often considered the treatment of choice for personality disorder, which may employ all varieties of psychological therapy, alongside a commitment to four guiding principles of democracy, permissiveness, community, and reality confrontation that govern the community (Lees et al. 1999). Within Therapeutic Communities, members are responsible for much of the daily running of the service, as well as being directly challenged and supported to change entrenched behavior, with agreed consequences if they lapse. Therapeutic Communities also importantly provide a social community to which members can belong, thereby reducing their isolation and increasing their potential for well-being and support. Notably for the purposes of this paper, specialist Therapeutic Communities for addiction are common and known to be effective (Ibid.).[3]

---

2. Yates et al. (1998) confirms this prediction with respect to self-harm: 27% of candidates for liver transplant in alcoholic cirrhosis (criterion [vii]) met the criteria for at least one personality disorder.

3. For discussion of the specific factors and mechanisms by which Therapeutic Communities may achieve positive outcome, see Pearce and Pickard (2012).

These treatments are united in conceiving of patients as agents, capable of controlling and changing the behavior associated with their diagnosis (Pearce and Pickard 2010; Pickard 2011a, 2013, forthcoming). Some interventions, like motivational interviewing, do this implicitly. The clinician adopts a submissive, nonchallenging stance, expressing empathy, and encouraging patients to see the unwanted consequences of their behavior as motivation to change. Other interventions, like those offered by Therapeutic Communities, are highly explicit. The language of agency and responsibility permeates the culture of the group: members are not only encouraged but also expected to see themselves in this light. Still other interventions, like emotional intelligence, fall in between. Patients are encouraged to distinguish emotions and behavior to allow them to take control over how they act when in the grip of strong emotions, even if they do not feel able to control the emotions themselves.

The Oxfordshire Complex Needs Service is a nonresidential National Health Service (NHS) Therapeutic Community for personality disorder.[4] Patients with personality disorder typically suffer from a range of problems, including suicidal ideation; self-harm; eating disorders; paranoid, obsessive, and depressive tendencies; impulsive and risk-taking behavior; anxiety; aggression; and severe and lasting difficulties in effectively managing negative emotions and interpersonal relationships. In line with the statistics above, many of them are also addicts. Before they can join the Therapeutic Community, they are required to stop, or adequately control, the use of alcohol, to stop the use of illicit drugs, and to stop taking certain kinds of prescribed medication, such as benzodiazepines, other sedatives, and hypnotics. Support for this requirement is provided by a weekly two-hour pretherapy group facilitated in part by members of the Therapeutic Community. It is noteworthy that patients manage to control or stop longstanding use with this minimal intervention (for the beginnings of an explanation see below, especially Factor Three). The primary reason for this requirement is that the use of alcohol and these drugs impairs the capacity to do the psychological work that the Therapeutic Community

---

4. Hanna Pickard is a therapist at the Oxfordshire Complex Needs Service (OCNS); Steve Pearce is the Clinical Director. The OCNS is currently conducting a randomized controlled trial to test outcomes. Initial results are expected in 2013. But outcomes have been monitored since the service started in 2004 via internal audits. A central part of the monitoring concerns patients' use of other services: people with personality disorder receive more medication, psychotherapy, psychiatric inpatient care, day care, and hospital care than people with major depressive disorder (Bender et al. 2001, 2006). Such service use typically declines steeply in those accessing the OCNS. Psychiatric inpatient bed-days drops by 70%, emergency department attendances by 45%, use of medication by 55%, and use of primary care services by between 45% and 70%. Finally, suicide attempts and self-harm events decline by over 80%. (Audit data from 2006, 2007, and 2008 audits.)

demands: in particular, the capacity to explore painful and difficult memo-ries and emotions and to learn new, healthier ways of coping with them. For personality-disordered patients, the use of alcohol and drugs does not only or even primarily provide pleasure. It is also a way of coping with psychological distress. As a result, patients are less able to learn new, healthier ways of coping, or develop better life skills, without first controlling their use.

The idea that alcohol and drugs are used to manage psychological distress is commonplace in our culture: we "drown our sorrows" or "hit the bottle" when in need. We routinely drink and use drugs to numb rage or sadness, for instance, or to control social anxiety. Within a practical clinical context, this idea is per-vasive (see, for instance, Boys et al. 2001; Khantzian 1997; Markou et al. 1998). Some psychological theories of addiction, like Social Learning Theory, use this idea to help explain the development of addiction and construct interventions that promote abstinence and prevent relapse. Certainly with respect to predic-tion of relapse, there is evidence in support of this theory. Negative emotion, stress, and interpersonal conflict are strong precipitant factors in relapse (Birke et al. 1990; Cummings et al. 1985; West 2006). Alternative coping skills are strong protective factors (Miller et al. 1996; West 2006).

This commonplace idea clashes with many popular and neurobiological depictions of addiction.[5] Herein, addicts are depicted as subject to irresistible desires: desires so strong and powerful that they are literally forced by these desires to use. These compulsive cravings are supposed to mean that, at least in most standard occasions of use, no alternative is available: there is no capac-ity for choice and control. A common metaphor is that the addict's brain is "hijacked" by the drug: "the compulsive drug-taking that defines addiction is a direct physiological consequence of dramatic neuroadaptations produced in the reward pathways of the brain" (Charland 2002: 40, 41; cf. Leshner 1997 and Hyman 2005). Such compulsions and cravings for drugs in addicts "nullify any semblance of voluntary choice" (Charland 2002: 41).

There is a priori reason to be skeptical about this picture at the very outset. Normally, we understand the difference between an action and a mere bodily movement, like a reflex or an automatic response, to depend on the capacity, however minimal, for choice and control. Most aspects of drug use appear to consist in actions, not mere bodily movements. If addicts are literally forced by their desires to use drugs, then it is not clear that their behavior can rightly count as agentive at all.[6]

---

5. Heyman (2009) is an important exception.

6. For discussion and defense of this conception of agency and action, see Alvarez (2009) and Steward (2009, 2012). Pickard (2013) argues that addiction does not provide an example of agents who act on irresistible desires and so lack the power to do otherwise.

Moreover, if addicts have no choice or control over their use, then it is unclear how it can be willfully abandoned (as required by the OCNS pre-therapy group alongside other forms of treatment) in favor of alternative, healthier coping mechanisms. The effectiveness of clinical interventions that target agency as a route to recovery would be puzzling, to say the least, if addicts were not agents with respect to their use. Before delineating the five rough-and-ready folk psychological factors that clinical interventions target, we briefly canvass the arguments offered in support of the claim that addicts are literally compelled to use.

COMPULSION

There are three common reasons offered in support of the picture of addiction as a form of compulsion: the nature of withdrawal, the neurobiological effects of drugs, and the testimony of addicts themselves.

The Nature of Withdrawal

Cultural portrayals of withdrawal, especially from alcohol and heroin, are dramatic: shakes, fever, retching, delirium. Heroin withdrawal is described as agony or torture: something no one should be asked to undergo, and which could break the will of the strongest of us (Arpaly 2006: 20). Equally, withdrawal from severe alcohol dependence, without medical monitoring, can be dangerous: people sometimes die. But withdrawal, even from alcohol and heroin, is rarely so extreme. Heroin withdrawal is typically similar to a bad cold or, at worse, the flu. Indeed, some addicts choose to abstain and suffer withdrawal simply in order to lower their tolerance (Ainslie 2000). Furthermore, the physical symptoms of all withdrawal can also now be minimized pharmacologically through the use of various drugs: benzodiazepines for alcohol withdrawal, and either a long-acting opioid, such as buprenorphine, or symptomatic treatment, such as antinausea drugs, for opioid withdrawal. If an addict wants to stop using, medication is available to make withdrawal a safe and physically manageable option.

It is thus simply not true that addicts are compelled to use drugs because of the physical need to avoid withdrawal. Of course, during withdrawal, addicts may yet have a strong, unfulfilled desire for the drug, which may be psychologically difficult to endure. But that is a different point: the physical effects of withdrawal can be medically managed, even if the psychological effects of abstaining remain.

The Neurobiological Effects of Drugs

Drug-associated cues are strong predictors of relapse. This is an established part of addictive lore: the rituals and obsessions of addictive behavior can verge on the fetishistic, and addicts are well aware of the association between cues and desire to use (Pates et al. 2005). But neurobiology has provided the skeleton of an explanation for why drug-associated cues would have such strong motivational force. Many drugs directly increase levels of synaptic dopamine, which may affect normal processes of associationist learning related to survival and the pursuit of rewards (for a review see Hyman 2005). Once drug-related pathways are thus established, the cues cause addicts to be motivated to pursue the reward of drugs to an unusually strong extent. Moreover, there is increasing evidence that as drug use escalates, control devolves from the prefrontal cortex to the striatum, in line with a shift from action outcome to stimulus-response learning (for a review see Everitt and Robbins 2005). In rats, drug use that is initially goal directed and sensitive to devaluation of outcome becomes increasingly habitual: triggered automatically and insensitive to (mild) devaluation.

There are at least four reasons to be skeptical of the claim that these neurobiological effects of drugs render drug taking truly compulsive. First, and most importantly, it suggests that not only spontaneous recovery but also motivated abstinence should be surprising and rare. Yet both are known to be not only possible but also common. As discussed above, large-scale national survey data establishes that addicts "mature out" of use: the majority of addiction resolves itself without clinical intervention by the late twenties or early thirties. Moreover, research suggests that the majority of addicts will abstain from using over prolonged periods of time when offered immediate but modest monetary incentives (Higgins et al. 1991, 1994, 1995).[7]

Philosophers often suggest that spontaneous recovery and motivated abstinence fail to establish that addicts are not compelled to use. The reason offered is that the capacity for control must be relativized to a motivational and epistemic context (cf. Mele 1990). Otherwise, as Levy puts it, "we get the absurdity that, say, agoraphobics are not compelled to remain indoors, since, given the appropriate incentives [e.g., the house is on fire], they would leave" (2011a: 271). Applying this lesson to addiction, the claim is that the fact that addicts refrain from use in particular circumstances (e.g., when offered immediate but modest monetary incentives, or when they secure a good job, or become parents) does not show that they have control over their use outside of these circumstances: all it shows is that they have control in these circumstances (cf. Levy 2011a). Control must always be relativized to circumstance.

---

7. This finding has led to the development of various forms of contingency management treatment for addiction. Such treatment is very simple: vouchers, money, or small prizes are given to patients who produce clean urine samples. Typically, patients submit urine thrice weekly, with increasing value for each clean sample. The samples are tested and the reward offered immediately. Contingency management treatment reduces risk of disengagement from treatment and increases periods of abstinence compared to other standard treatments (for a review, see Petry et al. 2011).

We should all agree that extreme circumstances affect people's capacities. In order to save a child from death, a parent may have the capacity to move a crushing weight even though in standard conditions they lack the requisite physical strength. After withstanding harrowing physical torture, a prisoner may lose the capacity to further resist the demand for information. Extreme circumstances no doubt affect what people can and cannot do. But this point should not bar us from holding that, in less extreme circumstances, behavioral change following motivational change provides strong evidence of a general capacity for behavioral control.

Consider, for instance, a man who "sees red" and routinely resorts to physical violence in drunken disputes—except when in view of a policeman. On such occasions, he is highly motivated not to hit, which he would otherwise do, out of fear of being detained and charged with common assault. Does his restraint in this context show only that he can control his aggression when in view of a policeman, but not necessarily otherwise? This is not our natural understanding of this man's behavior. The more natural understanding is that it shows that the man has a general capacity to control his aggression, but that he only exercises it when he wants to. As Michael Smith puts it, "capacities are essentially general or multi-track in nature, and...therefore manifest themselves not in single possibilities, but rather in whole rafts of possibilities" (2003: 26). We expect that the capacity to do something in one situation generalizes, even if there are some circumstances where a person genuinely lacks a capacity that they otherwise have, or possesses a capacity that they otherwise lack. There is a basic, common-sense distinction between what a person can do but won't (because they don't want do) as opposed to what they want to do but can't (because they lack the capacity). We must recognize extremes, but relativizing control too strongly to motivational and epistemic contexts threatens the cogency of this distinction.[8]

With respect to addiction, modest monetary incentives and the ordinary aspects of adult life that motivate "maturing out," such as securing a good job, or becoming a parent, are not extreme circumstances. They are standard, commonplace reasons for abstaining. They thus provide strong evidence that addicts have the general capacity to control their use, in a broad range of ordinary conditions, despite the neurobiological effects of drug use. Of course,

---

8. Note that contra Levy, from a clinical perspective, there is no absurdity in the claim that an agoraphobic can leave the house. Effective treatment for agoraphobia (or indeed any phobia) is likely to include a form of exposure therapy, which, in this case, involves nothing other than the patient leaving the house, with increasing duration and regularity, and decreasing support from the therapist (Gros and Antony 2006; Ito et al. 2001). Repeated exposure to anxiety-provoking stimuli reduces anxiety. The more you do it, the easier it gets; but you have to do it for exposure therapy to work. The clinical presumption in exposure therapy is that agoraphobics can leave the house. That is perfectly compatible with clinical recognition of the degree of the agoraphobic's anxiety, and the consequent difficulty for the agoraphobic in facing it.

addicts will only refrain from use if they want to. Equally, there may be particular circumstances, in the lives of particular individuals, when their general capacity cannot be exercised. But the link between motivation and abstinence should not cause us to hold that, unless motivated, addicts in general can't control their use. (For further discussion, see the discussion of testimony below and the section The Five Folk Psychological Factors.)

Second, although neurobiology may explain how cues associated with any substance that directly increases levels of synaptic dopamine strongly motivate behavior, it remains unclear why these mechanisms would be sufficient to render desires for drugs genuine compulsions: different in kind, and not simply in strength, from more ordinary appetitive or reward-driven desires.

Third, increasing striatal control and insensitivity to (mild) devaluation of outcome does show that the behavior becomes more automatic and habitual, but it does not show that control is fully lost. Automatic, learned habits can not only be deliberately altered over time but also, more simply, normally resisted in the moment when motivation is sufficiently strong. Moreover, human motivation is typically complicated and sensitive to more than (mild) devaluation of immediate outcome.

Finally, it is usually open to addicts, unlike experimental rats, to remove themselves from proximity of relevant stimuli: drug-associated cues and stimuli can be avoided if desired. For instance, alcoholics know that if they genuinely want to abstain, it is much better not to go to the pub in the first place: don't court temptation (for further discussion of the clinical significance of these last two points, see below, especially Factors Two, Three, and Four).

The Testimony of Addicts

The third reason offered in support of addiction as a form of compulsion is the testimony of addicts themselves. Louis Charland famously reports a conversation with a heroin addict named Cynthia, who treats the idea that heroin addicts have the capacity to consent to heroin prescription with utter disbelief: "if you're addicted to heroin, then by definition you can't say 'No' to the stuff" (Charland 2002: 37). Cynthia is not exceptional: especially when initially engaging with psychiatric services, it is not unusual for patients to say they "can't" control their drug-taking and other impulsive behavior. But it is generally recognized that there is good reason to treat self-reports of compulsive drug taking with some scepticism. First, not all addicts agree: for every story of compulsive use, there is a story of deliberate abstinence and hard-won recovery (cf. the first-person narratives in Heyman 2009). Second, not only does our cultural conception of addiction invite this self-image, but also adopting it can serve to excuse addicts from the stigma of addiction and responsibility for drug-related behaviors: addicts have reason to claim to be compelled (cf. Ainslie 1999; Davies 1997; Foddy and Savulescu 2006, 2010). Third and finally, clinical practice also lends support to such skepticism.

   Part of the clinical aim with patients who struggle to control problematic behavior is precisely to help them to see that it is not that they can't control their behavior, but that they don't. This change in self-image is an important step in the path to recovery. And indeed, a formulation of this distinction is found even in Edwards and Gross's seminal discussion of the Disease Model of Alcohol Dependence; they write that "it is unclear, however, whether the experience [of alcoholism] is truly one of losing control rather than one of deciding not to exercise control" (Edwards and Gross 1976: 1060). Self-control is hard: it is no small thing to require patients to control behavior that may be not only their habitual, but indeed their most effective and attractive, means of coping with severe psychological distress. No doubt, that is part of why they say that they can't. Indeed, this distress may offer an alternative reason for thinking that responsibility for drug-related behaviors is diminished: in absence of alternative coping mechanisms, we may hold not that addicts lack control, but rather that they are justified in taking drugs to relieve psychological distress, so long as whatever degree of harm their drug taking causes to others is minimal compared to the degree of harm the distress causes them. In effect, addicts may be excused by duress, not compulsion.[9] But questions of justification aside, the fact that the behavior is hard to control, especially in absence of alternative methods of coping and incentives to change, does not mean the desire is irresistible—that no choice or control whatsoever exists.

THE FIVE FOLK PSYCHOLOGICAL FACTORS

Once we recognize that addiction is not a form of compulsion, we can see how an explanation of addiction need not depart from the concepts employed in our basic folk psychological understanding of agency. In particular, we can identify five rough-and-ready folk psychological factors that explain why addicts struggle to control their use.[10] All five factors are targeted in treatment.

Factor One: Strong and Habitual Desire

The desire to use the drug of choice is strong and habitual. As suggested above, we are starting to understand some of the neurobiological mechanisms underpinning the formation of desires and the establishment of strong

9. For further discussion see Yaffe (2011) and Pickard (2011b) and (2013).

10. "Rough-and-ready" signals that there is no commitment to these factors carving human psychology at its joints. They may not prove to be the most accurate classification of folk psychological states; rather, they represent a natural and, from a clinical perspective, pragmatic grouping.

stimulus-response associations between cues and behavior. But even without this understanding, common sense tells us that strong habits are hard to break.[11] When desire is strong and one is in the habit of satisfying it, it is not easy to resist. Restraint requires a conscious effort at control: it requires will. It is also helped by replacement activities: by deliberate and repetitive engagement in alternative behavior when the inclination to use drugs is strong, so as to develop new associations and habits. One routine clinical intervention involves constructing and implementing concrete plans for what patients will do instead of using drugs when they experience a strong desire to use their drug of choice.

Factor Two: Willpower

There is increasing empirical evidence for what we might metaphorically construe as a faculty of willpower that acts much as a muscle does. It is effortful to exercise, and its exercise depletes its strength in the short term, although it can build it up in the long term (for a review see Muraven and Baumeister 2000). Self-control, especially in relation to strong habits, requires this faculty, which of course is typically not well exercised in addicts: conscious and sustained effort to resist the pull of the drug. Furthermore, it may also be that the conscious and sustained effort required to resist the pull of the drug can create "judgement shifts" whereby addicts, tired of resisting, reassess the value of abstinence and abandon prior resolutions in face of the present value of use (Levy 2011a, 2011b). The willpower and strength of resolve needed to break the habit is great.

One standard clinical intervention for all personality-disordered and addictive impulsive behavior is "the five-minute rule." When patients experience a strong desire to engage in whatever behavior they typically employ to cope with distress, they wait five minutes. After five minutes, they try to wait five minutes more, and so on until the desire abates. This technique may function to change problematic behavior in at least two ways. On the one hand, it empowers patients with the knowledge that they have resisted the desire for at least five minutes: if they can do that once, they can do it again. On the other hand, over time, it may build up willpower.

Factor Three: Motivation

As detailed above, addiction is associated with lower socioeconomic status, childhood abuse, psychiatric problems, and, of course, the problems attendant

---

11. William James expresses this point with typical verve, writing on "the ethical implications of the law of habit": "The great thing, then, in all education, is to *make our nervous system our ally instead of our enemy.... For this we must make automatic and habitual, as early as possible, as many useful actions as we can,* and guard against the growing into ways that are likely to be disadvantageous to us, as we should guard against the plague" (James 1890 vol. 1: 122, italics in original).

upon the acquisition and use of the drug itself. The life choices and alternatives available to addicts are typically meager: even if addicts manage to get control of their drug use, they will still need to pick up the pieces and squarely face some of the worst of life's various miseries. Bruce Alexander's infamous experiment "Rat Park" is instructive in this light (Alexander et al. 1978; Alexander et al. 1985). Caged, isolated rats addicted to cocaine, morphine, heroin, and other drugs will self-administer in very high doses, foregoing food and water, sometimes to the point of death. Alexander placed morphine-addicted rats in an enclosure called "Rat Park," which was a spacious, comfortable, naturalistic setting, where rats of both sexes were able to cohabit, nest, and reproduce. Rats were offered a choice between morphine-laced water and plain water. On the whole, they chose to forego the morphine and drink plain water, even when they experienced withdrawal symptoms, and even when the morphine-laced water was sweetened to significantly appeal to the rat palate. Recent studies complement Alexander's findings. Environmental enrichment protects against relapse in rats (Solinas et al. 2008) who even when addicted will typically choose not to self-administer drugs if provided with alternative goods (Ahmed 2010, 2012).

Addicts who try to control their drug use are not offered the immediate option of a human version of "Rat Park." The good life does not spring forth ready-made; help with housing, employment, psychiatric problems, and social community does not tend to be immediately available. The opportunities and choices available to many addicts may reasonably impede their motivation to control their use, for the alternative goods on offer are poor.

This is in all likelihood part of why it is possible for Therapeutic Communities and other group-based treatment programs to require addicts to control their use before commencing therapy. The existence of the program is an alternative good. It promises help with at least some of their problems and provides, very importantly, a stable, caring, social community that offers the possibility of strong interpersonal attachments and peer support.[12] It thus acts as an incentive: it increases motivation to control use through the offer of community and hope that a better life can be achieved.

Factor Four: Functional Role

Drugs and alcohol help people manage psychological distress.[13] Controlling use is thus very difficult until new ways of coping with negative emotions and skills

---

12. See Baumeister and Leary (1995) for a review of the importance of interpersonal attachment to well-being and motivation and Pearce and Pickard (2012) for further discussion of its importance within Therapeutic Communities.

13. For a review of the data see Muller and Schumann (2011).

for living have been learned: this functional role of alcohol and drug use needs to be fulfilled by other means. Most personality-disordered patients experience a period of severe struggle and doubt when they have succeeded in controlling their alcohol and drug use or other impulsive behaviors, but do not yet possess the constructive ways of coping and skills they need. They have no easily attainable alternative relief from the distress, or do not believe that another way is possible, which itself intensifies the desire to cope in habitual, harmful ways. During this period, patients need both willpower and trust in the treatment program if they are to succeed. New ways of coping and skills need at first to be learned deliberately and laboriously. With time, they become easier and more habitual, requiring less conscious effort and will to implement. Alongside the formation of attachments and the provision of peer support, most of the skills learned via Therapeutic Communities and group treatment program are common sense. Patients learn to recognize triggers for psychological distress and impulsive behavior, and to take steps to avoid these triggers. For addicts, as suggested above, this includes learning to recognize and avoid drug-related "cues." Patients learn to stop and think before acting, and to identify healthy activities that make them feel better. Patients use other group members for support and, with time, come to feel less alone and isolated. They speak about their feelings and past experiences in a safe and caring context, and develop a narrative understanding of themselves and their lives. It is striking how difficult these tasks are for patients: at first, many claim that they "can't" pick up the phone to call someone for support when in need, just as they "can't" not use their drug of choice. Indeed, the development of alternative methods of coping and new skills can sometimes seem to require more effort and will than does the restraint required to resist use.

Factor Five: Decision and Resolve

Controlling use typically requires not just willpower, but perseverance and resolve. Addicts must overcome any natural ambivalence they might feel about whether or not to stop using. They must decide to change, and they must form a resolution to stick with that decision in the face of future temptation. Techniques such as motivational interviewing can help patients overcome ambivalence (Rollnick and Miller 1995; Treasure 2004). Motivational interviewing helps patients to move through a cycle of change: from not being ready to contemplate it at all, to active contemplation, followed by resolution, planning, and implementation. The therapist adopts a nonjudgmental and subordinate position, drawing attention to discrepancies between the patient's values and their current behavior, while expressing empathy for the difficulties and dilemmas the patient faces in changing. The patient's autonomy and right to choose or reject the help offered is emphasized throughout.

Simply making a decision to change, never mind seeing it through, is a substantial undertaking for many patients. But, importantly, addicts cannot rationally make such a decision if they believe that they are powerless over their desire to use. If an addict, such as Cynthia above, genuinely believes that they are unable to resist the compulsion to use, then they cannot sensibly resolve to do otherwise, even if in fact this belief is false. One cannot rationally form an intention if one believes that one cannot succeed: that it is simply not in one's power to do so.[14] The cultural and clinical need to challenge and correct this belief is thus real: insofar as recovery depends on personal resolve, a belief that they are compelled to take drugs stands firmly in any addict's way.[15]

Central to recovery is the idea of hope: recovery is possible. Hope, as embodied in the belief that pathological behavior can be controlled and destructive patterns altered, is necessary if patients are to be able to resolve to change. Some patients may recover without forming such resolutions, but a more common path to recovery involves decision and will. Hope empowers patients to believe they can control their use of alcohol and drugs. Without this belief, they cannot resolve to do so. Without resolve, their chance of recovery is even less than it would otherwise be.[16]

Patients need clinicians to listen to them, and treat them with respect and compassion, but it is not in their interests for many of their beliefs about their drug use to be left unchallenged, let alone for psychiatric services and policies to be crafted according to the assumption that addicts are powerless to change. Cynthia is wrong that she cannot say no to heroin even if that is an apt way of expressing how she sometimes feels. Challenging such beliefs is often central to recovery.

14. Philosophers debate the nature and strength of the connection between intentional and belief: the connection suggested here is modest. For discussion of the philosophical debate see Holton (2009).

15. The success of 12-step programs such as AA may seem striking in this light, as addicts are asked to admit they are powerless and to turn to God, or a personally chosen higher power, for help in order to change. One natural thought is that resolutions formed in this way are simply irrational: the claim above is only that it is not rational to form an intention if one believes it is not in one's power, not that it is impossible. Another thought is that AA members are not really asked to admit they are powerless, but rather, asked to admit they are powerless *without the help of God or their higher power*. Having embraced him or it, it is then possible for them to believe they can change, and so to rationally resolve to do so.

16. Other factors connected to hope may be relevant to recovery, such as self-image. Robert West reports a study finding that within one week of quitting, half of all participating smokers thought of themselves as ex-smokers. This self-image is optimistic: on average 75% will be smoking again within the year. However, 50% of those who thought of themselves as ex-smokers were still abstinent at six months, as compared with 0% of those who did not immediately embrace the label (West 2006: 163; West expects to publish these and related findings more fully in the near future [personal communication]).

The Five Factors and the Struggle for Control

These five factors can explain why addicts struggle to control their use. Most chronic addicts come from backgrounds of poor opportunity and suffer from a range of comorbid psychiatric problems. The use of drugs and alcohol provides relief from consequent psychological distress. The desire to use is strong and its satisfaction habitual. Willpower and motivation are weak. Alternative goods and incentives may be few. Alternative way of coping have not yet been considered, let alone tried or learned. Resolutions have not been made. And belief in the compulsive nature of alcohol and drug use may stand in the way. The pieces of this explanation involve our ordinary folk psychological concepts. Neurobiology can shed light on the mechanisms underpinning habit, will, desire, motivation, and resolve. Environmental and genetic factors can help to explain their development in an individual. But folk psychology provides the basic structure for the explanation.

Clinical interventions target all five factors. Apart from the prescription of medication, such as buprenorphine, which can reduce craving, the interventions are common-sense techniques for developing agency. They presume addicts are agents: capable of control over their behavior, given motivation; willpower; a range of alternative, positive options; resolve; and, differently, but equally importantly, the care, support, and good regard of others in their group or community. It is difficult to see how such interventions could ever succeed if addicts were "hijacked" by irresistible compulsions: if the neurobiological effects of escalating drug use rendered drug taking wholly involuntary and the capacity for choice and control otiose.

DEGREES OF AGENCY

Personality-disordered patients and addicts are agents: they have the capacity for choice and control over problematic behavior. But, for all the reasons just sketched, their agency may be reduced compared to the general population. Agency comes in degrees. The capacity for choice and control develops throughout childhood and adolescence. It can be reduced by physical states like fatigue and pain, and emotional states like fear, anger, and anxiety. And it is arguably impaired in a range of psychiatric disorders. Reflection on the trajectory from addiction to recovery, as aided by clinical intervention, allows us to put flesh on the bones of this idea: to sketch an account of how the capacity for choice and control comes in degrees.

Before entering a Therapeutic Community or various other forms of therapy, addicts may be expected to stop or adequately control their use: to resist the temptation to use. And, given sufficient motivation, resolution, and will, they may succeed.

But this is, in a sense, a minimal capacity. On any particular occasion when they want to use, they have the power to refrain. They can choose to not give in to the temptation to use drugs now: to not perform that very act of drug use. But they do not yet have the skills to manage psychological distress and their desire to use by some other means: to choose to do something different instead. That is part of what clinical interventions aim to provide. If successful, it gets easier to resist temptation because, alongside increased motivation, willpower, and resolve, the addict develops a repertoire of alternative behaviors for managing psychological distress and cop-ing with temptation. The capacity for choice and control is thus augmented: patients come to possess a range of positive, alternative options, which, with time, can trans-form into a set of natural habits and inclinations. The clinical aim is thus to augment patients' capacity for choice and control: from a minimal capacity for mere restraint to a more generous capacity involving choice from a range of options.

In order for a piece of behavior to count as an action, it must be subject to the capacity for choice and control. But that capacity comes in degrees: there can be a greater or lesser number of alternatives available, and it can be easier or harder to avail oneself of them. As argued above, the fact that addicts routinely do control their drug use shows that they can. That is a good part of the evidence for holding they have at least the minimal capacity to refrain. So, if they use, that is a choice. But, for many addicts, they do not have many other, let alone better, options. Their psychological desire and distress are real. Restraint is hard. And their alternative choices are few. This is why their control is impaired. They have the capacity for choice and control, to a degree. But they lack the degree of agency and freedom that, ideally, we hope for all.[17]

TREATMENT AND PUNISHMENT

People who suffer from personality disorder and chronic addiction need treat-ment: they need care and therapy to recover. But equally, they are responsible

---

17. Following Bernard Williams, we might express this point by saying that, although free will does not come in degrees, freedom does: "Why does freewill, unlike freedom, not come in degrees? Presumably it is because its assertion consists only of an existence claim. How exactly that claim should be expressed is notoriously disputed, but it is something to the effect that agents sometimes act voluntarily, and that when they do so they have a real choice between more than one course of action; or more than one course of action is open to them; or it is up to them which of several actions they perform.... [This] merely requires that there be, in the appropriate sense, alternatives for the agent, and that it is indifference to their number, their cost, and so forth. That is why the freewill that it introduces is different from the freedom that comes in degrees and is opposed to constraint" (Williams 1995: 5). Addicts have free will: they have at least one alternative available given their capacity to refrain. But their choices are few and their control limited: they have less freedom than those with greater range of life options and coping skills.

before the law for offenses related to their disorder. In the case of addicts, these can include possession and trading, as well as crimes committed when under the influence of drugs or alcohol, such as theft or violence toward others. We have argued that addicts have the capacity for choice and control over behavior connected to their disorder, at least to a degree. Barring our emphasis on the notion of degree, this is in line with how the law treats addiction: it is not a form of compulsion that excuses from legal responsibility. Typically, people with personality disorder and addicts also have the capacity for knowledge of legal or moral wrong: they cannot appeal to insanity to avoid legal responsibility. Personality-disordered and addicted offenders are thus liable to prosecution, penalty, and imprisonment for criminal behavior that is connected to their disorder. In practice, the very same kind of behavior is in effect treated by clinicians and punished by law.

It is not straightforward to view treatment and punishment as complementary or indeed even compatible responses to the same kind of behavior (cf. Heyman 2009). One obvious reason is that they typically differ in intent. Treatment offers help to those in need: it is rehabilitative and caring. In contrast, the idea of punishment, whether by law or individual, is connected in part to attitudes such as blame and revenge for wrongdoing. We typically hold that people deserve to be punished when they knowingly and voluntarily do harm: punishment expresses justified anger and condemnation of bad behavior. It is thus natural to think that treatment and punishment must serve incompatible purposes.

This distinction is not codified in law. The UK Criminal Justice Act 2003 Section 142 states that the purposes of sentencing should include punishment, reduction of crime, reform and rehabilitation, public protection, and the making of reparation by the offender to those affected by the offense. Sentencing thus ideally aims to unite a host of purposes that can naturally appear incompatible, in particular, for our purposes, rehabilitation and punishment. How is it possible for the law to view these as complementary rather than inconsistent aims? Reflection on effective clinical treatment suggests how they can potentially be reconciled, in principle and in practice.

Effective clinical treatment suggests that negative consequences for behavior can deter and motivate, and accountability before others can encourage responsible agency, and with it the hope and expectation for change. The clinical key to effective treatment is the attitude with which the negative consequences are imposed. Good practice requires that patients be held responsible for problematic behavior but, crucially, not thereby blamed for it (Pickard 2011a, forthcoming). They must be treated with empathy and concern, as opposed to scorn and derision. And, importantly, interpersonal and communal relationships must be sustained: social bonds and the continued possibility of securing the affection, respect, and good regard of others provides reason to change problematic patterns of behavior and make amends. Only then is a demand for responsibility and the imposition of negative consequences therapeutic, as opposed to destructive to the individual.

Taking this clinical lesson into the realm of criminal law, the imposition of negative consequences that is typically part of punishment, such as community orders or imprisonment, can be effectively harnessed to treatment for behavior of personality-disordered and addicted patients if it is done with care and compassion, as opposed to blame, stigma, and revenge. Justice can be rehabilitative and genuinely reparative if it shows concern not only for the individuals or society who suffered the harm perpetrated, but also for the perpetrator. This possibility depends on the general attitude taken toward offenders: the nature of the intention in prosecuting and sentencing, the nature of the environment within the courts and institutions that punish, such as prisons, and the provision of appropriate therapy and socioeconomic opportunities for offenders.[18]

In practice, we may be far from such an outlook, let alone its implementation, but there are yet some promising developments. Initial research suggests that Therapeutic Communities for inmates, such as HMP Grendon, achieve at least two of the Criminal Justice Act's purposes in sentencing: they reduce recidivism rates and promote psychological well-being (Shine 2000; Newberry 2010). This is a small-scale example of the potential value in restorative as opposed to retributive justice, at least as it can be practiced within existing UK criminal legal institutions and prisons. There is strong evidence that societies that practice restorative justice have better crime rates and so are desirable on these grounds for all (Braithwaite 1989, 2002). But restorative justice also potentially has a great positive effect on the lives of offenders, many of whom suffer from personality disorder and addiction, and more often than not come from backgrounds of poor opportunity, with early environments characterized by severe psychosocial adversity. Addicted and personality-disordered offenders deserve to be held responsible for criminal behavior and harm done to the degree they are agents of that harm—but they also deserve help and compassion. With care, commitment, change in societal and individual attitudes, and no doubt practical reform in service provision, the law can potentially serve both these aims: it can hold addicts responsible and accountable before the law for harm perpetrated and impose negative consequences as part of a process of rehabilitation and treatment.

CONCLUSION

Understanding chronic addiction requires that we acknowledge that addicts tend to come from backgrounds of poor opportunity and suffer from a range

---

18. For a full discussion of the value and possibility of taking this dimension of clinical practice into criminal law, see Lacey and Pickard (2012).

of comorbid psychiatric problems. Although the use of drugs and alcohol is a problem in itself, it is also typically a way of managing consequent psychological distress in the face of limited choices, lack of alternative ways of coping, poor opportunities and mental health problems. It is not a form of compulsion but a choice. Only once this is acknowledged do the various psychological factors that explain ongoing addiction come clearly into view: (i) strength of desire and habit, (ii) willpower, (iii) motivation, (iv) functional role, and (v) decision and resolve. Effective clinical treatment targets all five factors and, in so doing, increases choice, improves control, and augments agency.

As reflection on the DSM criteria for substance dependence should make plain, there is no sharp line between addiction and more or less controlled use of drugs. Many of us use drugs, at different times, in different ways, with different degrees of control, without becoming chronic addicts (cf. Muller and Schumann 2011). Some people may see value in the lifestyle associated with addiction and see it as a choice, while others may despise themselves for their addiction and feel as if it controls them. And no doubt, these differences aside, most people who become addicts typically do so in part because of poor past choices, for which they may or may not be blameworthy (cf. Watson 1999).[19] But, that said, chronic addicts have problems other than their addiction. They come to psychiatric services because they want help. They want to live a more flourishing and fulfilling life, and their addiction, among other things, stands in the way. Sometimes clinical interventions help, sometimes not. Either way, we cannot understand chronic addiction unless we take seriously the psychological factors contributing to use, and we cannot help addicts unless we treat them as agents, capable of choice and control, and responsible for their behavior.

ACKNOWLEDGMENTS

We would like to thank Louis Charland, Bennett Foddy, Nicola Lacey, Andrew Mcbride, Jill Peay, Julian Savulescu, Gonzalo Urcelay, Walter Sinnott-Armstrong, and especially Neil Levy and Ian Phillips for extremely helpful comments and discussion of this paper. Hanna Pickard's research is funded by a Wellcome Trust Biomedical Ethics Clinical Research Fellowship.

REFERENCES

Ahmed, S. H. 2010. "Validation crisis in animal models of drug addiction: beyond non-disordered drug use toward addiction." *Neuroscience and Biobehavioral Reviews*, vol. 35: 172–184.

19. Note that blameworthiness is distinct from responsibility. For discussion see Arpaly (2006), A. Smith (2007), and Pickard (2011a, forthcoming).

Ahmed, S. H. 2012. "The science of making drug-addicted animals." *Neuroscience*, vol. 211: 107–125.

Ainslie, G. 1999. "Intuitive explanation of passionate mistakes." In J. Elster, ed. *Addictions: Entries and Exits (pp. 209–238)*. New York: Russell Sage.

Ainslie, G. 2000. "A research-based theory of addictive motivation." *Law and Philosophy*, vol. 19: 77–115.

Alexander, B. K., Coambs, R. B., and Hadaway, P. F. 1978. "The effect of housing and gender on morphine self-administration in rats." *Psychopharmacology*, vol. 58 (2): 175–179.

Alexander, B. K., Peele, S., Hadaway, P. F., Morse, S. J., Brodsky, A., and Beyerstein, B. L. (1985). "Adult, infant, and animal addiction." In S. Peele, ed. *The Meaning of Addiction* (pp. 77–96). Lexington, MA: Lexington Books.

Alvarez, M. 2009. "Actions, thought-experiments and the 'Principle of alternate possibilities.'" *Australasian Journal of Philosophy*, vol. 87 (1): 61–81.

American Psychiatric Association. 2000. *Diagnostic and Statistical Manual of Mental Disorders*, 4th edition, Text Revision (DSM-IV-TR) Washington DC: American Psychiatric Association.

Arpaly, N. 2006. *Merit, Meaning, and Human Bondage: An Essay on Free Will*. Princeton, NJ: Princeton University Press.

Baumeister, R., and Leary, M. R. 1995. "The need to belong: desire for interpersonal attachment as a fundamental human motivation." *Psychological Bulletin*, vol. 117: 497–529.

Bender, D., Dolan, R., Skodol, A., Sanislow, C., Dyck, I., and McGlasgan, T. 2001 "Treatment utilization by patients with personality disorders."*American Journal of Psychiatry* vol. 158(2): 295–302

Bender, D. Skodol, A., Pagano, M., Dyck, I., Grilo, C., and Shea, M. 2006 "Prospective assessment of treatment use by patients with personality disorders."*Psychiatric Services*, vol. 57(2): 254–257

Birke, S. A., Edelmann, R. J., and Davis, P. E. 1990. "An analysis of the abstinence violation effect in a sample of illicit drug users." *British Journal of Addiction*, vol. 85 (10): 1299–1307.

Blum, N., St. John, D., Bruce, P., Stuart, S., McCormick, B., Allen, J., Arndt, S., and Black, D. W. 2008. "Systems Training for Emotional Predictability and Problem Solving (STEPPS) for outpatients with borderline personality disorder: a randomized controlled trial and 1-year follow-up." *American Journal of Psychiatry*, vol. 165: 468–478.

Boys, A., Marsden, J., and Strang, J. 2001. "Understanding reasons for drug use amongst young people: a functional perspective." *Health Education Research*, vol. 16: 457–469.

Braithwaite, J. 1989. *Crime, Shame, and Reintegration*. Cambridge: Cambridge University Press.

Braithwaite, J. 2002. *Restorative Justice and Responsive Regulation*. Oxford: Oxford University Press.

Charland, L. 2002. "Cynthia's dilemma: consenting to heroin prescription." *American Journal of Bioethics*, vol. 2 (2): 37–47.

Coid, J., Yang, M., Tyrer, P., Roberts, A., and Ullrich, S. 2006. "Prevalence and correlates of personality disorder in Great Britain." *British Journal of Psychiatry*, vol. 188: 423–431.

Compton, W. M., Thomas, Y. F., Stinson, F. S., and Grant, B. F. 2007. "Prevalence, correlates, disability, and comorbidity of DSM-IV drug abuse and dependence in the United States: results from the National Epidemiologic Survey on Alcohol and Related Conditions." *Archives of General Psychiatry*, vol. 64 (5): 566–576.

Cummings, K. M., Jaen, C. R., and Giovino, G. 1985. "Circumstances surrounding relapse in a group of recent exsmokers." *Preventative Medicine*, vol. 14 (2): 195–202.

Davies, J. B. 1997. *The Myth of Addiction*, 2nd edition. Amsterdam: Harwood Academic Publishers.

DeJong, C. A. J., van den Brink, W., Harteveld, F. M., and van der Wielen, E. G. 2003. "Personality disorders in alcoholics and drug addicts." *Comprehensive Psychiatry*, vol. 34 (2): 87–94.

Edwards, G., and Gross, M. M. 1976. "Alcohol dependence: provisional description of a clinical syndrome." *British Medical Journal*, vol. 1 (6017): 1058–1061.

Everitt, B. J., and Robbins, T. W. 2005. "Neural systems of reinforcement for drug addiction: from actions to habits to compulsion." *Nature Neuroscience*, vol. 8 (11): 1481–1489.

Farrell, M., Howes, S., Bebbington, P., Brugha, T., Jenkins, R., Lewish, G., Marsden, J., Taylor, C., and Meltzer, H. 2001. "Nicotine, alcohol and drug dependence and psychiatric comorbidity: results of a national household survey." *British Journal of Psychiatry*, vol. 179 (5): 432–437.

Foddy, B., and Savulescu, J. 2006. "Addiction and autonomy: can addicted people consent to the prescription of their drug of addiction?" *Bioethics*, vol. 20 (1): 1–15.

Foddy, B., and Savulescu, J. 2010. "A liberal account of addiction." *Philosophy, Psychiatry, and Psychology*, vol. 17 (1): 1–22.

Fonagy, P., and Bateman, A. W. 2006. "Progress in the treatment of borderline personality disorder." *British Journal of Psychiatry*, vol. 188: 1–3.

Goleman, D. 1998. *Working with Emotional Intelligence*. New York: Bantam Books.

Gossop, M. 1976, "Drug dependence and self-esteem." *Substance Use & Misuse*, vol. 11 (5): 741–753.

Gros, D. F., and Antony, M. M. 2006. "The assessment and treatment of specific phobias: a review." *Current Psychiatry Reports* 8 (4): 298–303.

Hackman, D. A., Farah, M. J., and Meaney, M. J. 2010. "Socioeconomic status and the brain: mechanistic insights from human and animal research." *Nature Reviews Neuroscience*, vol. 11: 651–659.

Heyman, G. 2009. *Addiction: A Disorder of Choice*. Cambridge, MA: Harvard University Press.

Heyman, G. M., and Gibbs, S. P. 2006. "Delay discounting in college cigarette chippers." *Behavioural Pharmacology*, vol. 17 (8): 669–679.

Higgins, S. T., Budney, A. J., Bickel, W. K., Badger, G. J., Foerg, F. E., and Ogden, D. 1995. "Outpatient behavioural treatment for cocaine dependence: one-year outcome." *Experimental and Clinical Psychopharmacology*, vol. 3: 205–212.

Higgins, S. T., Budney, A. J., Bickel, W. K., Foerg, F. E., Donham, R., and Badger, G. J. 1994. "Incentives improve outcome in outpatient behavioural treatment of cocaine dependence." *Archives of General Psychiatry*, vol. 51: 568–576.

Higgins, S. T., Delaney, D. D., Budney, A. J., and Bickel, W. K. 1991. "A behavioural approach to achieving initial cocaine abstinence." *American Journal of Psychiatry*, vol. 148: 1218–1224.

Holton, R. 2009. *Willing, Wanting, Waiting*. Oxford: Oxford University Press.

Hyman, S. E. 2005. "Addiction: a disease of learning and memory." *American Journal of Psychiatry*, vol. 162: 1414–1422.

Ito, L. M., de Araujo, L. A., Tess, V. L., de Barros-Neto, T. P., Asbahr, F. R., and Marks, I. 2001. "Self-exposure therapy for panic disorder with agoraphobia: randomised controlled study of exteroceptive v. interoceptive self-exposure." *British Journal of Psychiatry*, vol. 178: 331–336.

James, W. 1890 (republished 1950). *The Principles of Psychology*, vols. 1 and 2 New York: Dover.

Khantzian, E. J. 1997. "The self-medication hypothesis of substance use disorders: a reconsideration and recent applications." *Harvard Review of Psychiatry*, vol. 4 (5): 231–244.

Kirby, K., Petry, N., and Bickel, W. 1999. "Heroin addicts discount delayed rewards at higher rates than non-drug using controls." *Journal of Experimental Psychology: General*, vol. 128: 78–87.

Lacey, N., and Pickard, H. 2012. "From the consulting room to the court room? Taking the clinical model of responsibility without blame into the legal realm." *The Oxford Journal of Legal Studies*. Published online November 19, 2012 doi: 10.1093/ojls/gqs028.

Lees, J., Manning, N., and Rawlings, B. 1999. *Therapeutic Community Effectiveness: A Systematic International Review of Therapeutic Community Treatment for People with Personality Disorders and Mentally Disordered Offenders*. York, UK: York Publishing Services.

Leshner, A. I. 1997. "Addiction is a brain disease, and it matters." *Science*, vol. 278 (5335): 45–47.

Levy, N. 2011a. "Addiction and compulsion." In T. O'Connor and C. Sandis, eds. *A Companion to the Philosophy of Action* (pp. 267–273). Oxford: Blackwell.

Levy, N. 2011b "Addiction, responsibility, and ego depletion." In J. Poland and G. Graham, eds. *Addiction and Responsibility* (pp. 89–111). Cambridge, MA: MIT Press.

Linehan, M., and Dimeff, L.2001 "Dialectical behavioural therapy in a nutshell."*The California Psychologist* vol. 34: 10–13

Markou, A., Kosten, T. R., and Koob, G. F. 1998. "Neurobiological similarities in depression and drug dependence: a self-medication hypothesis." *Neuropsychopharmacology*, vol. 18: 135–74.

Mele, A. 1990. "Irresistible desires." *Nous*, vol. 24: 455–472.

Miller, W. R. 1996. "What is relapse? Fifty ways to leave the wagon." *Addiction* vol. 91 (suppl): S15–S27.

Muller, C. P., and Schumann, G. 2011. "Drugs as instruments—a new framework for non-addictive psychoactive drug use." *Behavioural and Brain Sciences*, vol. 34 (6): 293–310.

Muraven, M., and Baumeister, R. 2000. "Self-regulation and depletion of limited resources: does self-control resemble a muscle?" *Psychological Bulletin*, vol. 126: 247–259.

National Institue of Mental Health in England (NIMHE). 2003. *Personality disorder: no longer a diagnosis of exclusion*. London: NIMHE.

Newberry, Michelle. 2010. "A synthesis of outcome research at Grendon therapeutic community prison." *Therapeutic Communities*, vol. 31 (4): 357–373.

Pates, R., McBride, A., and Arnold, K.eds. 2005. *Injecting Illicit Drugs*. Oxford: Blackwell.

Pearce, S., and Pickard, H. 2010. "Finding the will to recover: philosophical perspectives on agency and the sick role." *Journal of Medical Ethics*, vol. 36(12): 831–833.

Pearce, S., and Pickard, H. 2012. "How Therapeutic Communities work: specific factors related to positive outcome." *International Journal of Social Psychiatry*, published online July 20, 2012: http://isp.sagepub.com/content/early/2012/07/18/00207640124 50992. doi: 10.1177/0020764012450992.

Petry, N. M., Alessi, S. M., and Rash, C. J. 2011. "Contingency management treatment of drug and alcohol use disorders." In J. Poland and G. Graham, eds. *Addiction and Responsibility* (pp. 225–245). Cambridge, MA: MIT Press.

Pickard, H. 2011a. "Responsibility without blame: empathy and the effective treatment of personality disorder." *Philosophy, Psychiatry, Psychology*, vol. 18 (3): 209–223.

Pickard, H. 2011b. Review of *Addiction and Responsibility*, ed. J. Poland and G. Graham. *Notre Dame Philosophical Reviews* 11.01.

Pickard, H. 2012. "The purpose in chronic addiction." *American Journal of Bioethics Neuroscience*, vol. 3 (2): 40–49.

Pickard, H. 2013. "Psychopathology and the ability to do otherwise." *Philosophy and Phenomenological Research*. Published online April 8, 2013. doi: 10.1111/phpr.12025

Pickard, H. Forthcoming. "Responsibility without blame: philosophical reflections on clinical practice."In K. W. M. Fulford, M. Davies, R. T. Gipps, G. Graham, J. Sadler, G. Strangellini, and T. Thornton, eds. *The Oxford Handbook of Philosophy of Psychiatry*. Oxford: Oxford University Press.

Regier, D. A., Farmer, M. E., Rae, D. S., Locke, B. Z., Keith, S. J., Judd, L., and Goodwin, F. K. 1990. "Comorbidity of mental disorders with alcohol and other drug abuse. Results from the epidemiological catchment area (ECA) study." *JAMA: The Journal of the American Medical Association*, vol. 264: 2511–2518.

Robins, L. N. 1993. "Vietnam veterans' rapid recovery from heroin addiction: a fluke or normal expectation?" *Addiction*, vol. 88: 1041–1954.

Rollnick, S., and Miller, W. R. 1995. "What is motivational interviewing?" *Behavioural Cognitive Psychotherapy*, vol. 23: 325–334.

Shine, J. ed. *A Compilation of Grendon Research*. Aylesbury Bucks: HM Prison Grendon.

Skodol, A. E., Oldham, J. M., and Gallaher, P. E. 1999. "Axis II comorbidity of substance use disorders among patients referred for treatment of personality disorders." *American Journal of Psychiatry*, vol. 156 (5): 733–738.

Solinas, M., Chauvet, C., Thiriet, N. E., Rawas, R., and Jaber, M. 2008. "Reversal of cocaine addiction by environmental enrichment." *PNAS*, vol. 105 (44): 17145–17150.

Smith, A. 2007. "On being responsible and holding responsible." *Journal of Ethics*, vol. 11: 465–484.

Smith, M. 2003. "Rational capacities, or: How to distinguish recklessness, weakness, and compulsion." In S. Stroud and C. Tappolet, eds. *Weakness of Will and Varieties of Practical Irrationality* (pp. 17–38). Oxford: Oxford University Press.

Steward, H. 2009. "Fairness, agency, and the flicker of freedom." *Nous* 43: 64–93.

Steward, H. 2012. *A Metaphysics for Freedom*. Oxford: Oxford University Press.Thomas, H., Melchert, T. P., and Banken, J. A. 1999. "Substance dependence and personality disorders: comorbidity and treatment outcome in an inpatient treatment population." *Journal of Studies on Alcohol*, vol. 60: 271–277.

Treasure, J. 2004. "Motivational interviewing." *Advances in Psychiatric Treatment*, vol. 10 (5): 331–337.

Watson, G. 1999. "Excusing addiction." Reprinted in his *Agency and Answerability* (pp. 318–150) 2004. Oxford: Clarendon Press.

Weaver, T., Madden, P., Charles, V., Stimson, G., Renton, A., Tyrer, P., Barnes, T., Bench, C., Middleton, H., Wright, N., Paterson, S., Shanahan, W., Seivewright, N., and Ford, C. 2003. "Comorbidity of substance misuse and mental illness in community mental health and substance misuse services." *British Journal of Psychiatry*, vol. 183 (4): 304–313.

West, R. 2006. *Theory of Addiction*. Oxford: Blackwell.

Williams, B.1995. "How free does the will need to be?" In his *Making Sense of Humanity and Other Philosophical Papers* (pp. 3–21). Cambridge: Cambridge University Press.

Widom, C. S., Ireland, T., and Glynn, P. J. 1995. "Alcohol abuse in abuse and neglected children followed-up: are they at increased risk?" *Journal of Studies on Alcohol*, vol. 56 (2): 207–217.

Yaffe, G. 2011. "Lowering the bar for addicts." In J. Poland and G. Graham, eds. *Addiction and Responsibility* (pp. 113–138). Cambridge, MA: MIT Press.

Yates, W. R., LaBreque, D. R., and Pfab, D. 1998. "Personality disorder as a contraindication for liver transplantation in alcoholic cirrhosis." *Psychosomatics*, vol. 39: 501–511.

10

Are Addicts Akratic?

Interpreting the Neuroscience of Reward

GIDEON YAFFE

INTRODUCTION

We know that human beings like things; they find some things pleasurable and others painful and with various degrees and tones. We know that human beings value things; they take certain facts to be reasons for certain actions, and they take some facts to provide greater reasons for action than others. We know that human beings want things; they are more and less motivated to pursue some things rather than others. And we know that human beings act intentionally; they make choices and form intentions (where these mental states are understood to be distinct from desires) and they engage in bodily movements that accord with their choices and intentions. We can investigate, then, the systems that give rise to likings, valuings, wantings, and intentional actions. And we have learned a great deal about the nature of these systems. A great deal is known, that is, about the psychological states involved in such systems, about the environmental and genetic factors that influence them, about the social factors that contribute to them in various ways, and, importantly for our purposes here, about the brain structures and neural transmitters involved in them.

We even know something about how these systems interact. In a substantial class of normal, nonpathological cases, each of these systems provides an input to another and thereby influences its output. A person comes to like X; the liking of X contributes to making the person value X, or recognize a reason for acquiring X that is perhaps weightier than reasons that the person recognizes for not doing so; valuing X is part of what leads the agent to want X, or to be moved to act so as to acquire X; and this desire plays a role in the formation of a choice to pursue X and an intentional bodily movement aimed at acquiring X. There are, to be sure, quite complicated relations among inputs and outputs of the various systems that we do not begin to capture with this brief description. Sometimes, to give just one example, it is the wanting of X that leads to the valuing it, rather than the reverse; and sometimes there are complex feedback mechanisms: valuing X, you come to want it, which in turn leads you to value it even more strongly. The wiring diagram, as it were, describing the routes and gates connecting these various systems is likely to be very complicated. In fact, it is even possible that some of these systems are components of others, or have overlapping components. Further, even in normal, nonpathological cases, an input to one system can nonetheless be overridden and lead to an output discordant with it. Sometimes, for instance, we come to value what we do not like, come to want what we neither value nor like, and even come to intentionally pursue something we neither like, value, nor want. It seems likely, that is, that all of the various combinations of match and mismatch between the outputs of these various systems are possible.

I will focus here on one particular form of possible mismatch, namely, that between intentional action, particularly wrongful intentional action, and what the agent values. One form of failure of self-control—although it is not, by any means, the only sort—involves precisely such a mismatch. In this form of failure to control oneself, the agent ends up choosing contrary to what he values most and thereby chooses wrongful conduct. Let's call such conduct "akratic" conduct, recognizing that the label is sometimes used to refer to a wider range of failures of self-control than these. I focus on this form of mismatch for two reasons. First, it has been suggested by many people, among them Richard Holton in his terrific recent book, that addicts are often subject to such a mismatch. Holton writes,

> Standardly, if someone wants something—a clever device for peeling garlic, say—and then discovers it does not work, the want will simply evaporate. It is, as we might say, undermined. In contrast...in cases of addiction there must be an almost complete disconnection between judging an outcome good and wanting it, or, conversely, between judging it bad and not wanting it.[1]

Holton here suggests that what the addict values fails to match what he desires. His implication is that the addict nonetheless enjoys a match between desire

1. Richard Holton, *Willing, Wanting, Waiting*, Oxford: Oxford University Press, 2009, pp. 108–109.

and choice; he chooses what he wants, but does not want what he values, and so does not choose what he values. In short, if Holton is right, the addict is akratic.[2]

If this is the nature of addicts' failures to control themselves, then that's an important discovery that can direct further research into the causes of wrongful, not to mention self-destructive, behavior by addicts. And such research can potentially tell us a lot about how to intervene to keep addicts from hurting themselves and others. Helping someone to align what he chooses with what he values is a very different project from the project of, say, helping him to align what he likes with what he values as we do when, for instance, we try to teach someone who values truffles to enjoy them, or when we administer the recently developed "cocaine addiction vaccine," which, purportedly, prevents cocaine consumption from producing a high.[3] If Holton is right, for instance, it might turn out to be ineffective to try to help the addicted cocaine user, desperate to quit, to stop liking cocaine. The drug that stops cocaine from being pleasant to him will help him to align what he likes with what he values; he disvalues cocaine and the drug will prevent him from liking it, too. But unless he is also thereby led to align what he chooses with what he values (perhaps by aligning what he wants with what he values), he'll keep on using, if Holton is right. The drug might not intervene directly at the crucial place.[4]

The question of whether or not addicts choose in accordance with what they value at the time of action is important for another reason, as well. If, when the addict acts badly, he chooses contrary to what he values, then this fact is of immediate relevance to some forms of moral evaluation of the addict's behavior. It is relevant, in particular, to an assessment of the addict's blameworthiness for bad behavior. At least one of the things that modulates our blame of bad action, and should modulate it, is the degree to which that action is expressive of bad attitudes on the part of the agent of the act; and at least one of the

2. Holton's usage of the term "akratic" is different from that here. So, he may not endorse this way of summarizing his position. Still, in the sense in which the term is used here, Holton takes addicts to act akratically.
3. See Kosten, T., Rosen, M., Bond, J., Settles, M., St. Clair Roberts, J., Shields, J., Jack, L., & Fox, B. "Human therapeutic cocaine vaccine: safety and immunogenicity" in *Vaccine*, vol. 20, pp. 1196–1204, 2002.
4. In fact, such drugs probably *both* prevent the cocaine user from liking cocaine and decrease the likelihood he will choose it; what is unclear is whether they decrease the likelihood of choice *because* they decrease the degree to which cocaine is liked, or for some other reason. Such drugs work by producing antibodies that bind cocaine in the bloodstream before it enters the brain and so prevent cocaine from affecting either the liking system or the choosing system. It is therefore no surprise that we see decreases in consumption behavior in rats who have taken the vaccine. See Fox, B., et al., "Efficacy of a therapeutic cocaine vaccine in rodent models" in *Nature Medicine*, vol. 2, pp. 1129–1132, 1996.

reasons that we care about the attitudes of a person when he acted is because those attitudes indicate something of importance about what facts he took at the time of action to give him reason for action, and to what degree. An agent's modes of recognition, weighing, and response to reasons are deep facts about the agent that, arguably anyway, are of intrinsic moral importance. What facts agents take to be reasons, and with what weights, are facts about what the agent is like in a morally crucial respect. Wrongful akratic actions are not expressive of quite the same objectionable modes of recognizing, weighing, and responding to reasons that we find in those who do wrong nonakratically, and so the fact of akrasia mitigates blameworthiness. The akratic *merely seems* to care more about leisure than about work, or more about his own convenience than about physical harm to others. His conduct *seems* to be expressive of such distortions in his conceptions of what reasons he has, or what weights to give them, but is not in fact. This is not to say that the akratic is *excused* from blame; he is probably still blameworthy to some degree. But akrasia nonetheless *mitigates* blame; the akratic is less blameworthy than the otherwise identical agent who values what is gained through wrongdoing more than what is foregone. But then if we are to allocate blame to those who deserve it, and to the degree and in the way in which they deserve it, we need to know in which category to place the addict. Is the addict acting akratically, or not? This is not the only question that the proper allocation of blame requires us to answer about the addict, but it's one of them. But do addicts act contrary to what they value at the time of action? Or do they, instead, at least at the time of action, value that to which they are addicted more than those things that they forego in order to use? Does the heroin addict who leaves work in the middle of the day to use, knowing he'll be fired, value heroin, or the using of it, or the high that it gives him, more, at the time of action, than he values his job, or the money it pays, or the support that it provides to his family? Does the pregnant crack addict, who smokes crack, value what crack gives her more than she values the health of her unborn child, or more than she disvalues the punishment and censure that she expects her behavior to bring? Or, when she is using, is she doing violence, herself and through her own agency, to that which she values more than that which she pursues? These are empirical questions. And, in fact, we have empirical data from neuroscience that bears on them. The problem is that the data is difficult to interpret. This paper looks at two interpretations of some of the neuroscientific data that have been offered in the recent philosophical literature: Holton's and Timothy Schroeder's. For different reasons, although on the basis of some of the same data, Holton and Schroeder reach the conclusion that addicts are, indeed, acting akratically. The paper argues that the experiments that Holton and Schroeder mention show precisely the opposite of what Holton and Schroeder take them to show. They show, that is, that addicts ordinarily act in accordance with what they value at the time of action. This is probably often temporary—many addicts, that is, value use over abstention at the moment they choose to use, but value abstention over use moments before and even moments after. But, still, at the time of action they value what they choose. If this is correct, then addiction influences what people do intentionally by working through, rather than against, the valuing system.[5]

As we'll see in the final section of this paper, this result has implications for how a criminal defendant's addiction ought, or rather ought not, be considered when assessing his legal responsibility for a crime. It will be argued that addiction ought to be considered in a way quite similar to the way in which duress is considered in the criminal law. This claim, it will also be suggested, is consistent with denying what should be denied, namely, that addicts are under duress. They are not, but their condition bears sufficient similarity to the condition of those under duress to warrant treating them similarly under the criminal law. Like victims of duress, addicts find themselves valuing criminal conduct more than they value refraining from such conduct. And like those under duress, and unlike those with such values who are not under duress, addicts have the values they have thanks to the fact that they bear burdens that are not, themselves, reflective of morally or legally objectionable attitudes on their parts.

VALUING DEFINED

Before moving forward, it is important to head off a possible misunderstanding concerned with the verb "to value." To value X, for our purposes here, is not merely to say or believe that X is a good thing. It is, instead, to take oneself to have reason to do those things that promote X, or bring X about, or are believed to be necessary or even just useful to promoting X or bringing X about. To value X more than Y is to grant greater weight to the reasons one takes for promoting X or bringing X about than one grants to the reasons, if there are any, that one takes there to be for promoting Y or bringing Y about. To value something, in the sense in which the term will be used here, then, is to engage in a mode of recognition, weighing, and response to reasons. To believe that something

---

5. One implication of this is that there is something misleading in the idea of an "unwilling addict." (The term was coined in Frankfurt, H. "Freedom of will and the concept of a person" in *The Importance of What We Care About*, Cambridge: Cambridge University Press, pp. 11–25, 1988.) The unwilling addict is thought to take the drug to which he is addicted despite the fact that *even at the time of action* he does not value taking the drug. While such a creature is possible, if the argument of this paper works we have reason to believe that human addicts, with brains that function the way ours do, are not unwilling addicts in this sense. Consistent with having a brain like ours, however, it is possible, even common, not to value consumption both moments before and moments after the time of the decision to consume.

is a good thing often, maybe even always, goes along with valuing it; but it is nonetheless distinct. Insofar as it is conceptually possible to believe something to be a good thing while failing to recognize reasons for promoting or bringing it about, believing that something is good and valuing it are distinct. One's mode of recognition, weighing, and response to reasons is a function of the way in which one consciously deliberates, or of the way in which one would consciously deliberate in circumstances in which one does not. Say that one believes that a particular act would promote X; one believes, for instance, that boycotting British Petroleum, in contrast to Chevron, will promote the use of alternative sources of energy. Perhaps BP, unlike Chevron, actively lobbies against the expansion of research into alternative energy sources. To treat the fact believed as giving one reason to engage in the act is to deliberate in a way, or to be ready to deliberate in a way, that involves treating the fact that X would be promoted by the act as a reason to engage in that act. Someone who has the belief and who values the use of alternative sources of energy will deliberate, or be ready to deliberate, in a way that treats the fact that the boycott of BP would promote such use as a reason to boycott BP. It may be a reason that is outweighed by others, but it is still a factor given weight in deliberations about what to do, or would be were the agent to engage in relevant deliberations. By contrast, someone who believes that the boycott would promote the use of alternative energy but does not value the use of alternative energy sources will not grant the fact believed any weight in his deliberations about what to do. When deciding whether to fill his tank at BP or Chevron, he will consider and weigh a variety of reasons, but the fact that boycotting BP would promote alternative energy will not be among them.

To grant weight to certain facts in one's deliberations involves, among other things, being ready to recognize a failure to treat the fact as giving reason as involving an error in one's own deliberations. A mark of valuing, that is, is the acceptance of norms *governing deliberation* that would not be accepted by someone who did not value in the same way. To continue with our example, consider the person who values the use of alternative sources of energy and is deliberating about whether to go to BP or to Chevron to fill up his car's tank. If he ignores the fact that boycotting BP will promote the use of alternative sources of energy—he deliberates as though he granted that fact no reason to go to Chevron over BP— this will be a failure in his deliberations when they are held up *to his own standards*. Since he values the use of alternative sources of energy, he *ought* to take the fact that boycotting BP will promote it as a reason to shop at Chevron rather than BP. This "ought" applies to him and not to others who do not value as he does.

It is quite possible that the verb "to value" is used here as a term of art. Nothing is invested in the claim that there is perfect, or even approximate, overlap between one's modes of recognition, weighing, and response to reasons and ordinary usages of the term "to value." Perhaps they do not align, even if they do overlap. One reason to think that they diverge is that in some ordinary senses of the term "valuing," what a person values cannot be a local property of him, the possession of which at one time entails nothing about his properties at other times. In some ordinary usages of the term "valuing," that is, you cannot value something at one time unless there is a substantial period of time over which you value it. There are no fleeting valuings, in this sense of the term. By contrast, nothing in the way the term is being used here implies that. You may employ a mode of recognition, weighing, and response to reasons at one particular time and not employ that same mode at any other time at all. Valuing, in the sense in which the term is used here, could be a local property. This isn't to say that it typically *is* local. Typically, what one values at one time, one values at many other times, too. But this is not an entailment, instead, it is a contingent fact about most people.

A question arises, however, whether, in assessing people's blameworthiness, we are concerned with the local property for its own sake—with, merely, the person's modes of recognition, weighing, and response to reasons *at the moment of action*—or are concerned with the local property only because we assume it to be stable over time. Perhaps, that is, we think it more blameworthy to act harmfully and wrongfully while granting little reason-giving weight to the fact that one's act would be harmful to another only because we assume that a person who failed to grant sufficient rational weight to such a consideration at the moment of action fails in this regard generally. Perhaps, that is, valuing is important to blame only because of what it says about character, where one's character is understood as involving *stable tendencies* to recognize and respond to reasons in a particular way.

I suspect that sometimes what an agent values at the time of action matters for its own sake and sometimes it matters because of what it tells us about the agent's character. Judgments of blameworthiness are a diverse lot and there is little reason to expect uniformity in this regard. However, the criminal law, if not morality, has a particular concern with the very moment at which a defendant chose to commit a crime, and thus with the defendant's values at that moment, to the exclusion of other times. For the purposes of the criminal law, we care about the moment of action to a greater degree than moments before and after it for several reasons. One of the most important is that we typically don't allow prosecutors to bring in evidence about the defendant at other times unless it can be shown to say something about him at the moment of action. This is a fundamental principle of criminal law in a liberal state that underlies our practices of, for instance, excluding prior convictions from evidence except in special circumstances. We convict only for criminal conduct performed at a particular time and not for other features of the agent or his conduct that surround the conduct, but are not specifically proscribed by the state. But if the criminal law has good reasons to base its assessments of defendants on facts about them only at the time of criminal conduct, then the notion of valuing at work here, where valuing can be local, is potentially of importance to the criminal law, even if we grant that temporally distributed properties operative at the time of action are also potentially important.

In short, it is possible that the question of whether addicts act akratically is of relevance to only a subset of our judgments of blameworthiness; but, still, it is of importance to a large percentage of our judgments of *criminal* blameworthiness. If we are to treat addicts who commit crimes justly under the criminal law, if we are to blame them in a way and to a degree that matches their blame*worthiness*, we need to know if they act akratically or, instead, act in line with what they value at the time of action.

HOLTON ON BERRIDGE AND ROBINSON

Holton reaches the conclusion that addicts act contrary to their values largely on the basis of the well-known experiments on rats conducted by Robinson and Berridge and colleagues. Robinson and Berridge showed that amphetamine-addicted rats pursue a sugar reward far more zealously than do rats that are not addicted, despite the fact that the two groups of rats do not differ in the degree to which they like the sugar, at least by behavioral measures of liking. The addicted rats press a lever on hearing a tone that has been associated with sugar reward four times more frequently than unaddicted rats. Thus, the addiction seems to increase the desire for sugar that is prompted by the conditioned cue, and in turn increases the frequency of choices to consume sugar, despite the fact that the addiction has no effect on the degree to which sugar is enjoyed. The addicted rat receives no more pleasure from the sugar it zealously pursues than the unaddicted rat. But, still, it pursues it much more aggressively. Put in the terms in use here, addiction seems to increase desire, or want, but does not increase liking. The experiments do not show exactly how it is that addiction influences choice. But they do show that it does not do so by increasing the degree to which a substance is enjoyed. Its influence is on some system other than the system that gives rise to pleasure and pain.

In addition, the Robinson and Berridge experiments provide powerful evidence that this important behavioral change is linked to the dopamine system in rats. Amphetamines, as well as many other drugs of abuse, are known to cause immediate release of dopamine, and there is good reason to think that, after the cue has been associated with the reward, addicted rats, even when not treated with amphetamine at the time of the cue, have greater dopamine release on encountering the cue than do unaddicted rats. Thus, it appears that dopamine release plays an important role in the way in which the liking system modulates the outputs of the wanting system. The addicted rat is motivated to pursue the reward *as if* he liked it much more than the unaddicted rat likes it, despite the fact that he does not, in fact, like it any more at all. Addiction seems to weaken the normal connection between the liking system and the wanting system, and it seems to do so thanks to the way in which dopamine signals in addicts differ from those in unaddicted subjects. Since drugs of abuse have both temporary and long-term effects on dopamine release, they also have temporary and long-term effects in weakening the way in which liking modulates wanting.

What do these startling results show about human addicts? Since, as Holton notes, rats probably don't value anything—they do not recognize facts as constituting reasons in favor of certain courses of action and grant them weight in deliberation—the Berridge and Robinson experiments, as important as they are, do not speak directly to the question with which we are concerned here. To say that the wanting and the liking systems are disconnected from one another in addiction is not to say that the valuing system is disconnected from the wanting system. It is perfectly possible that while the addicted human being wants the drug much more than he likes it, he still comes to value it in a way that comports with his degree of desire for it. Holton thinks this unlikely largely because of the undeniable fact that addicts often pursue drugs in ways that directly conflict with what they judge to be good, or take themselves to have most reason to promote. The addict who prostitutes his child for drugs does not think this is a good thing. This is true. But what truth, exactly, does it register? The addict, to be sure, recoils at the prospect of selling his child for drugs when he is not craving, or is not in the presence of cues that prompt use; and he suffers powerful regret after having done this. His judgment that such behavior is an unqualified evil is real and is held by him for a much larger percentage of his time than any competing judgment. But it does not follow from this that, *at the time of decision*, he does not judge it best, overall, to sell his child; at the time of action, he may judge that to be the best of a number of bad options. The sense in which he acts contrary to what he judges to be best may just be that he acts contrary to what he *usually* judges to be best, and what he in fact judges to be best both before and after the time of action. But, still, his attitudes at the time of action matter and we have, as yet, no reason to believe that he does not, at that time, judge it less bad to sell his child than to go without the drug to which he is addicted. He may be locally, although not globally, just like the unrepentant child pimp.

How could we settle this question? How could we determine if the addict values what he chooses at the moment he chooses it, or values something else instead? In fact, we have a tool for making progress on this question already for much is known about the information that is carried by dopaminergic activity, which is what appears to be disrupted by drugs of abuse and addiction. As I will suggest, when we reflect carefully on what is known about the information carried by dopaminergic activity, we will see that disruptions of the dopaminergic system *are*, in human beings anyway, disruptions in the valuing system, and not just in the wanting system. If this is right, then precisely what we learn from experiments like Berridge and Robinson's is that addicts value, at the time of action anyway, precisely what they choose. I explain.

A crucial question is what the dopamine signal represents. Much of the most important work bearing on this question has been done with monkeys. In well-known experiments done by Wolfram Schultz and colleagues, for instance, dopamine is measured in monkeys at the time of a light cue, and at a time moments later when a reward is delivered.[6] There are important differences between the dopamine signal in the monkeys initially and the signal after the monkey has learned to associate the light with the reward. Initially, before the monkey has learned to expect a reward on seeing the light, the dopamine signal goes up when the reward is received. But after the monkey has learned that the light precedes reward, dopamine goes up when the light appears, and remains flat when the reward is obtained. In short, the signal increase moves from the time of the reward to the time of the cue, due to learning. (This fact by itself shows that the dopamine signal is not a measure of something like pleasure since the cue is never pleasurable and the reward always is.) Further, after the monkey has learned to associate the cue with the reward, when the light appears and no reward is given, the monkey's dopamine signal goes up initially on seeing the light, but goes down relative to its baseline when the monkey realizes that it will not receive a reward. That is, after the increase has moved from the time of reward to the time of the cue, the monkey shows a decrease in dopamine at the ordinary time of the reward when it does not receive a reward at that time.

What do these results show? A plausible explanation, which is the explanation favored by Schultz and his colleagues, is that the dopamine signal is modulated at least in part by the monkey's expectations. Initially, when the monkey does not expect the reward on seeing the light, it is the receipt of the reward, and not the appearance of the light, that shows the monkey's condition to be better than it expected it to be; and so the dopamine signal goes up on

6. See, for instance, Schultz, W., Apicella, P., & Ljungberg, T. "Responses of monkey dopamine neurons to reward and conditioned stimuli during successive steps of learning a delayed response task" in Journal of Neuroscience, vol. 13, pp. 900–913, 1993; Hollerman, J. R., & Schultz, W. "Dopamine neurons report an error in the temporal prediction of reward during learning" in *Nature Neuroscience*, vol. 1, pp. 304–309, 1998; Schultz, W. "Predictive reward signal of dopamine neurons" in *Journal of Neurophysiology*, vol. 80, pp. 1–27, 1998.

reward receipt. Later, when the monkey has learned to associate the light and the reward, it finds on seeing *the light* that its condition is better than expected, and so, again, the dopamine signal goes up on seeing the light. But, since the appearance of the light resets the monkey's expectations—having seen the light it now expects the reward—the dopamine signal remains flat when it receives the reward and its expectations are met. And the signal goes down when it does not receive the reward and things turn out to be worse than it expects thanks to its conditioning.

The last of these results is worth highlighting. It is widely believed, and not without reason, that the dopamine signal plays a role in the generation of choices. Decisions about what to do, that is, are influenced by the dopamine signal. But it is important to see how this comes to pass. It appears that the way the dopamine signal influences choices is by influencing future expectations, which then, in turn, influence choices. The dopamine signal represents something about the past; it represents the difference between how things actually came out and how they were expected to come out. But it influences *future decisions* by influencing expectations about the future. If things came out less well than expected, then future expectations ought to be different from past expectations, and the dopamine signal provides a guide for determining how different they should be. The larger the dopamine signal, the more need there is for having different expectations about the future when conditions are otherwise the same as they were at the time of the last prediction. The reason the primed monkey's dopamine signal goes down relative to the baseline when it is not given the reward following the cue is that it expects the reward *thanks to* the dopamine signal's representation of the world as just as expected on receipt of reward on the previous trials. The dopamine signal, then, is a representation of a fact about the past that influences future decisions by altering the subject's expectations about the future. What this implies, among other things, is that in a healthy animal that learns quickly from its mistakes a large dopamine signal will result, later, in flat dopamine signals in response to exactly the same experiences. The large dopamine signal will help the subject to learn to have expectations that match reality. And when expectations match reality, the dopamine signal is flat.

An important question remains when we accept that the dopamine signal represents the difference between expectation and reality: a difference in what respect? There is a powerful pull toward answering that the dopamine signal represents a difference in *the value* expected and *the value* actually received. In fact, it is believed that dopamine signals are unaffected by discrepancies in neutral differences between expectation and reality. Although the experiment has not been done, it is expected that when a monkey gets something different from what it expects, but of equal value, the dopamine signal remains flat. But we should be careful about characterizing the dopamine signal as representing a difference *in value*. What the experiments show is only that the dopamine signal represents a difference in *something* with the following property: more of it is better than less. To see the point, consider two competing hypotheses:

> The Likability Hypothesis: The dopamine signal represents the difference between the amount that the subject expects to like something and the amount that the subject actually likes it.
>
> The Desirability Hypothesis: The dopamine signal represents the difference between the amount of desire satisfaction that the subject expects to receive from acquiring something and the amount that he actually receives.[7]

The data just described—under which the monkey's dopamine signal varies with its expectations—does not allow us to discriminate between these two hypotheses. If both how much organisms like things, and how much they expect to like things, on the one hand, and how much desire satisfaction they experience on acquiring something, and how much they expect to experience, on the other, influence what choices they make, then *both* hypotheses are consistent with the data. And, importantly for our purposes here, given subsidiary assumptions of this sort, the data is also consistent with the following hypothesis about the dopamine signal in humans:

> The Value Hypothesis: The dopamine signal represents the difference between the amount that the subject expects something to be supported by reasons and the amount that it is actually supported by reasons.

How can a person's expectations diverge from reality in this respect? The obvious way this happens is when the facts turn out differently from expected. I expect the lock to turn when I insert the key and it doesn't, so I recognize myself to have had less reason to insert it than I expected to have. I had reason to turn the lock, and falsely expected the key to turn it. But there can be a discrepancy in expectation in this respect in other ways, too. Notably, there might be a shift in my standards about what counts as a reason between the moment of expectation formation and the later moment. If, after I insert the key, I come to the

---

7. Desire satisfaction is intended to be understood here as follows: When a subject is moved to acquire something, and acquires it, he enjoys a reduction in motivation. If he gets exactly what he was moved to acquire, then his motivation is reduced to zero. If he has residual motivation left over—he is not satisfied with what he acquired—then it is reduced to less than zero. Desire satisfaction is the amount of reduction in motivation that is enjoyed on acquiring the object. If the subject was highly motivated, there is greater potential for desire satisfaction, although there is also greater potential for disappointment.

view that turning the lock is not worth doing, but do not update my expectation in light of this change in view, then I will be disappointed in my expectations about what reasons I have when I find that the key turns the lock. Or, there can be a shift in the way in which I weigh reasons between the moment of expectation formation and the later moment. I expect myself to have more reason to turn the lock than to wait for the door to be answered, but my ordering of these two options swaps after I have inserted the key. Assuming that the swap in my attitude does not lead me to update my expectation, perhaps because there isn't time, I will find myself to have had less reason to insert the key than I expected. If how much a human subject expects available courses of conduct to be supported by reasons influences his choices, then the Value Hypothesis, too, is consistent with the data. We know that the dopamine signal represents the difference between what is expected and what is encountered. And we know that when the dopamine signal represents there as having been more of that, whatever it is, then the subject will more zealously pursue outcomes that are like those encountered; the signal is representing what was encountered as *better*, in some respect, than what was expected. But we don't know *in what respect* the expected and the actual world are represented as different by the dopamine signal.

What likability, desirability, and support by reasons have in common is that more of them is better than less. What the data about the dopamine signals shows is only that dopamine represents the difference in expectation and reality of *something* more of which is better than less. Let's call that something "X." X might be likability, desirability, or value, or perhaps something else entirely more of which is better than less. Further, what the Berridge and Robinson experiments show is that addicts choose as if they judged drugs to have a lot of X, under the assumption that what subjects choose is powerfully influenced by such judgements. And they do so thanks to the fact that drugs of abuse disrupt the dopamine signal.

Now, this much is clear: addicts do not act contrary to their judgments about how much X their acts promise. Precisely their problem is that they act *in line* with such judgments in circumstances in which *those judgements themselves* have been adversely affected by the disruptions of the dopamine signal from which addicts suffer. Why does the addicted rat press the lever so much more frequently than the unaddicted rat? It's not because he *actually* likes sugar more than the unaddicted rat. Nor is it because sugar gives him more desire satisfaction than it gives to the unaddicted rat. It's because the rat judges sugar to promise more X than the unaddicted rat judges it to promise. His judgment is different from the unaddicted rat's because his dopamine signal represents pressing the lever as far better, with respect to the amount of X it promises, than it was experienced as being last time he pressed it. But this last fact is consistent with, and in fact explains, the further fact that he represents pressing the lever as promising more X than any alternative. He judges it of his alternatives to be X-optimal, as it were, and that's why he pursues it so zealously. He seems, in fact, to judge it to be about four times better, with respect to X, than the unaddicted rats judge it to be.

To say that X must be something more of which is better than less is not to imply, all by itself, that in representing an act as promising more X than expected the organism is representing the act *as better* than expected. More vitamin C is better than less; but in representing the orange before me as containing more vitamin C than I expected it to contain, I am not necessarily representing it as better than expected. For that to be the case, I need to represent vitamin C *as good* in some respect. A dispassionate chart indicating the nutritional value of foods does not represent nutrient-rich foods as better than nutrient-poor foods; it merely represents how many nutrients the foods contain and leaves it to the reader of the chart to draw his own conclusions about which foods are better from the point of view of nutrition. What would allow us to distinguish between a mental representation of the orange as containing q milligrams of vitamin C and a representation of it *as worthy of pursuit in virtue of the fact* that it contains q milligrams of vitamin C? The answer is that the latter representation would play a role in both conscious deliberation and in the guidance of behavior that the former does not. Someone who represents q milligrams of vitamin C *as worth pursuing* will judge himself to have a reason to eat the orange, and will be motivated to pursue it. In short: it is thanks to its causal role in an agent's psychology that a representation of a fact *as reason giving* is distinguished from a representation of that fact that does not represent it as reason giving.

Now, a great deal is known about the causal role in our and animals' psychology played by the dopamine signal. As predicted by computational models of learning, so-called reinforcement models, biological organisms like human beings update their judgements in response to their calculations of the difference between expected and achieved X and they both deliberate and act in a way that accords with their updated judgements. [8] But, and here is the important point, the dopamine signal can play this role only if the organism represents things that are X as worth pursuing on those grounds. The dopamine signal itself needn't represent things that are X as things that there is reason to pursue on those

8. See, for instance, Waelti, P., Dickinson, A., & Schultz, W. "Dopamine responses comply with basic assumptions of formal learning theory" in *Nature*, vol. 412, pp. 43–48, 2001; Bayer, H. M., & Glimcher, P. W. "Subjective estimates of objective rewards: using economic discounting to link behavior and brain" in *Society of Neuroscience Abstracts*, vol. 28, p. 358.6, 2002; Berridge, K. C., & Robinson, T. E. "What is the role of dopamine in reward: hedonic impact, reward learning, or incentive salience?" in *Brain Research Review*, vol. 28, pp. 309–369, 1998.

grounds. It may represent only the fact that a particular thing promises more (or less) X than expected; it may be like the nutritional chart that represents the amount of vitamin C in various foods. But, still, a creature whose dopamine signal plays the crucial role in learning that the dopamine signals of rats, monkeys, and human beings play must also represent things as worth pursuing in virtue of the fact that they are X. Such organisms must represent X as reason giving. Given the information that the dopamine signal carries, that is, it must be part of *the valuing* system.

Is the claim just made consistent with the suggestion that animals like rats and monkeys, in contrast to human beings, do not think about what reasons they have for and against particular courses of action? Notice that there is one very important difference between the dopamine signal in animals like rats and monkeys and the dopamine signal in human beings. We have no reason to believe that rats and monkeys update *conscious judgements* about how much reason they have to pursue particular objects or courses of conduct in response to the dopamine signal. Because their psychologies are (probably) not as rich as ours in this respect, their dopamine signals play a relatively impoverished role in their psychologies compared with ours. Our dopamine signals lead us to update both conscious judgment *and* action-guiding preference, while theirs, since they probably lack the kinds of conscious judgements that we have, lead only to the second kind of updating. Whether both roles are required for a representation to count as a representation of a course of conduct as supported by reasons is a hard question. But, thankfully, it's not a question that we need to answer, for this much is clear: *in human beings*, conduct that makes sense in light of the dopamine signal makes sense in light of the person's values at the time of action. The dopamine signal represents something more of which is better than less, and thanks to the role that that representation plays in human psychology, it must be part of a system that represents acts, objects, and states of affairs as *worth* pursuing or avoiding. The result: addicts act in accord with, rather than in opposition to, their values at the time of action. Addicts do not act akratically.

SCHROEDER ON DESIRE AND THE REWARD SYSTEM

It helps to understand the argument just offered to contrast the position outlined here with Tim Schroeder's position as expressed in his recent book, and in an even more recent paper on addiction.[9] At least for the purposes of argument, Schroeder holds an instrumental conception of rationality. Under such a conception, what one has reason to do is a function of what one desires. If there are no

9. Schroeder, T. *Three Faces of Desire*, Oxford: Oxford University Press, 2004; Schroeder, T. "Irrational action and addiction" in *What Is Addiction?*, edited by D. Ross, H. Kincaid, D. Spurrett, & P. Collins, Cambridge: MIT Press, 2010, pp. 391–407.

desire-independent reasons, then the question of whether addicts act in accord with their desires seems directly relevant to the question of whether addicts act akratically, or contrary to their modes of recognition and response to reasons employed at the time of action.

So, *if* an instrumental conception of rationality is correct, and *if* it turned out that addicts frequently act contrary to their desires in the sense that they act contrary to the reasons that their desires supply, then that fact would turn out to be of relevance to our discussion here. Schroeder has argued that a proper appreciation of what is known about the effect of drugs on the reward system in humans supports the claim that addicts actually act contrary to their desires. If we think through what the neuroscience of reward *means*, we will see, thinks Schroeder, that addicts actually want that which they choose far less than it might appear.

Schroeder's argument takes the following theory of desire as a premise:

The Reward Theory of Desire: "[T]o desire something is for one's reward system to treat it as a reward. And for one's reward system to treat something as a reward is for the reward system to take representations of that thing as positive inputs into a calculation of how many rewards the world contains versus how many it was expected to contain." (Schroeder 2010, p. 395)

On this theory, it is not the case that everything a representation of which causes an increase in the dopamine signal is desired. Sometimes a representation of something will cause an increase in the dopamine signal even though the organism's *reward system* does not cause that increase. This is what Schroeder thinks takes place when one consumes a drug of abuse. The drug of abuse, not the reward system, causes an increase in dopamine. So the person who wants the drug and has a representation of it, on the one hand, and the person who does not want it but consumes it, on the other, have something in common: both have an increased dopamine signal in response to a representation of the drug. But they are also different: the first, and not the second, has *a reward system* that responds to a representation of the drug with an increase in the dopamine signal.

What does Schroeder take the dopamine signal itself to represent? He takes it to represent the degree to which the drug is desired. That is, where the object of desire is a thing in the world—a drug, say—that which is represented by the dopamine signal is actually a state of the organism: the state of desiring something in the world. So, when the dopamine signal is driven up by something other than the reward system's processing of a representation—when it is driven up, for instance, directly by consumption of a drug of abuse—the dopamine signal actually *misrepresents*: it represents the drug as strongly desired, when, in fact, it may not be desired at all. The result, Schroeder holds, is that insofar as an addict's conduct is dictated by his dopamine signal, he frequently pursues things *as though* they were strongly desired when, in fact, he does not desire them at all. But if he acts contrary to his desires, and if the reasons that he has are constituted by what he wants, then it follows that he acts contrary to what, given his desires, he has most reason to do. While this seems relevant to the question that concerns us here (namely, whether the addict acts akratically), it is not clear precisely what it implies in that regard. While Schroeder has provided us with a theory of desire, he hasn't provided us with a theory of valuing, and that's what's crucial to our question. If a person lacks a desire, but thinks he has one, and then acts as dictated by the desire he thinks he has, is he acting contrary to, or in line with, what he values? Put another way, is conscious deliberation responsive to our desires, or to what we think our desires are, or both, or neither? While I cannot claim to have an argument for this answer, I think we ought to hold that under a desire-based conception of reasons for action, a person takes himself to have a reason to A only if he has *both* a desire that is supportive of A-ing *and* a belief that he has a reason to A (which may be grounded in a belief that he has a desire that gives him a reason to A). Since, if Schroeder is right, the addict whose dopamine signal is driven up directly by the drug of abuse, and not by his reward system, lacks the desire, he also fails to value that which he pursues. He would not, that is, deliberate as though he took there to be reason to do those things that the desire he thinks he has provides. The result: if Schroeder is right, and if the accompanying theory of valuing just offered is adequate, then the addict acts akratically. He acts contrary to what he values, because he acts contrary to what he wants, and wanting is necessary for valuing given the desire-based view of reasons for action.

It is important to note a feature of Schroeder's position that might not be obvious. In saying that the dopamine signal represents the degree to which something is desired, Schroeder is not overlooking the evidence supportive of the claim that the dopamine signal represents the difference between expected and actual X associated with some object. Schroeder's idea is that the dopamine signal ordinarily covaries with two things: the difference between expected and actual X associated with an object, *and* the degree to which the reward system, when given a representation of the object as an input, causes the dopamine signal to go up. The dopamine signal covaries with the latter of these two things because, typically (although not when drugs of abuse are involved), the dopamine signal goes up *because* the reward system takes a representation of the object as an input and drives up the dopamine signal. Since the reward system's tendency to drive up the signal in response to a representation of the object is, under the Reward Theory of Desire, what it is to want something, Schroeder takes the dopamine signal to carry information about, or represent, the degree to which the object is desired.

To illustrate the point with an analogy, consider a camera that is used to take a photograph of an apple. The photograph represents the apple; but it also carries information about the camera. In particular, it will typically carry information about what kinds of representations the camera will produce when used in the normal way—namely, perspectival visual representations of those things at which its lens is pointed when the button is pressed. The photograph carries information of this sort because it is produced by the camera and has various properties—it is, in particular, a perspectival visual representation of that at which it was pointed when the button was pressed (namely, an apple). The dopamine signal represents the difference between actual and expected X associated with some object, but it also carries information about the reward system since it is typically created by the reward system. In particular, it carries information about how the reward system responds to certain kinds of inputs; and since what it is to desire something, Schroeder thinks, is for the reward system to respond in a certain way to certain kinds of inputs, it follows that the dopamine signal carries information about the organism's desires.

The analogy to the camera helps us to understand Schroeder's position, but it also helps us to see one of the problems with it. Imagine that I typically take pictures with a Nikon camera. I think the camera needs adjusting, so I bring a stack of pictures taken with it to the camera doctor so that he can diagnose the problem. Trouble is that I mistakenly include in the stack a picture of an apple taken with a different camera, a Canon. Does the picture taken with the Canon carry information about, or represent anything about, the Nikon? Of course not. The camera doctor might think it does because he thinks it was taken with the Nikon, but he's mistaken. Since the picture was taken with the Canon, it only carries information about the Canon, no matter what the camera doctor happens to think. Now consider the dopamine signal driven up directly by some drug of abuse. That signal is not the product of the reward system. Does it carry information about the reward system? No. In the first instance, it is a representation of the difference between actual and expected X analogously to the way in which the Canon photograph is a representation of an apple. We can grant that representations often carry information about the systems that created them. But since, according to Schroeder, it is not the reward system that created the dopamine signal when it is driven up directly by a drug of abuse, the signal does not, in such cases, carry information about the reward system. And, given the Reward Theory of Desire, it follows that the dopamine signal in such a case is not a representation of the subject's desire. But if the dopamine signal in such cases does not represent the subject as desiring its object, then nor does it *mis*represent that. Even when the dopamine signal is the product of a drug of abuse, the subject probably has representations of the degree to which he desires the object the signal represents, but the signal itself is not a representation of that desire.

While I believe that this is a problem with Schroeder's position—even given the Reward Theory of Desire, the dopamine signal is not a representation of the degree to which an object is desired when it is driven up directly by a drug of abuse—it is not a problem that interferes with the conclusion that interests us, namely, that addicts act akratically. So long as addicts really do act contrary to what they desire, then they act contrary to what they value; that conclusion can be reached without appeal to the claim that the dopamine signal in addicts represents the degree to which the object is desired. However, there is a more serious problem for Schroeder's position, and reflection on it suggests that his view fails to imply that addicts act akratically.

To see the problem, start by recalling that there is data supporting the idea that the effects of cues on the dopamine signal are found in heavy drug abusers even when they do not consume the drug. The amphetamine-addicted rats in Robinson and Berridge's experiments, for instance, press the lever for sugar much more frequently than unaddicted rats even when they are deprived of amphetamine. In such cases, the addicted rats would appear to represent the sugar—such a representation, after all, is what their perception of the tone causes in them—and then must suffer an increase in dopamine in response. Assuming that Schroeder wants to hold that the rats in such a case do not desire the sugar as much as they are moved to get it, he must hold that the effect of the representation of the sugar on the dopamine signal bypasses the reward system. He cannot hold, for instance, that the reward system is itself altered by heavy consumption of drugs resulting in an increase in the dopamine signal *caused by the reward system when a representation of sugar is given as an input.* If he were to hold that, then he would be holding that addicts actually want cued rewards more than nonaddicts want them, which is just what he hopes to deny. Why is this a problem for Schroeder? The reason is that to make this assertion is to overlook the most plausible explanation for the long-term effects of drugs of abuse on the dopamine signal.

We know that drugs of abuse drive up the dopamine signal directly. And, from independent experiments, we know that the dopamine signal encodes the difference between actual and expected X, where X is something more of which is better than less. But, further, we know from formal models of machine learning how a representation of the difference between actual and expected X helps an organism to learn: that representation *serves as an input* to the very system that generates expectations of the amount of X promised by a particular course of conduct. In other words, the representation of the degree to which the organism was mistaken last time in his expectation informs *his next expectation.* If he underestimated how much X a particular course of conduct promised last time, then, thanks to the fact that he has a representation of his degree of error, he will increase his estimate next time. The dopamine signal, that is, alters the way in which the reward system functions the next time it is fed a representation of the very thing that drove up the signal last time. But, if the Reward Theory of Desire is correct, it follows that the dopamine signal influences behavior *by* changing the organism's desires. The rat has a representation of amphetamine to come and expects it to promise a bit of pleasure. When he consumes it, the drug drives up the dopamine signal, which thereby represents the drug as actually yielding far more pleasure than it was expected to yield. Then, when the rat has a representation of amphetamine again, he uses this earlier dopamine signal to "learn" that he had it wrong last time, that he underestimated the amount of pleasure that amphetamine promised. The result is that his reward system responds with an expectation of a *greater* amount of pleasure. So, thanks to the way in which the drug drove up the dopamine signal, there has been a change in the way in which the reward system responds to a representation of the drug. It represents it now as more rewarding than it represented it as being prior to consuming it in the first instance. Thus, under the Reward Theory of Desire, the effect of the drug on the reward system has caused the organism *to want the drug*. So, when we appreciate the role that the dopamine signal plays in the reward system—it is an output now and an input tomorrow—we can see that under Schroeder's own theory of desire, the opposite conclusion from the one he reaches is the correct one. Things are just as we would have thought they were before any fancy theorizing: addicts want drugs and that's why they pursue them. Therefore, Schroeder's remarks ought not to lead us to think that addicts act akratically, even if we accept that all reasons for action derive from our desires.

LEGAL IMPLICATIONS

What lesson, if any, should the criminal law take from the fact that addicts do not act akratically? It is important, in thinking about this question, to separate the question of what should be done with addicts who commit crimes, generally, from the question of what should be done with addicts who commit *the crime of drug possession*. Although no shortage of addicts find themselves in trouble with the criminal law solely because they possess illegal drugs, there is also no shortage who, instead, commit other, independent crimes—sometimes violent crimes—solely so that they can feed their addictions. Possession of drugs is almost an intrinsic feature of addiction; what drug addict has never possessed drugs? And so, it can seem that when we criminally punish an addict for possession we are, in the end, merely punishing him for being an addict.

That is little different from punishment on the basis of status, a practice that is abhorrent. The point for our purposes, however, is this: whatever objections one might make to punishing addicts for possession are independent of the question of whether addicts are akratic. Criminal behavior performed in order to come into possession of drugs, or in order to make use possible, is importantly different from possession itself. Such behavior is not an intrinsic feature of addiction and punishment of it is not punishment for status. Still, it can seem as though the fact of addiction is relevant in such cases. Our question, then, is what the criminal courts should do with addicts who have committed crimes other than possession. Should the courts treat two people who do the same bad thing for the same reasons in the same circumstances differently when one, but not the other, is an addict? Compare, for instance, two people both of whom leave a young child in a very hot car for two hours so as to buy drugs from a dealer inside a nearby house. Should the fact that one is addicted, and the other merely wants the drugs for recreational use, matter to the assessment of their criminal responsibility for child endangerment? Does the fact that addicts are not akratic help us to answer questions of this kind?

To see how it helps, start with a distinction between two different kinds of reasons that might be given for less severe treatment of a defendant with feature F in comparison to a duplicate differing only in that he is not-F. First, we might claim that thanks to the fact that he is F the defendant lacked the power to comply with the law, or had a severely diminished ability to do so. A delusional and religious defendant who believes that God has ordered him to kill is capable of compliance with laws against murder only to the degree to which he is capable of mustering the courage and fortitude to defy a divine command. Alternatively, we might cite some burden that the defendant would bear, thanks to the fact that he is F, that made compliance with the law particularly costly for the defendant. A delusional defendant who believes that God will punish him severely if he does not kill would, he believes, have to bear such punishment were he to comply with laws against murder. Or, more prosaically, a defendant who robs a bank when the mob threatens to kill his child if he does not would, he believes, bear a severe burden—namely, the loss of his child's life—were he to comply with the law. Call features of defendants that ground an argument in their favor of the first sort "Can't factors" and features of the second sort "Can't-Be-Expected factors." To cite a Can't factor is to say that the defendant's path to compliance was blocked (or he believed it to be). To cite a Can't-Be-Expected factor is to say that the defendant's path to compliance would involve severe hardship on the defendant's part (or he believed it would) of a sort that he cannot be expected to suffer. As the two examples of delusional defendants with deific visions indicate, a single factor—for example, that the defendant has deific visions—might be a Can't factor or might be a

Can't-Be-Expected factor, depending on the details. The person who cites the factor, that is, might take it to be relevant because it diminishes or eliminates the defendant's power to comply or might take it to be relevant because it results in compliance involving severe burdens that the defendant should not be expected to bear in order to comply.

One set of Can't factors produce a mismatch between conduct and the defendant's values; they produce akrasia and do so inevitably. In such cases, what the agent cannot do is to guide his conduct in accordance with his values; something else determines what he does. Consider someone, for instance, who kills someone he loves while in a rage. What he does—namely, kill another—fails to align with what he values, we can imagine, even at the moment that he does it. But his rage takes over. In this case, the wanting system controls conduct thanks to the influence of emotion, and bypasses the valuing system. Thanks to his rage, that is, the agent is motivated to kill and does so, despite the fact that he does not value killing. We would need to know much more about the case before we could know whether the defendant's rage, understood as a Can't factor, actually diminishes responsibility. If the defendant is a hothead, then it does not; if he had a good reason for being so angry, then perhaps it does diminish responsibility, as under the law of manslaughter, even if it does not eliminate it entirely.[10] But the point for our purposes isn't whether such a factor diminishes responsibility; the point is that if it does so it does so in part because it inevitably induces akrasia: it causes conduct that is in violation of the law, is not valued by the agent, and in circumstances that make it impossible for the agent to have avoided akratic conduct.

So, what we learn from the fact that addicts are not akratic is that addiction is not this kind of Can't factor. Perhaps it is another kind. Nothing said here rules out that possibility. But it seems more likely that it is, instead, a Can't-Be-Expected factor. Addiction is relevant to responsibility, that is, because for addicts to comply with the law they must bear burdens that unaddicted duplicates need not bear, burdens that suffice to make it inappropriate, or less appropriate, to hold them responsible for bad behavior.

What burdens must they bear? As I want to briefly suggest, the fact that addicts are not akratic helps us to identify the particular burden that compliance with the law would require them to bear. The key is to recognize that addicts are inevitably subject to periods in which they will value violating the law over complying with it. When they are in such a state, *compliance with the law would require them to act contrary to the dictates of their valuing system.*

---

10. Under the *Model Penal Code*, for instance, a homicide is a manslaughter, rather than a murder, if it was performed "under extreme mental or emotional disturbance for which there is reasonable explanation or excuse" (*Model Penal Code* §210.3(b)).

The reason that they violate the law is, precisely, that they are built, as we all are, to avoid suffering this burden; we are built to, as much as possible, guide our conduct in accordance with our conception of our reasons for action. And a substantial burden it is, for part of what it is to be a fully functioning, autonomous adult is to act in accord with what one values. To have to give that up in order to comply with the law would be no less than to have to give up part of what makes one a citizen of a state equipped to be the target, not to mention the beneficiary, of exercises of state power.

Consider an example. D has a legal obligation to deliver his child to his former spouse by 3:00 PM on Saturday following his weekly court-approved visit. He's an addict and he's craving and he knows that if he drives himself and his child to his former spouse's home, he will come to judge that he has greater reason to stop to use than he has to deliver the child on time. The result will be that he will not deliver the child on time and will violate the law. What is he to do? Notice that he *can* comply with the law. He merely needs to ask a friend to drive. But if he asks a friend to drive, then during the course of the trip there will be a time when he is doing something—foregoing use—that he values less than the alternative. He can anticipate, that is, that compliance with the law will come with a price: akratic action. Now imagine that D does not ask the friend to drive and so violates the law. He stops for a hit and so delivers the child late, in line with his values at the time of use, although not in line with his values at earlier and later times. Is the fact that he is addicted relevant to his responsibility for this failure? The answer is yes. He should be treated less harshly than a nonaddict who is late because he stops for a hit. D, unlike the nonaddict, would suffer the burden of engaging in akratic conduct were he to take the path to compliance that was available to him (namely, having a friend drive). Now, we can debate how much of a break D warrants for his bad behavior given this burden—perhaps a great deal, perhaps very little—but the point is that it is that debate that we must have if we are to make progress on the question of the relevance of addiction to legal responsibility. The discovery that addicts are not akratic when they act badly helps us to see, then, what burdens they would need to bear in order to act as the law demands. Often, they would have to bear the burden of performing akratic, nonautonomous action; they would have to bear the burden of taking steps to bypass their own valuing systems and give control of their conduct over to something else. What exactly this *means*, in practice, about how addicts are to be treated under the criminal law is hard to say. To determine that we need a theory of the degree to which a burden associated with compliance ameliorates responsibility for noncompliance. Lacking such a theory, we must settle at this point for less: we now have a better idea of what question needs to be answered.

CONCLUSION

Our attitudes toward addicts are deeply ambivalent. To have an addicted friend, or family member, who (inevitably) acts badly and harmfully is to find oneself torn between the conception of his behavior as a symptom of a disease, on the one hand, and as a sign of distortions in his fundamental values, on the other. It is to be torn between pity and resentment. What has been suggested here is that both reactions are appropriate. Addicts should be resented for their bad behavior. The addict who hurts another to feed his addiction typically cares more, when he acts, about himself than he cares about the injury he inflicts. Addiction influences behavior not by bypassing what the addict cares about, but, instead, by influencing it and shaping it, at least over short periods of time—short, but long enough to lead to very bad behavior. This is one of the things that we learn when we recognize what the neuroscience of addiction, and particularly the influence of drugs of abuse on dopaminergic systems, means. Given what dopamine signals represent, what information they carry, we can deduce that drugs of abuse cause us to recognize greater reasons to use drugs than we recognize for promoting the things that we hold most dear most of the time. But, at the same time, to be subject to such distortions in one's values is a deep and terrible burden to bear, one that no one should have to bear in order to comply with the law. To be in such a condition is, indeed, to be worthy of pity and to be worthy also of some special consideration from the courts. We should not be ambivalent in our attitude toward addicts, vacillating between conflicting points of view. Instead, we should recognize that our conflicting attitudes have an equal and legitimate basis in addiction's nature.

ACKNOWLEDGMENTS

Thanks to Pamela Hieronymi, Neil Levy, and Walter Sinnott-Armstrong for comments on earlier drafts.

11

Addiction and Blameworthiness

TIMOTHY SCHROEDER AND NOMY ARPALY

In David Carr's addiction memoire, *The Night of the Gun*, there is the story of how, late one cold November night in Minneapolis, Carr put his infant twin girls into snowsuits, bundled them into his car, and drove to a house that specialized in dealing cocaine for intravenous use.

> I could not bear to leave them home, but I was equally unable to stay put, to do the right thing. So here we were, one big, happy family, parked outside the dope house. It was late, past midnight.
>
> Then came the junkie math; addled moral calculation woven with towering need. If I went inside the house, I could get what I needed, or very much wanted. Five minutes, ten minutes tops.... .
>
> Sitting there in the gloom of the front seat, the car making settling noises against the chill, the math still loomed. Need. Danger. A sudden tumbling? Naw. Nothing to it, really. In that pool of darkness, I decided that my teeny twin girls would be safe. It was cold, but not *really* cold. Surely God would look after them while I did not.[1]

Carr ends up leaving the girls in the car for hours; when he returns they are still alive, sleeping peacefully. Though he gets lucky, it is obvious that his leaving them was a terrible act. Any theory of moral blameworthiness should agree, with Carr himself, that he is to blame for what he did. At the same time, it needs to be acknowledged that what Carr did happened because of his addiction

---

1. Carr (2008, chapter 28).

to cocaine. Back when he was familiar with the pleasures of cocaine but not addicted, he would not have acted in this way.

It has seemed to many that the addict's blameworthiness for acts like Carr's is mitigated by the fact that he is addicted: that addiction, specifically, mitigates blameworthiness for bad acts. If Carr had been a big fan of the Minnesota Vikings football team, and had abandoned his infant daughters in the car on an equally cold night in order to use a free ticket to watch the Vikings play, he would seem far worse. There is something special about addiction that is different from having strong desires in general. At the same time, it appears that the blameworthiness of addicts for the bad things they do because of addiction is only mitigated, not eliminated. Addicts can stop using (many do, eventually), and when faced with opportunities to do what is wrong many of them do not do what is wrong on many occasions, even to service their addictions. So there is no reason to think of addicts as subject to irresistible compulsions. And because there is not, it seems (to many addicts and many observers) that there is room for blame on many occasions.[2]

To give a systematic account of why this response to the blameworthiness of addicts is warranted requires both a theory of blameworthiness and a theory of addiction. We offer both.

BLAMEWORTHINESS

To be blameworthy for an action is, not surprisingly, to warrant blame for it. For one to be blameworthy is thus for an attitude of blame to be appropriate or justified given what one has done and why one has done it.

To be blameworthy for an action is not the same thing as others having moral license or an obligation to condemn, censure, shun, or otherwise punish the blameworthy person. In the first instance, this is because blaming someone is a matter of holding an attitude toward the person and what he has done, not taking an action: blaming Hitler for the war requires only an attitude, not a denunciation. In the second instance, blameworthiness is not being a licensed or obligatory object of punishment because it is conceivable that someone not be a licensed or obligatory object of punishment while still being blameworthy. Perhaps condemnation of Hitler for his role in the war would have been impermissible for someone on a given occasion because of

---

2. Some philosophical theories leave the addict with no blameworthiness at all for bad acts carried out in service of the addiction, or no blameworthiness so long as they are appropriately distanced from their addictions (as with Frankfurt's unwilling addict; Frankfurt 1971). We obviously disagree, but for this paper will just presuppose that Carr is blameworthy for some of what he does (and by extension that all addicts are), rather than argue for this.

Hitler's likely reaction; even if so, Hitler would have been blameworthy on that occasion.[3]

What, then, is it to be worthy of blame? As we argue elsewhere,[4] to be blameworthy for an action is to act badly as an expression of one's ill will or one's moral indifference.

Ill will: an intrinsic desire for that which is wrong or bad.[5] Ill will is greater the stronger the desire.

Moral indifference: a lack of an intrinsic desire for that which is right or good. The weaker the desire for the right or good, the greater the moral indifference.

Blameworthiness: To be blameworthy for a wrong or bad action A is to do A out of ill will or moral indifference. All else being equal, one is more blameworthy the more ill will one's act expresses, or the more moral indifference one's act expresses.

We will not repeat our defense of these claims here, but a little clarification is in order. We use the phrase "that which is wrong or bad" to refer to the substantive content of the correct normative theory, whatever that turns out to be.[6] If Millian utilitarianism is correct, then what is wrong or bad is that overall happiness decrease. If Kantian deontology is correct, then what is wrong or bad is that people be treated as mere means to ends. And so on. Thus, being morally indifferent (for example) is a matter of having a particularly weak intrinsic desire that people be happy (if Millian utilitarianism is correct), or having a particularly weak intrinsic desire that people be treated as ends in themselves (if Kantian deontology is correct), and so on.

To act out of ill will is for one's ill will to be the cause of the action in the ordinary manner[7] in which intrinsic desires cause actions along with instrumental beliefs. To say something cruel in order to make a rival feel bad is a paradigmatic

<hr/>

3. See Arpaly (2000) for a fuller argument.

4. Arpaly (2002, 2003); Arpaly and Schroeder (in preparation).

5. What is sometimes called what is wrong or bad "*de re*," though we think this is a somewhat misleading use of jargon from the philosophy of language; see Smith (1994). We clarify the idea below.

6. Obviously, we presuppose that there is a correct normative theory. This is not much of a presupposition—it is compatible with cultural relativism about morality, Moorean realism, and everything in between—but it does presuppose the falsity of expressivism.

7. We here assume that there is some adequate causal theory of action. We contribute to such a theory in Arpaly (2006) and Arpaly and Schroeder (in preparation).

way in which one can act out of ill will: one intrinsically desires the misery of the rival and sees that particular words will cause misery in the rival, and so one says the words. But moral indifference is a little different, because moral indifference is a matter of an absence. To act out of moral indifference is for one's moral indifference to be an important part of the cause (or, if absences cannot cause, then causal explanation) of one's action.[8] Of course, if that action involves anything other than limply lying still, there will be some other desire that is also an important part of the cause and explanation of one's action. But this need not preclude appeal to the absence of a strong moral desire as well. To sell a mortgage that will almost certainly become unpayable in three years to a very unsophisticated buyer, just to earn a commission, is a paradigmatic way in which one can act, in part out of a desire for enrichment, but also in part out of moral indifference—because, had one cared more about people's happiness, or treating them as ends, one would not have sold the mortgage under those conditions.

One other point of clarification: we assume that when figuring out how much a person cares about something we look at her preference ranking; that is, we turn to the question of what the person cares about *more*. Caring about money more than about morality is a bad thing even if one's concern for morality seems quite strong overall. Thus, on our view, the mortgage dealer mentioned above who is accused of moral indifference cannot defend himself by saying, however truly, "I'm not morally indifferent because my concern for morality is very strong, it's just that my desire for money is even stronger." Prioritizing money over what is moral is the very nature of (some degree of) moral indifference.

Return now to David Carr's story of leaving his infant daughters alone in a car (at night, in a Minnesota winter) in order to use cocaine intravenously. It seems obvious that Carr is blameworthy for doing so, and our theory of blameworthiness agrees. An intrinsic desire to use cocaine, or to have a particular experience characteristic of cocaine use, is Carr's main positive motivation to go into the house. This desire is not (we take it) for something that is necessarily contra-moral; it is not a form of ill will. There are possible situations in which the satisfaction of this desire is entirely morally permissible. However, in leaving his daughters behind and entering the house, Carr acts wrongly. And he acts wrongly because of a deficiency of moral concern: he does not desire his daughters' happiness, or their treatment as ends in themselves, as much as he might, and his deficiency is part of the explanation of why he acts

---

8. Again: the moral indifference must be a cause of behavior in the ordinary way in which not desiring things leads us to act indifferently to them, as when Tim's indifference to the music of a pop singer is part of the cause of his discarding a flyer about a coming performance. We again assume that there is an adequate account of what this amounts to, though we defend the idea in Arpaly and Schroeder (in preparation).

wrongly. Had he cared enough, he would not have left his daughters behind in order to consume cocaine. Hence Carr displays moral indifference, and is blameworthy.[9]

Our difficulty in discussing the case comes in accounting for the fact that addiction is a mitigating factor when considering Carr's blameworthiness. Yes, Carr demonstrates a certain amount of indifference to something of tremendous moral importance, but he would not have abandoned his daughters in order to see the Minnesota Vikings play football, or to finish work that might be important for his career. His addiction is something that has a special hold upon him, and in assessing the way in which he is blameworthy the addiction should be recognized. Within our theory of moral blameworthiness, however, doing so appears to be difficult. Our theory is focused entirely on the intrinsic desires of people who are blameworthy. Do they intrinsically desire what is right or good, or are they conatively indifferent to it? This is the only question the theory asks about people like Carr. It does not ask about the origin of his desire for cocaine,[10] it does not ask about the ease with which he might resist his desire,[11] it does not ask about his attitude toward his desire for cocaine[12]—it does not, in other words, take into consideration the various facts that other desire-friendly moral psychologists have appealed to in explaining what is special about people who do what is wrong because they are addicts. As a consequence, our theory appears unable to make a distinction between the case of David Carr and the case of the imaginary fan of the Minnesota Vikings who faces a parallel situation and who makes the parallel choice. The fan who leaves his infant children alone in the cold car in order to see some football—who does so with as clear a vision of the stakes as Carr seems to have—strikes us as horrifyingly indifferent to his children's fate. His moral indifference is grotesque: he is willing to leave his children to risk death by exposure just in order to watch a football game. And because he is not (by stipulation) an addict or otherwise psychologically disturbed with respect to his enthusiasm for the Vikings, he has no excuse for his behavior, not even a partial excuse. Carr deserves a partial excuse, because his behavior is driven by addiction, while the fan of the Vikings does not. But if we look only at the desires that explain their actions, it is hard to see how a principled difference could be found from within our theoretical perspective. Carr seems to desire cocaine much more than he desires what he ought regarding

9. Perhaps Carr is also blameworthy for being indifferent to the law, or to the enrichment of criminals, but we set these issues to one side. They complicate, but do not fundamentally change, the assessment of Carr's blameworthiness.

10. E.g., Fischer and Ravizza (1998).

11. E.g., Fischer and Ravizza (1998).

12. E.g., Frankfurt (1971).

his daughters, and from our perspective this would seem to make him just the same as the football fan who desires to see football much more than he desires what he ought regarding his daughters.

What our theory needs is for the fact of Carr's addiction to make a difference to his desires, and so to the verdict of moral indifference. This needs to be a difference that distinguishes Carr from the fan of the Vikings who performs parallel acts because he really wants to see his team play and does not much care about his daughters' lives. But this cannot be found within our theory of blameworthiness. If it is to be found anywhere, it will be in the theory of addiction. And so we now turn to addiction.

THE SCIENCE OF ADDICTION

Early research on addiction in human beings focused on phenomena such as dependency, withdrawal, and tolerance.[13] However, in more recent years scientific thought has been redirected toward other phenomena.[14] A striking fact about addiction is that the condition persists even once use has stopped, dependency has ended, withdrawal is over, and tolerance is gone. The abstinent addict who has ceased to show these signs of addiction nonetheless remains extremely vulnerable to poor decisions to return to using the addictive good, and this vulnerability decreases only very slowly as abstinence continues over the years.[15]

If addiction were to end with the end of withdrawal or the like, then the treatment of addiction would be a simple matter: hospitalize people until their withdrawal symptoms end, and then send them off cured.[16] As recognition has grown that this is not a successful method of treating addiction, theoretical work on the nature of addiction has come to focus on the condition that exists both in actively using addicts and in abstinent addicts. This work is on addiction itself.

Research on addiction has come to focus on the way that addictive goods "hijack"[17] the brain's reward system. This hijacking affects the reward system

---

13. This can be seen in, e.g., the lingering focus on these issues in the psychiatric diagnostic criteria for addiction-type disorders in the *Diagnostic and Statistical Manual of Mental Disorders*, and is commented on in Hyman (2005).

14. Representative scientific papers illustrating this include Robinson and Berridge (2002), Hyman (2005), and Schultz (2011).

15. One nice discussion of the theoretical importance of the abstinent addict is found in Gjelsvik (1999).

16. This point is made succinctly by Hyman (2005, 1414), whom we paraphrase here.

17. We take this apt expression from a philosophical work written in response to the neuroscience: Elster (1999), but it can also be found in use by scientists, e.g., in the abstract for Schultz (2011).

in a way that other, nonaddictive, goods do not. There are long-term effects of this hijacking, and several have been identified as central to the persistence of addiction beyond withdrawal and into even prolonged abstinence. We will say a little about this research on its own terms in this section. In the next, we will consider what it means for a philosophical theory of addiction.

To understand the science of addiction, we begin with the reward system.[18] The brain contains a small collection of nerve cells (found deep in the brain, near the top of the brainstem) that are distinctive in that they release dopamine when they fire.[19] Normally, this dopamine is released in a light, steady trickle, but there can be surges in the release of dopamine, and its release can also drop off to nothing. The dopamine released in these ways reaches many different parts of the brain, but it is particularly influential on parts of the brain that realize the experience of pleasure and parts of the brain that directly control behavior.[20]

The brain's reward system has been thought of as a pleasure system,[21] a motivational system,[22] and even an attention-for-action system,[23] but in our view (and that of many scientists) the best way to think about the reward system is that it is, in itself, a learning system.[24] Dopamine release causes a specific form of unconscious associative learning known as "reward learning," in which the ability of one mental event to cause another is increased when one instance of the first mental event causing the second is immediately followed by an increase in the amount of dopamine received.[25] So, for example, if perception of a light

18. Another valuable discussion of the neuroscience of the reward system and addiction—one that is perhaps more accessible to philosophers than some others, while still being more technical than what follows—can be found in Gardner and David (1999). Other discussions of the reward system by philosophers—to more conventionally philosophical ends—can be found in Morillo (1990) and Schroeder (2004). This section and the next receive an extended treatment on their own in Schroeder (2010).

19. These are the cells of the ventral tegmental area and the substantia nigra, pars compacta. See, e.g., Kandel, Schwartz, and Jessell (2000) for an overview.

20. See, e.g., Kandel, Jessell, and Schwartz (2000) for the textbook basics. An extended discussion of this idea can be found in Schroeder (2004, ch. 2).

21. Morillo (1990), though a philosophical work, makes the best case for this position based on scientific evidence.

22. See the discussion of the reward system in Robinson and Berridge (2002), for example.

23. Berridge and Robinson (1998).

24. For our full argument to this effect, see Schroeder (2004, ch. 2). For key experiments, see Romo and Schultz (1990), Schultz and Romo (1990), and Bao, Chan, and Merzenich (2001). Theoretical papers sharing this position include Schultz, Dayan, and Montague (1997); Dayan, Montague, and Sejnowski (1996); and many of the papers in Houk, Davis, and Beiser (1995).

25. A lucid scientific presentation of reward learning can be found in White and Milner (1992).

coming on (mental event one) causes a rat to attempt to press a lever (mental event two), and that causal sequence is immediately followed by an increase in the dopamine received (perhaps because some food appeared, and perception of the food triggered an increase in dopamine release), then the causal power of the perception of a light coming on to cause the specific action to be attempted—the pressing of the lever—will be increased. The rat will become more likely to attempt to press that sort of lever when that sort of light is on in the future, and to attempt to press the lever just because the light is on—no further inference required (in whatever sense rats are capable of inference). It is from processes like these that behavioral inclinations and habits can be built.[26]

The above example, with its behavioristic cast, is much too simple to convey the whole range of effects of reward learning. Distinct perceptual events can change how they influence each other through reward learning,[27] and there is strong evidence that spontaneous thought dispositions[28] and problem-solving techniques[29] are also changed through reward learning, not to mention preferences.[30] The effects of reward learning are widespread throughout our minds.[31]

Ordinarily, increases in the release of dopamine are generated by perceiving and thinking about the world. A monkey perceiving a burst of sweet juice in its mouth has an increase of dopamine release in its brain,[32] and a human being who realizes that she will be getting money for what she has just done in an experiment also has an increase in the dopamine released in her brain.[33] Dopamine has been shown to increase its release in human beings in response to listening to favored music,[34] seeing an image of a loved person,[35] understanding that one is being cooperated with in a prisoner's dilemma–type

26. See, e.g., Knowlton, Mangels, and Squire (1996).

27. Bao, Chan, and Merzenich (2001).

28. Greenspoon (1955).

29. Saint-Cyr, Taylor, and Lang (1988).

30. Johnsrude et al. (1999).

31. If nothing else, the mere fact that there are dopamine receptors throughout an enormous part of the brain must render this true. On the distribution of neurons disposed to react specifically to reception of dopamine, see, e.g., Kandel, Schwartz, and Jessell (2000).

32. Schultz and Romo (1990). It should be noted that, of all the findings described in this list, this is the only very direct observation; for the rest the finding that it is dopamine release that is being observed is more inferential. But the inferences have been widely accepted within neuroscience.

33. Knutson et al. (2001).

34. Salimpoor et al. (2011).

35. Aron et al. (2005).

situation,[36] and many other things. It is also known to increase when hungry animals receive food and thirsty animals receive water.[37]

As might be suggested by these examples, not every perception or cognition produces an increase in dopamine release. Only things that are, intuitively, "positive" generate increases in dopamine release when they are perceived and thought about. A monkey seeing that the wind is stirring the leaves on a tree will not experience a change in dopamine release, nor will an ordinary person who sees that a blue car has just gone by on the street. A monkey deprived of some expected juice actually has a drop in dopamine release when it perceives that the expected juice has not arrived.[38] And so on. That is, "neutral" and "negative" events do not promote reward learning. Only "positive" events do—normally.

What is special about addictive drugs is that they all promote dopamine release, or promote dopamine reception, or simulate the immediate effects of dopamine release. And they do this independently of perception and cognition. They work directly on the dopamine-releasing cells, or on other neurons that are directly connected to these cells. This is where the metaphor of hijacking comes from. There is a normal process by which dopamine release leads to reward learning, and that process goes via perceiving or conceiving things that have come (through natural development or through learning) to be promoters of dopamine release—that have come to be "positive" things. The "positive" thing is perceived or grasped cognitively, and then under certain conditions there is an increase in dopamine release, leading to the characteristic sort of unconscious learning. Addictive drugs circumvent this process. They promote unconscious learning and all of its consequences, regardless of how their use is perceived or conceived. A person who hates Imelda will not have dopamine release promoted in her by seeing Imelda. But a person who hates cocaine in just the same way, with just the same neural connections between the idea of cocaine and the reward system as her counterpart has between the idea of Imelda and the reward system, will nonetheless get a strong surge of dopamine-type effects if that person consumes cocaine. This is the way in which addictive drugs hijack the reward system.[39]

36. Rilling et al. (2002).

37. See, e.g., Stellar and Stellar (1985).

38. Schultz and Romo (1990).

39. It should be noted that different addictive drugs fit this pattern more or less well. The connection between cocaine, amphetamines, and MDMA ("ecstasy") is all much as one would think from the above description. The route by which opiates (including heroin) affect the reward system appears to be a little more indirect, and perhaps also involves a hijacking of a

It might be imagined that the foregoing makes a key mistake, that of neglect-ing the role of pleasure. While cocaine is not "positive" for some addicts, plea-sure is "positive" for everyone. Since cocaine use induces pleasure (and so, too, for other addictive drugs), perhaps it is true that cocaine simply produces something that is very "positive"—pleasure—and then the pleasure is respon-sible for a powerful release of dopamine, and so a great deal of reward learn-ing, and motivation, and so on. However, this would be to misunderstand the causal sequence. Dopamine release is a direct cause of pleasure,[40] and drugs such as cocaine are direct causes of increased dopamine release, reception, or other effects very closely linked to dopamine release. Thus, the drugs cause the dopamine-related events that cause pleasure; the dopamine comes first, and the pleasure comes second.[41]

Cocaine and other addictive drugs thus stimulate the same effects as things that are naturally very "positive"—sporting victories, trips to Hawaii, finally winning the love of one's beloved—regardless of how "positive" one's attitude toward the drugs themselves. This is a key step in explaining addiction. This is the hijacking.

In and of itself, hijacking is not sufficient to explain addiction. People can feel and act as though they very much want trips to Hawaii without feeling and act-ing as though they are addicted to trips to Hawaii. Why is it that the immediate effects of cocaine, which are like the immediate effects of going to Hawaii, lead to addiction?

To understand what is most distinctive about addictive drugs, it is neces-sary to understand a few more details of the unconscious learning brought about by increases in dopamine release. The key fact is this: dopamine release is not increased every time one perceives or thinks of getting something that is "positive" for one—every time one perceives or thinks of a "positive" thing. Dopamine release is sensitive to not only what is perceived or thought but also

---

parallel punishment system, though this has not been substantiated. Nicotine, alcohol, and THC (marijuana's active ingredient) have all been demonstrated to have purely chemical effects on the reward system (i.e., not mediated by perception or cognition of one's ingestion of these compounds), but the ways in which these effects are related to addiction appear to require fur-ther study. At this point, however, scientists generally hold out hopes for reward system–based explanations of addictions to all these substances.

40. Not, however, the only one. See Berridge (2003) and Berridge and Robinson (1998).

41. Interestingly, this same pattern holds in a nonpathological way for sweet tastes and other sensuous pleasures. That is, perception of the sensuous state (this taste, that odor, the other sound) is such that it does or does not stimulate dopamine release, and the dopamine release then causes learning, motivational, hedonic, and attentional effects. So it is not the pleasure of sweet tastes that makes us pursue them; it is their being wanted that makes us pursue them, and getting what we want is what makes us pleased. This is argued for in Schroeder (2004, ch. 3).

to the extent to which one is jaded or hardened with respect to a given experience: the extent to which one takes it for granted. Perceiving or thinking that one might or will get a grade of A, when one is not jaded, can increase dopamine release in a way that reflects how "positive" an event this is for the student. Perceiving or thinking that one might or will get an A, when one is jaded about getting A's, does not increase dopamine release even when the A is very "positive" for the student in question (that the A is still "positive" can be seen in the fact that getting an A– when an A is expected will result in a drop of dopamine release for the student).

Scientists describe this state of being jaded regarding "positive" things, and being hardened against "negative" things, as a matter of what is called "prediction," as found in the term "prediction error"—the difference between what was actual at a given moment and what was predicted for that moment. But this is prediction in a very technical sense: prediction, not at a conscious level or as a matter of rational belief, but at an unconscious level not sensitive to an agent's full information—at the level, that is, at which one becomes jaded to the "positive" things in life ("I knew I would get an A, so why would I get excited?") and at which one becomes hardened to the "negative" things in life ("I never expected to get an A, so why should I be disappointed?").

The way in which unconscious prediction features in generating an increase in dopamine release is worth illustrating. In a well-known experiment that is the foundation of recent work on the brain's reward system, a monkey was given a sip of sweet juice one second after a light turned on.[42] Initially, the turning on of the light had no effect on the monkey, but the arrival of the juice had a strong effect, and greatly increased the release of dopamine (for a moment; the effect is in general a very short-term one). As the light continued to be paired, after a one-second delay, with the juice, the release of dopamine started to change in the monkey. Soon the turning on of the light caused the same strong increase in dopamine release that the juice had initially, while the juice itself caused no change in dopamine release. The monkey had come to predict (unconsciously) that the juice would follow one second after the light. Now it was the light that brought the news, the unpredicted information, that something "positive" (the juice) was to happen; the juice itself added nothing unpredicted: the monkey "took for granted" that there would be juice one second after the light came on. Finally, the experimenters turned on the light but did not deliver any juice. When the light was perceived dopamine release increased in the monkey's brain. One second later, when the unconsciously predicted juice was not received, dopamine release in the monkey dramatically *decreased*. The absence

42. See Schultz and Romo (1990) and Romo and Schultz (1990), published back to back, which brought a new level of precision and insight to research on dopamine and reward learning.

of what was "taken for granted" caused a drop in reward signaling, which is (in terms of unconscious learning) a form of punishment.

These experiments demonstrate a pattern that conforms to what would be expected on a theoretical basis from a system that implements reward-based learning. From a theoretical perspective, a reward learning system should calculate the difference between how "positive" the world appears to be at present and how "positive" the world was, a moment ago, predicted to be at present. And it should then broadcast the difference between these values as its learning signal: an increase when what seems actual is more "positive" than predicted, no increase when what seems actual is just as "positive" as predicted, and a decrease when what seems actual is less "positive" than predicted.[43]

The reason to have a reward learning signal express only the difference between what is actual and what is unconsciously predicted is illuminating: it is required to prevent overlearning of connections between kinds of mental events. Imagine a creature that gets water when it performs a certain action under certain conditions. The first time the creature performs the action, its getting water is unpredicted, and so it undergoes some reward learning and its propensity to perform the action under the conditions will go up. But at a certain point, the action will be bringing about the predicted result—getting water—when it is performed under the relevant conditions. When this point is reached, it would actually be harmful to continue the behavioral learning further. At this point, further behavioral learning will make the action more and more likely to be performed under the certain conditions, even though all that will be gained is a set amount of water. As this disposition to take this one action increases in strength, the creature will lose the ability to look for food, explore, or flee predators under the water-related conditions, because its behavior will be totally dominated by the tendency, when in those conditions, to perform the water-securing action. The creature will have overlearned, have become excessively likely to perform one action, because its unconscious link between perceiving the conditions and performing that action was forced to grow stronger and stronger without limit.

What goes for our imagined creature goes also for human beings. Suppose that for Tim it is "positive" that his father be healthy. If every occasion on which Tim asked after his father's health, and on which he received the "positive" news, were an occasion on which he would undergo unconscious reward learning, then soon he would do little other than ask after his father's health (so long as that health remained good). Regardless of what else Tim could be doing, the power of his idea of asking after his father's health to cause that action—asking

---

43. The difference between these two values is commonly called the error in reward prediction. See, e.g., many of the essays in Houk, Davis, and Beiser (1995).

after his health—would be so great that whenever Tim thought of his father's health he would be very unlikely to do anything other than ask after it. And since many things can make Tim think of his father's health, many things would lead to this particular behavior. Tim's day would be dominated by asking after his father's health. It is for this sort of reason that there are natural limits to reward learning, implemented through unconscious prediction of "positive" and "negative" events.

Return now to addictive drugs. Because they hijack the reward system, addictive drugs can keep producing powerful reward learning effects long after trips to Hawaii, sips of water, news of good familial health, and the like would have produced weaker reward signals and eventually stopped producing them at all. Because these drugs hijack the reward system, the reward system always reacts to them as though more "positive" things happened than were unconsciously predicted—no matter how "positive" the unconscious prediction system was predicting consumption of the addictive drug to be. The result is very close to the above-imagined scenarios in which nothing can shut off the reward learning caused by one kind of event.[44] The result of consuming addictive drugs is that they generate reward learning in a pattern that would only be appropriate if addictive drugs were infinitely "positive"—if, no matter how "positive" the reward system predicted cocaine consumption to be, cocaine consumption would be more "positive" than that. This is the source of the problems. The natural activators of the reward system slowly diminish in their power to generate more reward learning; the hijackers of the reward system never do, because they circumvent the normal process by which a reward signal is generated.

The immediate effects of a sharp increase in dopamine release are, most saliently, pleasure and motivation (to do what seems needed to secure the "positive" thing, if there is something still to be done; if not, then the motivation might be expressed by just bouncing around excitedly, talking a mile a minute, and so on). These effects, in themselves, would not have to be problematic. After the health scare, Tim will at first be pleased and motivated by news that his father's health is improving, but eventually (with luck) he will come to take it for granted again, and this sort of news will not be particularly pleasing or motivating. But it would not be a disaster for Tim if he continued to get pleasure from this news every time, and to find it invigorating (both an impetus to maintain that good health, when possible, and to just bounce along excitedly when not). The characteristic effect of addictive drugs is that one never becomes jaded to their effects, because they cause these effects by hijacking the

44. It appears that the brain has some mechanisms that adapt, to some extent, to the continually overpowering reward learning generated by the addictive drugs—but this amounts to only weak resistance to the effects of the hijacking. Some tolerance effects would be an example of the action of such mechanisms.

reward system. But in itself, this would not have to be any more problematic than Tim never taking his father's health for granted. But of course, the problems quickly begin to accumulate.

The problem is that the immediate effects of an increase in dopamine release—the pleasure and motivation—are accompanied by a long-term effect on unconscious learning. And this long-term effect on learning appears to be the main source of the central phenomena of addiction—the phenomena in common between addicts who are still using and abstinent addicts, and also between people who wholeheartedly hate the drugs they abuse and people who wholeheartedly love these same drugs.[45]

The first important effect caused by the runaway reward learning that addictive drugs induce is an effect on unconscious behavioral dispositions—on habits and their relatives. Habits and related unthinking behavioral tendencies appear to be realized in a region of the brain that is crucial in action production, and that is an important recipient of dopamine. Runaway reward learning induces increasingly strong habits and related unthinking behavioral dispositions. Long-time smokers often report smoking cigarettes unthinkingly, even when they have already consumed so much nicotine that more nicotine will make them feel ill. This appears to be the result of the strong habits and habit-like behavioral dispositions inculcated through the effects of reward learning upon the smoker.

It is easy to denigrate the importance of habits. After all, it seems easy enough to override habits when one is paying attention. But this is a mistake. For one thing, it is possible to exaggerate how easy it is to override habits. For some habits, it only takes a little attention to override them, but for others it can be extremely difficult to do so. An informant reports to us an experience of being trained to throw grenades in the Israeli armed forces. An important part of grenade-throwing technique is to not watch whether the grenade falls where one has thrown it, since this leaves the thrower open to injury. Trainees were lined up with mock grenades, and required to take turns lobbing the mock grenades at mock targets. A menacing instructor stood over the trainees and threatened to hit them with a stick if they should watch where the mock grenades fell. And many trainees were struck on the first try. Our informant reports that he focused his mind on the task, so that he would not be humiliated or hit with the stick when his turn came—but, sure enough, when his turn came he threw his grenade, watched it fly, and got hit with the stick.

For another, it is possible to exaggerate how easy it is to pay attention to whether or not one is acting on an unfortunate habit at any given moment. It can be easy enough for a drug addict to not use the drug on any one given occasion,

45. To pick up a Frankfurtean theme (Frankfurt 1971).

but abstinence requires not using the drug on every occasion. And insofar as not using requires not being subject to temptation, abstinence also requires never going anywhere out of habit, never talking to anyone out of habit, never agreeing to do something out of habit—if doing so might lead to temptation. People rely on their unconscious behavioral dispositions to guide them successfully through the day; we do not constantly monitor ourselves. But many of a would-be abstinent addict's unconscious behavioral dispositions have become untrustworthy, and these actions need to be monitored, or the abstinent addict will do things without thinking about them at the time, only to find a difficult situation arising. "Why did I agree to go to that party where everyone will be using?" "Why did I turn down this street that leads me close to the dealers, and not down the next street?" "Why did I end up calling my old drug buddy when I was bored?" Questions like these are often answered by an addict's unconscious behavioral tendencies. While we all have these tendencies, in the addict the effect of the addictive drug has been to strengthen them out of all proportion to what one would expect.[46]

The second important effect caused by the runaway reward learning induced by addictive drugs is the effect on the unconscious prediction system. The unconscious prediction system has the job of predicting how "positive" the world will look in a moment. Because addictive goods induce runaway reward learning in this system, the system responds to perceptual and cognitive signs of coming cocaine (or whatever the addictive drug of choice might be) by predict-ing that the world will look enormously "positive" soon. If the addict consumes the addictive drug, then the predicted "positive" nature of the next moment is apparently confirmed (and exceeded) given how the reward system responds to the drug. But suppose the addict does not consume the drug. There will be a sudden drop in the release of dopamine: the predicted "positive" feature of the next moment is missing. This affects the addict's feelings and motivations in just the way having any "positive" thing snatched from a person would affect her. The addict feels tremendously denied, restless, motivated to find some way to recapture the predicted "positive" event.

It might be thought that this problem of absent but unconsciously predicted "positive" events would be restricted to situations in which the addictive drug

---

46. Though the above examples are all behavioral, it is also important to note that we also have habits of thought, and there is the above-cited evidence that dopamine release, and so reward learning, is important to shaping habits of thought just as it is important to shaping habits of action (e.g., Greenspoon 1955; Saint-Cyr, Taylor, and Lang 1988). We are not aware of the effect being documented in addicts, but we would not be surprised to learn that Carr's "junkie math" was influenced by habits of considering certain things, rehearsing certain excuses, avoiding thinking about things in terms likely to lead to not using, and so on, mental habits developed and powerfully reinforced by prolonged cocaine use—or that Carr's case generalizes to that of many addicts.

is right in front of the addict but not consumed. But the unconscious predictive system, though not tied to the sorts of evidence recognized in conscious reasoning, is still much more sophisticated than this. Just as a light came to be a predictor of juice for a monkey, so too do things associated with addictive drugs come to be predictors of the "positive" event, the acquisition of the drug. Anything substantially statistically associated with the addictive drug should come to cause unconscious prediction of drug acquisition, given what is known about the unconscious predictive system. The abstinent addict who can talk to an old friend who was also a drug buddy will, on seeing the old friend or thinking about the opportunity to talk to her, unconsciously predict a coming "positive" event, consumption of the addictive drug, and feel motivated to reach out. To go on to talk to the friend keeps the world looking as good as predicted (it unconsciously "looks" like the addictive drug is still coming), but to not talk to the friend feels disappointing, demotivating, and like a problem in need of a solution. It does so because this is how it feels when one experiences a sudden drop in dopamine release generated by suddenly abandoning an unconsciously predicted "positive" event. Thus, the addict feels good about talking to the old drug buddy, and motivated to do so, and actions to prevent this interaction feel bad and induce motivation to find some way around this decision. Under these circumstances, it is no surprise that abstinent addicts often unwisely get in touch with old drug buddies, even before habits are taken into account. And what goes for talking to friends goes also for visiting old hangouts, listening to music that is strongly drug associated, going to drug-associated sorts of events, and so on.

Additionally, all of these effects can be generated (probably, to a lesser degree) by mere perception or cognition of things that are merely fictional or imaginary instances of things associated with addictive drug consumption. Watching someone pretend to inhale cocaine on television is something that elicits strong feelings in cocaine addicts, even though the act is known to be fictional and even though there is no change in the availability of cocaine.[47] The unconscious prediction system does not seem to typically make sophisticated discriminations between what is merely depicted or imagined and what is real. As a result, the effects on feelings and motivations that can be generated by the presence of the addictive drug, or a friend or a place associated with that drug, can also be generated (perhaps more weakly) by pictures of these things, people, and places; by talking about them; by seeing films and television programs reminiscent of them; and so on. For the abstinent addict, these feelings and motivations are often just around the corner. And because the immediate trigger need only be something associated with the addictive drug, it need not be obvious to the

47. One experiment relying on this effect is Berger et al. (1996).

addict what the ultimate source is of her longing to talk to this person, or of her disappointment at missing that event, or the like.

The effects just described are sometimes called "cravings" or "cue-conditioned cravings" by scientists working on addiction.[48] Cravings (in this literature) are negative feelings experienced when an addict is exposed to cues—things and images of things—associated with past consumption of addictive drugs. While anything one imagines having but is denied can cause a craving in the ordinary sense of the term, drug addicts are particularly vulnerable—because of the runaway reward learning to which they have been subjected—to particularly strong and persistent cravings felt in the presence of even modest cues associated with former addictive drug use. Cue-conditioned cravings in addicts are associated with motivations to consume the addictive good, or take steps (not necessarily regarded as such) toward such consumption.

The generation of powerful behavioral tendencies and habits, on the one hand, and powerful cravings, on the other, are two effects generated by the runaway reward learning generated by addictive drugs. In the absence of these effects, abstinent addicts would be much harder to distinguish from nonaddicts who are merely familiar with the effects of the addictive drugs.

THE PHILOSOPHY OF ADDICTION

The previous section paints a picture of how the reward system works, and how it induces problematic effects in drug addicts that seem particularly associated with addiction. For a philosopher interested in blameworthiness, the next thing to do is to understand these problematic effects in terms that have some meaning in moral psychology. And for our purposes, what this amounts to is trying to understand how these problematic effects are related to desires.[49]

We will consider the two effects in turn.

First, there is the effect on unthinking behavioral tendencies and habits. Addictive drugs strongly inculcate behavioral tendencies and habits that lead to increased probabilities of drug consumption by addicts. How should this be understood?

One way in which to interpret the phenomenon is to say that this effect is a matter of the addictive drugs inducing very strong desires to do the things that drug addicts are inclined to do. After all, strong behavioral tendencies sound, almost by definition, like strong desires.

We think that the obvious interpretation should be resisted here. This first phenomenon is a matter of the inculcation of strong habits and habit-like

48. E.g., Lowenstein (1999), Berger et al. (1996).

49. For a longer discussion along similar lines, see Schroeder (2010).

tendencies. And habits, however strong or weak, are distinct from desires. What is done out of habit need not be done out of a desire to do it.

Consider the way in which acting out of habit is commonly treated. "Did you want to turn left here?" asks the confused passenger. "No," answers the bemused driver, "I think I just did that out of habit." This ordinary way of making the distinction seems to be supported by the phenomenology: when one does not do something one wanted to do, there is often a little disappointment or regret. But when one does not make a habitual left turn, there is no disappointment or regret that coincides with not acting out of habit. And then, consider also what the putative content of the desire would have to be. A person in the habit of making a left turn at a given intersection does not have a desire to make a left turn at that intersection—at least, such a person neither longingly thinks of making the left turn when at other intersections, nor is behaviorally disposed to get into a position to make the left turn. The habit only has influence upon behavior, and only has influence upon it when the habit's triggering conditions are met. And in the case of driving habits, the triggering conditions are sometimes very specific: that one is approaching a given intersection from a given direction while driving, and seeing that the way is clear for a left turn, then one is inclined to turn left. It could be suggested that this odd content, cut off from all feelings normally associated with desires, is nonetheless a desire: a desire that, when one finds oneself approaching the given intersection from the given direction, and so forth, one turn left. But at this point, the putative desire is so far divorced from ordinary examples of desires that it seems better to put it in a separate category: the category of habit. Unlike desires, habits do not influence our feelings or guide our attention (unless they are specifically habits of attention) or lead us to motivated irrational belief or motivate us under varied conditions to bring about a certain kind of result. Habits incline us to respond to particular prompts (in perception, thought, or both) with particular responses, nothing more.

If part of what is distinctive in the motivation of addicts is habit, then that part of what is distinctive does not entail that addicts have unreasonably strong desires for the drugs to which they are addicted. An addict with a moderately strong desire for an addictive drug might nonetheless be extremely strongly motivated to act to get that drug, if the required action is also one that is habitual (or one that involves habitual components), because the behavioral force of the unusually strong habits generated by addictive drug use would in those circumstances combine with the desire for the addictive drug to generate a much stronger behavioral inclination to use the drug than would exist if the desire alone existed, or if the desire and a habit of strength appropriate to the desire were to exist.

Second, there is the effect that addictive drugs have on unconscious prediction of how "positive" the world is about to appear to be. Since we characterized this as amounting to how addictive drugs generate cravings for those drugs, this would seem to be an obvious point at which desires enter the picture. But the picture is more complicated than that.

Consider first the unconscious prediction system, and its proclivity for predicting extremely "positive" events upon being presented with cues (real or imagined) that are statistically associated with consuming addictive drugs. Insofar as it is correct to treat it as a *predictive* system, it is impossible to see it as instantiating desires. Predictions are true or false; they make claims about how the world will be. Desires are neither true nor false, and they make no claims about how the world will be. And given that the unconscious prediction system is required to have a predictive role within the computational models of the reward system that form our basis for understanding it, we assume we are on safe ground in holding that the unconscious predictive system does not, itself, instantiate desires.

The unconscious prediction system gives rise, in addicts, to cue-conditioned cravings. These cravings are states in which the addict feels bad (deprived or denied) and is highly motivated to do something that will redress the apparent state of deprivation or denial. Are cue-conditioned cravings desires? Is this where desires distinctive of addiction can be found?

Cue-conditioned cravings appear to be very like desires. A person who has a cue-conditioned craving to go to a familiar old bar where she used to get drunk, or to go into the house dealing cocaine while his daughters wait in the car, appears to be a person with a strong desire. The person in this situation feels highly motivated, feels good about the prospect of doing the thing in question and bad about the prospect of not doing it, and would describe herself as very much wanting to do what she craves doing.

To address cue-conditioned cravings, we need to return briefly to the neuroscience of the previous section. As we said, the reward system treats certain states of affairs as "positive," "neutral," or "negative," by responding to representations of these states of affairs by increasing, leaving the same, or decreasing the likelihood of an increase in dopamine in response to each. Under normal conditions, the reward learning generated by representation of "positive" states of affairs leads to certain changes in the unconscious predictive system, changes that level off over the course of reward learning because the reward system treats the states of affairs as being finitely "positive." At some point, on average the predicted "positive" events will match the actual "positive" events and reward learning will stop.

How should all of this be understood psychologically? This is a difficult question, but a strong case can be made that it should be understood in terms of desires. "Positive" states of affairs are appetitively desired ones, "negative" states of affairs are ones that are aversive (roughly, the agent desires that they not obtain), and "neutral" states of affairs are neither. When one desires a state of affairs, this affects how one feels about it and one's motivations regarding it; it also influences the ways in which this state of affairs influences one through the unconscious process of reward learning.

The case for understanding the reward system as realizing desires has three main components. First, the reward system is the unique common cause of both behavior associated with desiring things and feelings associated with desiring things. It is natural to think that desires are the unique common cause (in ordinary human beings) of the behavior and feelings associated with desiring things. And this suggests that the reward system realizes desires: the reward system is the only thing that does what desires do. Second, the reward system mediates our behavior and feelings regarding food and water and sweet tastes. These contents are paradigmatic contents of desires. So if these desires are realized anywhere in us, it is apparently in our reward systems. Third, the structure of our reward system, and its connections to feelings and behaviors, is something we share with other mammals. Likewise, desires are the motivational states that are most reasonably thought to be shared with other mammals. If we have some desires that other mammals do not (e.g., that the Montreal Canadians win the Stanley Cup), that is because we have the ability to conceive of things that other mammals cannot. But having conceived it, there is no fundamental structural difference between desiring victory for the Montreal Canadians and desiring to have enough water. Thus, this structure shared with other mammals is probably best interpreted as realizing an attitude we credibly share with other mammals, such as desire. Other possible interpretations of the system, say, in terms of treating things as reasons for action, would be harder to sustain when applied to other mammals (and would also have less clear connections to pleasure).[50]

If we interpret the reward system as realizing desires, then this affects how we think about desire strength, and this is where these general considerations once again make contact with the moral psychology of addiction. If a state of affairs is treated as "positive" to a certain degree by the reward system—representations of that state of affairs contribute to the calculation of reward learning with this weight or that weight—then that is the best candidate for how much a state of affairs is desired. If a strongly desired state of affairs fails to have a strong motivational or emotional effect on a given occasion, it might be because the individual is jaded, but this would not diminish the claim that the state of affairs was strongly desired. Tim can strongly desire that his father be healthy but be rather jaded about it and so not typically feel strongly about his father's health, nor be much motivated to act to protect that health. And similarly with

50. See Schroeder (2004) for a full defense of our view of the relation between the reward system and desire.

a weakly desired state of affairs having a strong effect on motivations or feelings on a given occasion: a soda might only be weakly desired, but if one was fully expecting a soda only to be denied it at the last second, one can feel strongly about it anyway, and motivated to rectify the situation (while acknowledging that "it's only a soda," perhaps). In addition to these normal ways in which the strength of a desire might not match the strength of its effects on motivation or feelings, there might be abnormal ways in which there might be a mismatch. Perhaps extreme sleep deprivation can reduce the motivational and felt impact of a desire without thereby changing the strength of the desire or the jadedness of the person who desires, for example.

If this is credible, then the same should be said about desires for addictive drugs. Addicts desire to consume the drugs to which they are addicted, but do they desire them as much as one would think given how strongly they feel about them and are motivated by them? Given, that is, how strongly they crave them? Following the above reasoning, the answer has to be no. The cravings addicts have—the motivations and feelings generated by images and ideas associated with their drugs of choice—are not proportional to the strength of the addicts' desires for their drugs. This will be true because these cravings follow (largely or entirely) from the unconscious prediction of a very "positive" event when the addict sees or thinks about things associated with the addictive drug, and as we saw in the previous section, it is a distinctive feature of addictive drugs that the unconscious prediction will always become excessively "positive." Regardless of how positively the reward system responds to the idea of cocaine, the consumption of cocaine will always "teach" the reward system that it should have predicted that the event would be more positive than that. Thus, the effects of the unconscious predictive system—the cravings—will be effects that are out of proportion to how positively the reward system treats the addictive drug. Thus, the cravings will have effects out of proportion to how much the addictive drug is desired, and similarly for the motivations to use that stem from habits engendered by the hijacking of the reward system.

THE BLAMEWORTHINESS OF ADDICTS

With the theories of moral blameworthiness and addiction just presented, we can now give a full account of the blameworthiness of an addict who does something wrong or bad because of the addiction.

Return to the case of David Carr. Carr left his infant daughters in the November cold of Minneapolis in order to consume cocaine. His motive—the consumption of cocaine—is not one of ill will. But to act on that motive in that circumstance is to act wrongly in part because of an absence of needed good will. It is to act with moral indifference. And this is the source of Carr's blameworthiness. This far we got at the outset. But what puzzled us was the explanation of how Carr's blameworthiness is reduced or mitigated in some way by the fact that he did what he did because of his addiction. He is not the cold-hearted monster who could abandon his children for hours in order to see a football game. He does not deserve the same blame that such a monster would deserve. Carr was gripped by an addiction to cocaine, and that matters.

After the previous section, we can say what is special about an addiction to cocaine or to any other drug. Carr's addiction appears to be instantiated in an extremely strong desire for cocaine. He very powerfully craves cocaine at the moment at which he makes his terrible decision, and this craving is a key part of the explanation of his action. But this is only half right. It is true that, if he had not experienced his lack of cocaine as a "towering need" for more, he does not seem like the sort who would have left his daughters alone in the car in the cold. His craving, and perhaps also certain habits of thought and action, is a key part of the explanation of his behavior. But the "towering need," the immense craving, is not indicative that there is an equally towering desire for cocaine motivating Carr. There is a desire—a strong one, perhaps—that is having enormously outsized effects on Carr's feelings and motivations.

As a result, Carr's leaving his daughters is not an expression of the monstrous moral indifference we might have thought—the sort we would have rightly attributed to him if he had done the same thing in order to watch football. Carr credibly cares for his daughters as much as he should. But caring as much as any decent parent should, while desiring cocaine no more than any fan of a sports team desires his team to win, does not lead to Carr doing the right thing, as it would in the responsible sports fan. And this is because there is, in an addict like Carr, a motivational force to the idea of cocaine out of proportion to how much it is desired. This motivational force, added to the force that is proper to the desire given that it is (presumably) a strong one, leads Carr to do something terrible. And given that there is no question about his understanding of the situation, this makes him a suitable candidate for blame. But Carr does not demonstrate monstrous moral indifference in his act. He demonstrates something lesser. A true moral hero, a parent of colossal concern, might have done otherwise in the circumstances. So Carr appears to demonstrate that he is much less than perfect in his desire for what is right and good in the circumstances. A true paragon would have seen that the bottom was hit before getting out of the car; the transformation that eventually takes root in Carr and leads to his breaking free of cocaine would have flowered right there. But Carr is not this paragon, and his action shows it. In doing what is wrong he shows he is to some degree less than perfectly concerned with the right and the good, and since he acts wrongly he is blameworthy. But all his action shows is that he is less than a paragon. It does not show that he is less than an ordinary parent; it does not show that he is a cold-hearted monster. And for this reason, Carr is less blame-worthy than he might have been had this strength of motivation come from something other than his addiction.

This sort of result, in which addicts can be found variably blameworthy for what they do out of addiction depending on how much of their bad actions can be attributed to what they care about and how much can be attributed to impulses to act that do not reflect what they desire, is one we think is correct. It does not absolve addicts from all responsibility for what they do out of addiction, but it also does not treat them on a par with people doing equally lamentable things without addiction or any other disorder playing a role in their acts. In doing so, it treats addicts the way many addicts think of themselves.

REFERENCES

Aron, A., Fisher, H., Mashek, D., Strong, G., Li, H., and Brown, L. 2005. "Reward, Motivation, and Emotion Systems Associated with Early-Stage Intense Romantic Love." *Journal of Neurophysiology* 94, 327–337.

Arpaly, N. 2000. "Hamlet and the Utilitarians." *Philosophical Studies* 99, 45–57.

Arpaly, N. 2002. "Moral Worth." *Journal of Philosophy* 99, 223–245.

Arpaly, N. 2003. *Unprincipled Virtue*. New York: Oxford University Press.

Arpaly, N. 2006. *Merit, Meaning, and Human Bondage*. Princeton, NJ: Princeton University Press.

Arpaly, N., and Schroeder, T. In preparation. *In Praise of Desire*. New York: Oxford University Press.

Bao, S., Chan, V., and Merzenich, M. 2001. "Cortical Remodelling Induced by Activity of Ventral Tegmental Dopamine Neurons." *Nature* 412, 79–83.

Berger, S., Hall, S., Mickalian, J., Reid, M., Crawford, C., Delucchi, K., Carr, K., and Hall, S. 1996. "Haloperidol Antagonism of Cue-Elicited Cocaine Craving." *Lancet* 347, 504–508.

Berridge, K., and Robinson, T. 1998. "What Is the Role of Dopamine in Reward: Hedonic Impact, Reward Learning, or Incentive Salience?" *Brain Research Reviews* 28, 309–369.

Berridge, K. 2003. "Pleasures of the Brain." *Brain and Cognition* 52, 106–128.

Carr, D. 2008. *The Night of the Gun: A Reporter Investigates the Darkest story of His Life— His Own*. New York: Simon and Schuster.

Dayan, P., Montague, P., and Sejnowski, T. 1996. "A Framework for Mesencephalic Dopamine Systems Based on Predictive Hebbian Learning." *Journal of Neuroscience* 16, 1936–1947.

Elster, J. 1999. *Strong Feelings: Emotion, Addiction, and Human Behavior*. Cambridge, MA: MIT Press.

Fischer, J., and Ravizza, M. 1998. *Responsibility and Control: A Theory of Moral Responsibility*. New York: Cambridge University Press.

Frankfurt, H. 1971. "Freedom of the Will and the Concept of a Person." *Journal of Philosophy* 68, 5–20.

Gardner, E., and David, J. 1999. "The Neurobiology of Chemical Addiction." In J. Elster and O. Skog, eds. *Getting Hooked: Rationality and Addiction*. Cambridge, Cambridge University Press. 93–136.

Gjelsvik, O. 1999. "Addiction, Weakness of the Will, and Relapse." In J. Elster and O. Skog, eds. *Getting Hooked: Rationality and Addiction*. Cambridge, Cambridge University Press. 47–64.

Greenspoon, J. 1955. "The Reinforcing Effect of Two Spoken Sounds on the Frequency of Two Responses." *American Journal of Psychology* 68, 409–416.

Houk, J., Davis, J., and Beiser, D. 1995. *Models of Information Processing in the Basal Ganglia*. Cambridge, MA: MIT Press.

Hyman, S. 2005. "Addiction: A Disease of Learning and Memory." *American Journal of Psychiatry* 162, 1414–1422.

Johnsrude, I., Owen, A., Zhao, W., and White, N. 1999. "Conditioned Preference in Humans: A Novel Experimental Approach." *Learning and Motivation* 30, 250–264.

Kandel, E., Schwartz, J., and Jessell, T. 2000. *Principles of Neural Science: 4th Edition*. New York: McGraw-Hill.

Knowlton, B., Mangels, J., and Squire, L. 1996. "A Neostriatal Habit-Learning System in Humans." *Science* 273, 1399–1402.

Knutson, B., Adams, C., Fong, G., and Hommer, D. 2001. "Anticipation of Increasing Monetary Reward Selectively Recruits Nucleus Accumbens." *Journal of Neuroscience* 21, 1–5.

Lowenstein, G. 1999. "A Visceral Account of Addiction." In J. Elster and O. Skog, eds. *Getting Hooked: Rationality and Addiction*. Cambridge, Cambridge University Press. 235–264.

Morillo, C. 1990. "The Reward Event and Motivation." *Journal of Philosophy* 87, 169–186.

Rilling, J., Gutman, D., Zeh, T., Pagnoni, G., Berns, G., and Kilts, C. 2002. "A Neural Basis for Social Cooperation." *Neuron* 35, 395–405.

Robinson, T., and Berridge, K. 2002. "The Psychology and Neurobiology of Addiction: An Incentive-Sensitization View." *Addiction* 95, 91–117.

Romo, R., and Schultz, W. 1990. "Dopamine Neurons of the Monkey Midbrain: Contingencies of Responses to Active Touch during Self-Initiated Arm Movements." *Journal of Neurophysiology* 63, 592–606.

Saint-Cyr, J., Taylor, A., and Lang, A. 1988. "Procedural Learning and Neostriatal Dysfunction in Man." *Brain* 111, 941–959.

Salimpoor, V., Benovoy, M., Larcher, K., Dagher, A., and Zatorre, R. 2011. "Anatomically Distinct Dopamine Release During Anticipation and Experience of Peak Emotion to Music." *Nature Neuroscience* 14, 257–262.

Schroeder, T. 2004. *Three Faces of Desire*. New York: Oxford University Press.

Schroeder, T. 2010. "Irrational Action and Addiction." In D. Ross, H. Kincaid, D. Spurrett, and P. Collins, eds. *What Is Addiction?* Cambridge, MA: MIT Press. 391–407.

Schultz, W. 2011. "Potential Vulnerabilities of Neuronal Reward, Risk, and Decision Mechanisms to Addictive Drugs." *Neuron* 69, 603–617.

Schultz, W., Dayan, P., and Montague P. 1997. "A Neural Substrate of Prediction and Reward." *Science* 275, 1593–1599.

Schultz, W., and Romo, R. 1990. "Dopamine Neurons of the Monkey Midbrain: Contingencies of Responses to Stimuli Eliciting Immediate Behavioral Reactions." *Journal of Neurophysiology* 63, 607–624.

Smith, M. 1994. *The Moral Problem*. Oxford: Blackwell.

Stellar, J., and Stellar, E. 1985. *The Neurobiology of Motivation and Reward*. New York: Springer-Verlag.

White, N., and Milner, P. 1992. "The Psychobiology of Reinforcers." *Annual Review of Psychology* 43, 443–471.

12

Addiction Between Compulsion and Choice

RICHARD HOLTON AND KENT BERRIDGE

Despite a wealth of recent empirical findings, the debate on addiction remains polarized along traditional lines. In one camp stand those who see the characteristic actions of addicts as driven by something very much like a disease: by a pathologically intense compulsion that they can do nothing to resist. Over a century ago William James apparently quoted an alcoholic giving expression to this approach:

> Were a keg of rum in one corner of a room, and were a cannon constantly discharging balls between me and it, I could not refrain from passing before that cannon in order to get at the rum.[1]

At the same time this understanding of addiction was finding its way into literature. Oscar Wilde described the lure of opium on Dorian Gray in very similar terms:

> Men and women at such moments lose the freedom of their will. They move to their terrible end as automatons move. Choice is taken from them, and conscience is either killed, or, if it lives at all, lives but to give rebellion its fascination and disobedience its charm.[2]

---

1. (James, 1890) Vol. II p. 543. It is unclear from the text whether this is a real quotation or whether James simply made it up. And the case that follows it—of an alcoholic who supposedly chopped his hand off with an axe so that he would be given brandy—is very hard to credit.

2. (Wilde, 1891) Ch. 16. In describing it this way Wilde says he is "following what psychologists tell us." Admittedly, there is much more going on in Dorian Gray than simple opium addiction; but into those depths we do not venture.

Modern expressions tend to be less dramatic, but the basic conception remains much the same. Many contemporary theorists insist that addicts are in the grip of a brain disease that removes control over their actions and so requires treatment rather than condemnation.

In the other camp stand those who see addictive behavior as involving normal choices, and so as something that takes place within the domain of ordinary intentional action. This is to see an addict's decisions to take drugs as motivated by a standard structure of beliefs and desires and still subject to self-control. Such an approach harks back to a traditional understanding of addiction, but in recent years has received new impetus in the hands of certain economists and behavioral psychologists.[3]

Members of the disease camp point to the extraordinarily self-destructive behavior that addicts exhibit, and to the burgeoning literature that suggests that their brains are functioning in abnormal ways. Members of the ordinary choice camp point to findings that show that addicts often respond to incentives in normal ways. For example, most succeed in getting over their addictions by their mid-thirties, often with minimal help.[4] Further, many addicts beyond that age stop taking drugs if the incentives are great enough and clear enough. Anesthesiologists and airline pilots who, having been once detected in their addiction, are required to pass random and frequent drug tests on pain of dismissal, are remarkably good at giving up.

The two approaches are typically seen as quite incompatible. If addiction is a brain disease, then there is no role for willpower or self-control. To take a representative example, the book from a recent television series lists as one of the "seven myths of addiction" the idea that "addiction is a willpower problem," and goes on to say:

> This is an old belief, probably based upon wanting to blame addicts for using drugs to excess. This myth is reinforced by the observation that most treatments for alcoholism and addiction are behavioral (talk) therapies, which are perceived to build self-control. But addiction occurs in an area of the brain called the mesolimbic dopamine system that is not under conscious control.[5]

---

3. The classical understanding of alcoholics saw them as people who were simply too fond of wine; the idea that addiction involved some kind of compulsion doesn't really take hold until the 18th century. For discussion see (Sournia, 1990).

4. This point is made very forcefully in (Heyman, 2009), Ch. 4. He draws his conclusion from examination of national population surveys—not just surveys of addicts. He argues that most of those who remain addicted do so because they suffer from other psychiatric illnesses.

5. (Hoffman and Froeke, 2007) p. 37 (accompanying an HBO TV series).

We agree with the last sentence here; we agree that the mesolimbic dopamine system is centrally involved in addiction, and that the workings of that system do not appear to be under direct conscious control (in the sense that there doesn't seem to be much that one can deliberately do to directly affect the workings of that system). But it is one thing to say that people cannot control their mesolimbic dopamine system, and quite another to say that they cannot control how it influences their actions. In a parallel way, there isn't much that people can deliberately do to influence their perceptual system, but that doesn't mean that there is nothing they can do to control its effects on their actions.

Our aim is to present a middle path. The findings from brain science are solid enough. There is good evidence that the brain of an addict is importantly different from that of a normal nonaddicted individual—indeed, there is even some reason to think that the addict's brain might have started out with a vulnerability to addiction. Certainly once addiction is under way, the desire for the addictive drug takes on a life of its own, with an intensity that is particularly, perhaps uniquely, high.[6] The desire becomes insulated from factors that, in normal intentional behavior, would undermine it, and so persists even when the addict knows that acting on it would be highly damaging. The addict may recognize that taking the drug again will incur the loss of family, friends, job, and most of what makes life worth living, and yet still continue to take it. More surprisingly, addicts need not even like the thing that they are addicted to: they need gain no pleasure from it, nor anticipate that they will. Nor need they be motivated by a desire to avoid the horrors of withdrawal. Alcohol or heroin addicts often relapse long after withdrawal is over, and cocaine addiction is no less potent for having a relatively mild withdrawal syndrome. Addicts may relapse when they see nothing good in their drug whatsoever. They may see it as nasty, damaging, and worthless in every respect. Yet they may still want it, and want it, moreover, in a particularly immediate and intense way—perhaps more immediately and more intensely than most other people ever experience.

There is another way in which an addictive desire does not typically function like a desire to see the Pyramids or to get a paper finished before the weekend. It does not serve as an input to deliberation, something to be weighed, along with other competing desires, in deciding what to do. Instead, addictive desire functions as something more like an intention: as something that, unless checked, will lead, in a rather direct way, to action. This combination of features—the insulation of addictive desires from factors that should undermine them, and

6. We speak in terms of "drugs" here as a shorthand for "addictive substances," even though some such substances—most obviously alcohol—are not typically thought of as drugs outside the biomedical community.

their tendency to lead directly to action—means that addictive behavior is very different from ordinary behavior that results from deliberation.

Nevertheless, the intensity and power of addictive desires do not mean that addicts are automata, standing as powerless spectators as they are moved by their desires. For while addictive desires are very strong, the human capacity for self-control is also highly developed—much more developed, it seems, than in rats. Addicts do not actually cross into the paths of cannonballs or their equivalents, despite William James's colorful assertion. They go around or wait for a lull. Smokers on airplanes postpone their urge to smoke until the flight is over.

So addictive urges are not entirely uncontrollable: as these cases show, they can be controlled, at least for a short while, and sometimes for longer if the stakes are high enough and clear enough. The experience of self-control that everyone has at certain moments is a veridical one: self-control is a real phenomenon, something that can be used to control acting on addictive desires, even if at a considerable cost and, for most addicts, subject to occasional failure. We should thus not be thinking of addictive desires as things that are impossible to resist, but as things that are very difficult to resist.[7] Our moral evaluations should reflect this fact, and our scientific account of addiction should explain why resistance is difficult and why failure happens on the occasions it does.

Our aim here is to articulate such a model, one that explains why addictive desires have the distinctive features they have, but that also explains how they can be controlled. We start by outlining what we think is wrong with the two extreme positions, the pure choice model and the pure disease model.

ORDINARY CHOICE MODELS

We cannot hope to survey all of the different ordinary choice models here, but some brief comments will serve to show why we think that they cannot provide a complete explanation of addiction. An ordinary choice model can, of course, easily explain the behavior of those who willingly and knowingly take addictive drugs. But addicts frequently say that they have been somehow captured by the addiction—that they wish they could escape it but that something is making it very hard for them to do so. Some listeners might dismiss these comments as disingenuous or self-deceived, but we think there is something in what they say.

How can ordinary choice models make sense of this capture? They have two approaches. One is to ascribe to addicts abnormal desires; the other is to ascribe to them mistaken beliefs. Advocates of the first approach typically see

---

7. Could they sometimes be truly irresistible? It seems rash to rule that out, although it is hard to be sure quite what the claim means: That no incentive *would* overcome it? That no incentive *could*?

addicts as having steep temporal discount curves—they see them as having much stronger desires for the present and immediate future than for the more distant future. Since addictive drugs normally involve a nasty period of withdrawal, already addicted agents whose focus is on the immediate future will want to avoid embarking on the suffering that such a process will involve, even if they know that the long-term effects will be beneficial. Of course, they might well prefer not to have started consuming the drug in the first place—in this way advocates of this approach can make sense of the idea that they are really addicted and are not simply willing consumers—but given the state that they are in now, continuing to take the drugs is preferable to withdrawal.[8]

Advocates of the second approach typically see addicts as mistaken, at least initially, about the effects of their drugs (they believe that they will not become addicted, or that addiction will not be so bad); or they see them as failing to take into account the consequences of current consumption for their future state: by focusing only on their current options, addicts fail to see that consuming addictive drugs now will lower their overall well-being in the future.[9]

The two approaches may be combined: mistaken beliefs might explain why addicts fall into addiction, and then the steep discount curves might explain why they stay there; and elements from these approaches might be used to supplement other accounts. Indeed, we ourselves are inclined to think that there are important insights to be had here. In particular, there is good evidence that ignorance has an important role in the process of acquiring an addiction. But we do not think that an ordinary choice account can provide the fundamental explanation of what is distinctive about addiction, for if it were right, then former addicts who had been through the pains of withdrawal should be the least likely to consume again. They would no longer have the cost of withdrawal to endure; and they, of all people, would be well informed of their own vulnerability to addiction, of how nasty it is, and of the cost of not looking to the future. We are not talking here of those who really prefer to be addicted; they will just start consuming again, although they would be unlikely to have put themselves through the process of withdrawal in the first place. But those who genuinely wanted to be free of the drugs should be uniquely well qualified to ensure that they remain so.

8. The most influential presentation of this line is from Becker and Murphy; for a simplified presentation see (Skog, 1999). Becker and Murphy give no explanation of how addicts get into the state of addiction; that is left to be explained by exogenous factors.

9. See (Loewenstein, 1999) and (Herrnstein and Prelec, 1992) for versions of the first approach,, and (Heyman, 2009) Ch. 6 for a detailed development of the second. Addicts, understood on Heyman's lines as those who fail to think about their future, will be behaviorally equivalent to the steep discounters who don't care about it; but this will derive from features of their beliefs rather than of their desires.

Yet that is not what we find. People who have come through withdrawal, and gained much self-knowledge in the process, are much more likely to take up drugs again than those who never started, a process that is typically triggered by cues that are associated with the previous addiction. Indeed, withdrawal seems largely irrelevant in the process of maintaining addiction. It is not just that people consume again after having gone through it; in addition cravings are experienced long before it comes withdrawal, and some highly addictive drugs—most notably, cocaine—have minimal withdrawal symptoms. A pure choice model struggles to explain these features. So let us turn to the disease models that do better with them.

DISEASE MODELS

There are many disease models of addiction. To get some traction on the debate, we divide these into four, at the cost of some simplification. The first, exploiting classical behaviorist mechanisms, sees addiction as a habit: drug-taking actions are triggered automatically in particular situations, independently of the subject's beliefs and desires. The second sees it as involving distorted pleasure: addictive drugs "hijack" the subject's pleasure circuits, and it is this that causes the skewed behavior. The third, using reinforcement learning theory, sees the distortion as affecting not the pleasure itself, but the subjects' *beliefs* about what will give them pleasure. The final account, which we shall endorse (while denying that this provides the *whole* story about addiction), involves desire: consumption of addictive drugs gives rise to pathologically intense desires or cravings, states that are largely insulated from the subject's beliefs and other desires. We start by briefly outlining those with which we disagree.

Habit Accounts

In its simplest form the habit model follows the classic stimulus-response account that was laid down in the early 20th century by Thorndike, and that became the staple of behaviorist models. An agent explores its environment, gets a positive reaction to some things and an aversive response to others, and subsequently comes to repeat those behaviors that produced the positive outcomes. In its early behaviorist guise, this approach was linked with skepticism about positive/aversive mental states altogether; but such an approach has few supporters now, and we shall say nothing about it. More interesting is the idea that habits stand alongside, but independent from, the agent's beliefs and desires.[10] Contemporary versions of habit theory hold that drugs induce brain

10. For accounts along these lines see (Wise, 2004) and (Everitt et al., 2008).

systems of action (e.g., in the neostriatum) to form the tendency in the presence of drug cues to perform particular behaviors, behaviors that have been established during previous drug-taking episodes—much like a shoe-tying habit but even more strongly automatic.

If addictive states were understood this way that would provide some explanation of why they are insensitive to the addict's desire to stop. But the habit account assumes that drug taking is unmotivated, and most likely to surface when the addict's attention is distracted elsewhere. That belies the intensely motivated nature of addictive urges, and turns upside down the observation that attentively thinking about drugs is the most dangerous situation for an addict—more dangerous than thinking about something else. While some aspects of habitual behavior might be important in addiction—reaching unthinkingly for a cigarette—the account cannot easily explain how agents will take a drug in full awareness of what they are doing, while this is quite contrary to their views of what is best.[11]

Pleasure Accounts

So let us move to the second class of accounts, those premised on excessive pleasure.[12] Clearly many addicts do get great pleasure from the drugs they take. If drugs can "hijack" the pleasure circuit, giving a disproportionate amount of pleasure to those who consume them, then this would give rise to a very strong learned desire for them.[13] And if the pleasure per unit decreased over time, as tolerance developed, the agent would want more and more of the drugs to compensate.[14]

This account was once thought to be bolstered by the finding that the addictive drugs have an impact on the mesolimbic dopamine system: either by stimulating the release of dopamine (in the case of amphetamine, nicotine, and caffeine); by reducing the release of substances like GABA that themselves reduce the amount of dopamine released (opiates and perhaps THC); by reducing the level of substances that break down dopamine (alcohol); or by reducing the

11. For work on the areas in which pure habit accounts do provide good explanations see (Wood and Neal, 2007).

12. Thorndike's original account of learning was in terms of pleasure, though he later came to talk purely in terms of stimulus and response. Historically, then, pleasure-based accounts represent something of a reversion to an earlier idea.

13. We speak of "hijacking" and "disproportionate pleasure" here, but of course accounts that think that there is no rational constraint on what gives one pleasure will find it hard to make sense of this. To that extent, this approach will lapse back into a rational choice account, in which the agent acts on desires for their strongest pleasure.

14. See, for instance, Roy Wise's earlier work: (Wise, 1980, 1985).

activity of the system that reabsorbs dopamine (cocaine and perhaps amphet-amine). Add the premise that the mesolimbic dopamine system is the pleasure system, and we have what looks like a compelling picture.[15]

Simple and straightforward though the pleasure account is, it doesn't fit the empirical findings. It assumes that the dopamine system is concerned with lik-ing. But a host of findings have now shown fairly conclusively that the primary role of the dopamine system is not to do with liking. In rats, suppressing the dopamine system does not result in a lack of pleasure responses to sweet sub-stances; we shall discuss cases of this shortly. Likewise, human subjects whose dopamine systems are suppressed artificially, or as a result of Parkinson's dis-ease, give normal pleasure ratings to sugar. Conversely, elevated dopamine levels in rats do not result in greater pleasure. And elevated dopamine levels in human subjects do not give rise to increased subjective pleasure ratings.[16] Dopamine thus does not seem to be directly concerned with the production of liking. We will suggest that it is concerned with the creation of wanting.

This might not matter if there were nonetheless a very tight correlation between liking and wanting: if liking invariably resulted in wanting, and if wanting were invariably the result of prior liking. But the very results that show that they are distinct states also show that, while they might *typically* be linked by causal connections, sometimes those connections will fail. We will argue that this is crucial for understanding addiction.

Learning Accounts

So let us move to those models that see addiction as resulting from *learning*. Admittedly, in a simple behaviorist model learning is not a very contentful notion: there isn't much more to it than the idea that subjects' behavior changes as a result of what happens to them, and hardly anyone could disagree that that is true of addiction. But in more cognitivist models, the idea of learning is much more specific: it is the idea of forming predictive associations, that is, *beliefs*.[17]

---

15. For a recent popular presentation of such an approach by a neuroscientist, see (Linden, 2011) Ch. 2. Linden writes, "Addictive drugs, by co-opting the pleasure circuitry and activating it more strongly than any natural reward, create deeply ingrained memories that are bound up in a network of associations," p. 53.

16. For details, see (Berridge, 2012) p. 1132.

17. At least, this is the core notion of learning that is present when one says that a subject learns *that* something is the case, or learns *who*, or *what*, or *where*. In all such cases the subject acquires a belief. We also speak more broadly of learning *to* do something, and in this sense our account could be phrased in terms of *learning to want*. But to avoid confusion, we'll talk only about acquiring wants. A further linguistic complication: in most ordinary talk, "learning *that*"

These accounts see addiction as stemming not from heightened pleasure itself, but from mistaken *belief* about pleasure. Addictive drugs hijack not the pleasure circuits, but the circuits that *learn* about pleasure, and so they distort the memories that are used to guide future desires. One popular theory of reward learning holds that dopamine spikes indicate "reward prediction errors": dopamine is released whenever an outcome is better than expected.[18] Applied to addiction, the idea is that dopamine-stimulating drugs cause an exaggerated prediction error: it is as though the drugs were much more pleasurable than expected.[19] Consumption of the drug itself doesn't have to be especially pleasurable—though it may be—since the effect on the dopamine system is to trigger a large prediction error *as if* it were pleasurable, with the result that the "memory" of the pleasure can greatly exceed the actual pleasure. This in turn gives rise to the extreme desires that characterize addiction. On this approach, then, the addict's fundamental desire is a desire for pleasure. Since, at some level, addicts mistakenly believe that consumption of the drug will give them pleasure, this results in a strong instrumental desire for the drugs.[20]

We think that this is mistaken. We will present instead a model—the incentive salience model—that sees addiction as driven by desires that have no essential connection with beliefs about what will be liked, or about what will be beneficial in other ways. The key idea here is that the dopamine signals are not learning signals, in the sense that they do not give rise to beliefs, predictions, or memories (real or apparent) at all. Instead, they give rise to desires directly—or, more accurately, to a sensitivity to experience desires when cued with appropriate stimuli. The desire felt is not an instrumental desire, driven by an intrinsic desire for pleasure; instead, it is an intrinsic desire for the drug, a desire that may lead to action even in the face of contrary desires, and in the face of beliefs that consumption will have bad consequences. While the incentive salience account can embrace a parallel formalism to that employed by

---

and "learning *who*" are factives: the belief that is formed must be true. We'll follow the standard psychological use and talk of learning even when the resulting belief is false.

18. (Sutton and Barto, 1998).

19. (Schultz et al., 1997); (Redish, 2004).

20. We say "at some level," since many proponents of the prediction error approach insist that their account is "model free," by which they mean that subjects do not have full-blown representations or cognitive maps of the world and of their own preferences within it. Nonetheless, we insist that if talk of "prediction" is appropriate, there must still be beliefs, even if they are of a partial, local, or implicit form; otherwise we would simply have a habit account. The other possibility is to understand the relevant states as desires, the approach that we develop below. Of course, treating predictions as beliefs is compatible with the idea that subjects also have more explicitly articulated beliefs about their own preferences.

the prediction error model—we explain how below—it uses that formalism to explain the formation of desires and not of beliefs.

Before we explain the evidence for such an account in any detail, let us get clearer on the distinctions we have just outlined: that between wanting and liking, and that between the formation of beliefs and the acquisition of desires.

DISTINGUISHING WANTING AND LIKING

In one sense it is obvious that wanting and liking are distinct, at least if we think of liking in terms of pleasure: wanting typically comes before one gets the thing wanted, whereas the pleasure typically (though not invariably) comes once one has got it.[21] And liking and wanting can also come apart as a result of false beliefs. We can want something that we believe we will like, even though we won't in fact like it: perhaps we haven't tried it before, or have forgotten that we didn't like it, or believe for some reason that our reaction will be different from last time.

For parallel reasons we can like something and not want it: we might not realize that we like it, or we might have other reasons for foregoing it. Indeed, those disciplines that have not traditionally made much of the distinction between wanting and liking—behaviorist psychology, say, or revealed preference economics—have not normally identified them. Rather, they have thought that they could make do with one (typically wanting) while discarding the other (typically liking) as illusory or scientifically intractable.

So the real issues do not concern the *identity* of wanting and liking. Instead, we think that they are twofold. One concerns the *causal* relations between wanting and liking, and their embodiment in particular brain mechanisms. The second concerns the relation of wanting to *expected* liking. We take these in turn.

Causal Relations Between Wanting and Liking

Does liking invariably cause wanting (i.e., is liking causally *sufficient* for wanting)? Are increases in wanting always preceded by incidents of liking (i.e., is liking causally *necessary* for wanting)? It is commonly supposed that there are some such relations here. Indeed, even so implacable an opponent of hedonism as G.E. Moore wrote that he was "ready to admit that pleasure is always, in part

---

21. In discussing the incentive salience model, one author (KB) has in previous writings been careful to distinguish the notions of wanting and liking that are involved from our ordinary folk notions. For that reason he has placed them in quotation marks. The other (RH) has no such scruples, and he has prevailed here. But note that the kind of wanting involved here needs to be distinguished from other kinds that have equally good claim on the term, and that certain features that might be expected—that one knows what one wants, that one judges it to be worthwhile—will often be absent.

at least, the *cause* of desire."[22] But that is a substantial claim. While we think that brain activations that cause increases in liking *typically* cause increases in wanting, too, we think that these mechanisms are in principle separable, and that under some conditions liking can in fact be generated without wanting.

When we turn to the converse question of whether wanting is always preceded by liking, our answer is more straightforwardly "no". Many brain activations that cause wanting are not accompanied by increased liking; wanting without liking occurs frequently in addicts. The evidence here came originally from studies of the brain activity and behavior of rats. Since rats can't talk, we need to have some nonverbal behavioral indicators of wanting and of liking. Wanting is straightforward: rats want something if they try to get it. (This is where we assume that issues of self-control will not intrude; things are more complicated with human beings as we shall see later.) Liking has been traditionally viewed as harder to identify. But a set of results indicate that a range of evolved facial expressions—including tongue protrusions and lip sucking—are correlated with liking for the sensory pleasure of tastes across a wide range of species including rats, monkeys, and human infants.[23] In the past decade, the distinction between liking and wanting has also been confirmed in a number of human studies based on ratings of their own experience of sensory pleasures, such as cocaine and other addictive drugs.[24]

Once we have distinct criteria for wanting and liking, we find that one can be induced without the other. If rats' dopamine levels are suppressed, they are no longer prepared to work to gain food rewards that they would previously have worked for. At the extreme, they will not eat pleasant foods that are freely available, even though they still display strong liking for them once the foods are placed in their mouths. Indeed, rats who had 98% of the dopamine neurons in their nucleus accumbens and neostriatum chemically destroyed would have starved to death had they not been intragastrically fed, yet their normal liking reactions indicated that pleasure in the food was unchanged. So liking is not sufficient for wanting. Conversely, by boosting rats' dopamine levels, we find that their wanting can be increased without their liking being increased—we will discuss an example of this shortly.[25] So increased liking is not necessary for increased wanting. Indeed, wanting can be artificially engendered in rats without any signs of liking.[26]

---

22. (Moore, 1905) §42.

23. (Berridge, 2000); (Berridge and Kringelbach, 2008). The reaction seems to be suppressed in humans after early infancy, but can recur in those suffering from Alzheimer's.

24. (Leyton, 2010); (Lawrence et al., 2003).

25. See also (Berridge, 2007); (Smith et al., 2011).

26. (Peciña et al., 2003); (Wyvell and Berridge, 2000); (Faure, et al., 2010); (Smith et al., 2011); (Tindell et al., 2005); (Berridge and Valenstein, 1991).

Relation of Wanting to Expected Liking

The second issue concerns the relation of wanting to expected liking. Can subjects want something while believing they will not like it? And conversely, can they believe that they will like something and not want it? This is where the talk of learning fits in: can subjects come to learn that they like something, and yet not go on to form a desire for it? And conversely, can they come to learn that they dislike something, and yet go on to form (or at least maintain) a desire for it?

Here again the empirical evidence suggests that wanting without expected liking is indeed possible, and so the two cannot be identified, nor are they invariably causally connected. There are two kinds of consideration. First, wants fluctuate in ways that are hard to mesh with the idea that belief is also fluctuating. Second, what we know about the formation of belief suggests that it uses quite different mechanisms to those involved in the formation of wants.

On the first point, consider a set of experiments done by Cindy Wyvell, which produced momentary pulses of elevated wanting for rewards that exceeded both liking for the rewards and learned memories and expectations of the reward's value. The initial stage was to get rats to associate a random stimulus (a noise) and an activity (lever pressing) with each other by pairing each with a sugar reward. As a result, the noise tended to trigger the lever pressing. The experiment was then to see the effect of changes in the dopamine level on this triggering, even when the sugar was not present.[27]

On some days the rats were trained to press a lever to gain sugar (instrumental training). On others a conditioned stimulus was created: a sound heralded freely available sugar, which resulted in the rats associating the sound and the sugar (Pavlovian training). Their facial responses showed that they liked the sugar.

Cannulas were inserted into the rats' brains, enabling their mesolimbic dopamine systems to be affected directly by microinjections of tiny droplets of drug. A control group received an inert substance through this cannula, while the other group received amphetamines, which greatly increase dopamine release. The effects of the action of the mesolimbic dopamine system could then be determined by observing the differences between the two groups.

Both groups continued to like the sugar. As expected, they liked it to the same degree: the amphetamine group did not show an increased facial pleasure response when given it, further evidence that dopamine does not produce pleasure. Importantly, though, the amphetamines did not seem to increase anticipated pleasure from the sugar: when given the lever to press, the amphetamine

---

27. See (T. Robinson and Berridge, 2003) pp. 41–43, for further discussion of why this feature is important.

group did not press it any more frequently than the controls when freely allowed to without any distraction.

The difference came when the rats heard the noise that they had been conditioned to associate with sugar. Now both groups increased their lever pressing. But rats in the amphetamine group pressed the lever dramatically more: more than four times as frequently as before, and more than 50% higher than the rats in the no-amphetamine group who heard the same noise. And this effect was switched on and off as the cue went on and off.[28]

What was happening here? It appears that the increased dopamine levels resulted in a massive amplification of the conditioned response that was already present. Hearing the cue signal caused the control rats to press the lever. But the presence of high levels of dopamine caused the group that was receiving the amphetamines to press it far more.

It is very hard to explain this result in terms of changes in expectation, for we have no reason to think that hearing the signal caused change in the rats' beliefs about how pleasurable the sugar would be, and since the amphetamine rats did not elevate their effort to earn reward in the absence of the particular noise. The rats were not learning anything new, and the effects fell off as soon as the tone ceased.

In general, learning seems to be different from wanting. For example, the rats discussed above who have lost nearly all of their mesolimbic dopamine due to neurochemical 6-OHDA lesions are still quite capable of learning new values about food rewards. When a previously liked food is made unpalatable by inducing nausea, the dopamine-depleted rats will learn to react to it with signs of disgust, in just the same way as normal rats. Similarly, mice who have been genetically engineered to lack dopamine are still able to learn basic Pavlovian reward associations.[29] When learning and "wanting" are made to diverge by manipulating a second input to "wanting" (physiological state/trait), levels and roles of dopamine and mesolimbic brain activations all track "wanting" outputs much more faithfully than learning inputs.[30] Learning, in the sense of the

---

28. It's an interesting question why the sight of the lever didn't itself work as a cue. Clearly not all cues are created equal.

29. For summary see (Berridge, 2012) pp. 1139–1140.

30. (Flagel et al., 2011); (Tindell et al., 2005); (Smith et al., 2011); (M. Robinson and Berridge, 2010); (Saunders and Robinson, 2012). There are a number of highly influential papers by Schultz and others that appear to demonstrate that dopamine firing does track learning: see, for instance, (Schultz et al., 1997) and (Schultz, 2002). We suggest that these finding may have been flawed by an experimental confound. Those studies allowed only the learning input to vary, while clamping the second physiological input as stable. Under those conditions, wanting and dopamine as outputs naturally track the only input that was allowed to vary: learning. The wanted output then mimics the learned input, the two signals cannot be told apart, and an observer can confuse one with the other. For further discussion see (Berridge, 2012) p. 1132.

formation of new beliefs or of the formation of new behaviors, does not seem to be essentially dependent on the dopamine system.

So what exactly is dopamine doing? As we saw from the Wyvell experiments, it is involved in the generation of desire at particular moments. But as those experiments showed, this is not blanket desire. Dopamine seems instead to be involved in producing specifically targeted desires in response to certain stimuli. To see what it might be doing, let us start by employing some relatively a priori considerations about creatures like us and about the kind of wanting system that we would need. This is not to tell an evolutionary just-so story—we think that the account we give is independently well supported by the empirical evidence. Rather, we tell it because a good way of understanding a complex mechanism is by understanding its function.

MODELING THE WANTING SYSTEM: SOME A PRIORI CONSIDERATIONS

Some creatures are tightly locked into a specific pattern of consumption: an insect that eats the leaves from a single plant species, or a koala that eats the leaves from four. Such creatures can have their tastes hard-wired. Other creatures are more opportunistic, adapting their consumption patterns to what is available. Human beings, like rats, are at the far end of this continuum. Although some of our desires are perhaps hard-wired, most are highly plastic.

Let us think in the abstract about how a creature with plastic desires will structure its consumption. We assume that it has some way of telling, when it samples a given food, how good that food is in providing it with what it needs. It might do this largely by means of a pleasure mechanism—the better the food, the more pleasure it gives—although in fact we think that, for reasons we shall discuss shortly, pleasure is not always involved. So let us just say that the creature can register how good the food is for it. Suppose, then, that the goal of the creature is to maximize its consumption of things that are good for it. How could it go about that?

One way would be for the creature simply to try each thing that it comes across to see how good it is and then consume it if it is; but obviously that would be highly inefficient, since it would involve constantly retrying things that had already been shown to be bad. A second would be to learn what is good for it, in the full sense of that term: the creature would develop beliefs about which foods are good for it, and then, given a desire to consume what is good, it would form instrumental desires for those foods.[31] A third possibility would be to avoid forming the beliefs at all. Instead, the creature could directly

---

31. (Dickinson and Balleine, 2010).

form its desires on the basis of what it had discovered to be good. That is, it could form intrinsic desires for the good foods, without recourse to any beliefs or predictions about them.

This third possibility would have some advantages. It could be simpler and easier to implement than a belief-based system, and in some ways more robust. So let us consider how it might work. The creature we will consider will need to do two things. First it will need to form its desires for certain foods; then it will need to act on them in the presence of those foods. To do this it will need to make use of two systems, a desire formation system that creates intrinsic desires for foods, and a consumption system that regulates the creature's consumption in accord with those desires. We should keep these systems conceptually distinct, even if, for reasons we shall come to shortly, there may be some overlap of function. So spelling this out, we have:

(i)   A desire formation system. This will need to identify each sample as belonging to a certain food type; to determine how much goodness it gets from that type; and, on the basis of that determination, to send a signal to the consuming system that will regulate its subsequent desire for foods of that type. Let us call this the *A-signal*.

(ii) A consumption system. The settings of this system will be determined by the A-signal. Presented with a potential food, it will need to identify it as belonging to one food type or another, and then it will respond to this by sending out, in accordance with its setting for that food, a signal that regulates consumption of that food. Let us call this the *B-signal*.

Quite how to use the term "desire" here is delicate (so far we have fudged it). The term could be used to label the *dispositional state* of the consuming system: its tendency to respond to a certain food in a certain way, as determined by the A-signal. Alternatively, it could be used to label the state that comes about as a result of the triggering of that dispositional state: the *occurrent state* that is the B-signal or that is brought about by the B-signal.[32] Both uses have good philosophical and ordinary language pedigree. To mark the distinction, let's call the first the *dispositional desire*, and the second the *occurrent desire*.[33] The desire formation system is thus

32. We won't broach the question of whether the B-signal will actually be the desire (or its neurophysiological correlate, if that is meant to be different). We don't see any compelling arguments, other than an appeal to ontological economy, for or against that claim. But to keep things simple, and to avoid getting involved in issues of the nature of phenomenal states and so forth, we will just talk about the B-signal as the immediate cause of desire, with the thought that the identity claim may be substituted. Obviously if the B-signal is the desire, it is rather misleading to call it a "signal."

33. As we shall see, dispositional desires understood in this way are rather different from dispositional desires as they have normally been understood in philosophy, since they have a very

in the business of forming dispositional desires, and the consumption system is in the business of forming occurrent desires when the dispositional desires are triggered.

Let us inquire a little further into how these systems might work. Since there is likely to be considerable variation in the goodness of different samples of the same food (as we all know, while some strawberries are delicious, others are quite tasteless), an obvious strategy will be for the creature to sample each food several times over, to compute the mean goodness it gets from the set of samples of each food, and then to proportion its desire to that mean. How would it do this?

We'll first address the issue of how it computes the mean from a given set of samples of a certain foodstuff. It could, of course, record the value of each sample taken so far, sum them, and divide the result by the number of samples. But keeping on computing the mean in that way would involve keeping track of a lot of data that aren't needed, which would be far from easy for a biological system to implement; and it would mean that there would be no provisional result until the sampling period was over.

A far simpler method, which does provide provisional results, is to keep a rolling mean and a record of the number of samples taken. Then the creature can update the mean with each new sample recorded. Suppose it has so far examined n samples, has identified the value (V) of each, and has computed their mean (mean_n). Now it takes a further sample, n+1, with value V_{n+1}. To compute the new mean (i.e., mean_{n+1}), all it needs to do is to see how much the value of the current sample differs from the existing mean, give this difference the right weight by dividing it by the total number of samples, and then add it to the existing mean. Or more concisely:

$$\text{mean}_{n+1} = \text{mean}_n + (1/(n+1) [V_{n+1} - \text{mean}_n])^{34}$$

This update-rule, which looks at the difference between the current sample and the previous mean—or, in other words often used in the literature, at the error between the prior prediction and the current sample—provides the core of most reinforcement learning methods; and certainly a mechanism based on it can be used to acquire new beliefs. These are the learning systems that we mentioned above when discussing the learning interpretations of the role of dopamine. But such a rule need not be tied to a learning system. The very same rule can be used in this framework to form new desires directly.

specific cue. Without the cue they have no force. In that sense, then, they are more like disposi-tions to have desires than like dispositional desires as traditionally conceived.

34. See (Sutton and Barto, 1998) pp. 36–37 for the simple proof that this is equivalent to the more normal way of defining the mean.

To employ this rule the desire formation system will (i) need to recognize the sample it is encountering as belonging to a certain foodstuff; it will (ii) need to retrieve the mean level of goodness for that foodstuff ($mean_n$) and the previous number of samples (n); it will (iii) need to register the level of goodness gained from the current sample (V_{n+1}); and then it will (iv) need to perform the computation. In fact, the desire formation system doesn't need to send the mean on to the consumption system. All it needs to do is to send the new information gained from each new sample, so that the consumption system can modify its dispositional desires in light of this. To do this it need only to send a signal corresponding to ($1/(n+1)$ [V_{n+1} − $mean_n$]). In the learning literature this is commonly termed an "error signal" or a "learning signal," but since we are working with a desire-based system, rather than a belief- or prediction-based system, and hence are not concerned with learning in the strict sense, we will stick with our earlier stipulation and just call it the *A-signal*.

The consumption system will now employ the A-signal to regulate its activity by setting its dispositional desires. How will it do this? One possibility would be for the desire formation system to send, in addition to the A-signal, information about the identity of the thing that had been sampled. But sending such information would be a complicated business, and, besides, it would be largely redundant. If it is to employ the information sent to it, the consumption system will anyway need to be able to categorize potential food as belonging to one of the food types. So, rather than requiring additional information about the identity of the food sampled, it could instead use a basic associative mechanism. On receiving the the A-signal, it would form a desire for whichever food it identified as being currently consumed. This of course will mean that it is vulnerable to a certain kind of error: if it receives the A-signal at the same time that it identifies a given food as being consumed, it will impute the information to that food even if it is not in fact the source of the signal, or not the source in the standard way. This fact will be crucial to our account of addiction.

Let us summarize then: the consumption system will set its dispositions—its dispositional desires—on the basis of two inputs, the strength of the A-signal and its own identification of what is being consumed at the time it gets the A-signal. On the basis of these dispositions it will send out an appropriate B-signal whenever it recognizes a food as belonging to a certain group. That B-signal will in turn determine the pattern of consumption.

The model that we have presented sounds much like a simple version of an actor-critic model: the consumption system is the actor, and the desire formation system the critic.[35] Rival models combine the two roles. Such an approach might seem attractively economical. In particular, couldn't a single signal serve

35. See (Sutton and Barto, 1998) pp. 151ff.

both to lay down dispositional desires and to induce occurrent desires? We don't mean to rule out such an approach, but we will persist with the two-system model for three reasons. First, as we mentioned before, even if the systems are not realized distinctly, it is useful to keep them conceptually distinct. Second, there is some good evidence that rats employ an actor-critic model; we will come to this in the next section. Third, there is a real advantage to a creature in keeping the two systems—and hence the A-signal and the B-signal—distinct.

To see this, consider the role of appetite. No creature will gain by going on consuming even when it no longer needs to. Once it has eaten to capacity it should stop. Better still, it could regulate its appetite depending on its current needs. If it has plenty of one nutrient and not enough of another, it should increase its desire for the latter relative to the former. The advantage of the two-system model is that it enables the creature to do this while still gaining useful information. A simple—doubtless oversimple—example will make the point. Suppose that our creature's sugar needs are sated, but that it still needs water. It samples a new foodstuff and finds it rich in sugar but quite without water. It shouldn't form an occurrent desire for the food; it should go on searching. But it would be good if the information that this food is rich in sugar could have some impact on its dispositional desire for it; after all, next time it comes across it, it may be short on sugar. Having a system that keeps separate the A-signal and the B-signal enables it to make just this distinction. The idea is that appetite is regulated at the level of the consumption system, that is, by controlling the B-signal. So when the creature in the water-deprived state encounters the sugar-rich substance, its A-signal can still fire, laying down the dispositional desire. But because it is not hungry for sugar, the B-signal will not fire, and so there will be no occurrent desire. In contrast, if both dispositional and occurrent desire were regulated by a single signal, it is hard to see how one could be triggered without the other.

But there is a further issue that is potentially important. The model that we have presented is good, if a little slow, at responding to relatively stable changes— a food getting better or worse, and staying that way for some time. In addition, though, the world is likely to exhibit some unstable changes—different samples of the same food fluctuating, sometimes wildly, in their goodness (a phenomenon most of us are all too familiar with from tomatoes and strawberries). Thus, suppose that a creature has tried a certain foodstuff many times in the past and found it middling good: worth consuming if there is really nothing else available, but not so good that the creature should keep consuming it rather than exploring elsewhere. Now it tries the same food again and finds it extremely good. How should it respond? Clearly it should increase its desire for future samples of the foodstuff, though not precipitously: its prior experience suggests that this will be an anomaly, and that future samples will not be as good as this. But at the same time it would be crazy not to make the most of this exceptionally good sample. It should consume all it can of it here and now, rather than moving on to explore elsewhere, or to consume a different food that it has found on average to be slightly better but that is likely to be considerably worse than this sample.

This requires, then, that the creature have a two-part response—a large but short-lived burst in desire for this particular sample, and a smaller but more stable increase in desire for future samples of the same type. But if, for the reasons we have discussed, occurrent desire is regulated by the B-signal and not by the A-signal, how can this be achieved?

We see one possibility. Even if the A-signals do not directly cause occurrent desires, they might nevertheless boost the effectiveness of the signals that do. So even if only a B-signal can cause an occurrent desire, the degree to which it does is regulated by the strength of the current A-signal. The higher the current A-signal, the higher the effectiveness of the B-signal. Call this the "accelerator" approach. It might be implemented in different ways. One particularly simple way would be to make the change imparted to the dispositional desire by the A-signal into a temporally stepped one. Suppose that the initial impact of the A-signal on the dispositional desire is comparatively large, but that this decays rapidly to a reach a new lower equilibrium after a short while. That would give us the accelerator approach, and would be quite compatible with standard Hebbian models.[36]

We have gone about as far as we can go using a priori considerations. But before we return to consider the empirical findings, let us summarize. A creature with a flexible wanting system can change its intrinsic desires so that they are focused on the things that have given it pleasure, or have otherwise benefited it, in the past. If this system employs two separate signals, an A-signal that forms the dispositional desires and a B-signal that gives rise to occurrent desires when these are triggered, it will be able to change its dispositional desires even when it is not hungry. And if the A-signal can also boost the power of the B-signal, it can work to avail itself of an unrepresentatively good sample of a food, without changing the dispositional desire disproportionately. We don't want to be tied to the details of this account. But the empirical evidence suggests that something along these lines is correct.

EMPIRICAL EVIDENCE FOR THE WANTING SYSTEM

We start by returning to the findings of Cindy Wyvell and to some related experimental results. As discussed above, she found that injection of amphetamine

---

36. (McClure et al., 2003) also give dopamine two different roles, but the second is not the same as that suggested here. Rather than serving to regulate dispositional desires, it is involved in "learning to predict future rewards."

into rats' mesolimbic dopamine systems caused, in the presence of the reward cue, huge increases in short-term wanting. But this was not all. She also ran a parallel set of experiments on rats who had received earlier amphetamine injections, rather than infusions into their brains at the time of the stimulus. She found that this sensitized their brains in an apparently permanent way. Despite being free of the drug for ten days, the conditioned stimulus of the sound still elicited twice the frequency of lever pressing from these rats as it did from a control group who had not received the sensitizing injections. This behavior could not have resulted from the elevated dopamine levels caused directly by amphetamines, since the rats received no amphetamines when they heard the sound; it looks instead that it was caused by the structural changes produced by the earlier administration of amphetamines.[37]

So here we have exactly the evidence of exactly the kind of model that we suggested would be beneficial. Injection of amphetamine does not cause increased occurrent wanting on its own. Rather, it increases dispositional wanting (i.e., increases long run sensitivity to the cues), and it increases occurrent wanting when the cue is also present. This is what we suggested would be the function of the A-signal. Amphetamines are thus boosting the naturally occurring A-signal; and since what they are boosting is dopamine, we conclude dopamine is the A-signal.[38]

What of the B-signal? The evidence here is far from overwhelming, but we suggest that the most likely candidates are phasic glutamate corticolimbic signals that reach the nucleus accumbens. These signals come to the nucleus accumbens from the prefrontal cortex and from the basolateral amygdala, the thalamus, and the hippocampus. It is well established that these signals interact with dopamine;[39] our suggestion is that the acceleration effect results from

37. (Wyvell and Berridge, 2001). See also (Tindell et al., 2005); (Smith et al., 2011).

38. There is some very striking evidence that creatures can gain evidence that has an effect on subsequent consumption even when it does not like or need that thing. A rat who is exposed to highly concentrated saline solution, akin to swallowing a mouthful of the Dead Sea, that it neither wants nor likes, will, if subsequently deprived of salt, show both wanting and liking for the solution without needing to do any further exploration; see (Tindell et al., 2009); (Berridge, 2012); (M. Robinson and Berridge, 2010). One of the current authors (RH) is tempted to understand this as the formation of a dispositional desire at the time when the rat is first exposed to the saline, a disposition that is only triggered by the later salt deprivation. The other (KB) thinks it far more plausible that the rat's initial exposure to the saline causes it merely to learn that the solution gives a salty sensation (as well as a nasty one), a case of sensory-based learning that gives rise to a dispositional desire only when the rat is salt deprived. Resolution of this would require finding out whether the initial exposure did elicit the A-signal. What is not controversial is that creatures can form dispositional desires for things that they enjoy even though they will not currently consume them because they are sated.

39. See, for instance, (Kalivas et al., 2009).

the dopamine magnifying the impact of the glutamate signals on the nucleus accumbens neurons. The glutamate signals are the primary cause of the occurrent cravings, but the level at which they do this is determined by the level of dopamine present.[40]

An accelerator effect along these lines also explains how foods can prime for their own consumption—the familiar cocktail party effect, where taking just one peanut can lead you to take many more. The dopamine release from the initial consumption in turn boosts the effectiveness of the glutamate signal and hence of the occurrent desire. This effect is equally familiar to those working with laboratory animals, where often a free taste of a reward is necessary to get the animals working again. Such effects can be very specific: human subjects who have already eaten a full sandwich lunch will be induced to consume further pizza by being primed with a small sample of pizza, or to consume further ice cream by being primed with a small sample of ice cream.[41] Importantly for our topic, such effects are generated by addictive drugs: a small dose of cocaine will increase future cocaine craving, and a dose of alcohol will increase alcohol consumption.[42]

While the desires generated by cues are specific in this way—a specific cue gives rise to a specific desire—there is some tendency for desires to generalize in the other direction; that is, there is a tendency to develop intrinsic dispositional desires for any of the cues that heralded a particular dopamine release. This is just what we would expect if the formation of the dispositional desires result from an associative mechanism as described above. Thus, for instance, pigeons will come to peck an illuminated piece of plastic that has heralded the delivery of food or of drink, and will do it, moreover, with the distinctive forms of pecks that correspond to what has previously been delivered, an eating peck or a drinking peck.[43] Likewise, human cocaine addicts will "chase ghosts," scrabbling for white specks that are only sugar grains or pebbles, and

---

40. We suggest that this is what is happening in the famous Schultz electrophysiology experiments (Schultz, 1998). Unlike the Wyvell experiments, which involve elevated tonic (i.e., relatively enduring) dopamine levels, Schultz found that cues could elicit phasic (momentary) dopamine neuronal firing (and presumably firing-induced release), which has been widely interpreted as the phasic cause of the occurrent wanting. But here, too, the brain could be releasing phasic dopamine that amplifies the phasic glutamate signal triggered by the cue, thereby amplifying the cue-triggered "wanting" engendered. Of course, if both dopamine and glutamate signals are necessary for occurrent wanting, then it won't do to speak of the glutamate as itself the cause, but the point will remain that the dopamine is not sufficient on its own.

41. (Cornell et al., 1989).

42. (Jaffe et al., 1989); (de Wit and Chutuape, 1993).

43. (Jenkins and Moore, 1973); (Allan and Zeigler, 1994).

some smokers will prefer to puff on nicotine-free cigarettes rather than receive intravenous nicotine.[44]

There is much more evidence that we could draw on here. But rather than pursuing it, let us apply the model to an account of what it is that goes wrong in cases of addiction.

ADDICTION AS MALFUNCTION OF THE WANTING SYSTEM

Now that we have the model in place, our account of addiction can be quick. Let us assume, then, that when it is functioning properly dopamine works as the A-signal. What would happen if a subject consumed a substance that caused an artificial boost in that signal? The effect on the subject would be twofold. First, it would likely experience a large boost in occurrent desire for the substance. Second, there would be a large boost in its dispositional desire for the substance. Given the associative nature of the system, that desire would be cued by the substance itself, or by other cues that were around at the time that the substance was consumed. If the dopamine signal was strong enough, the ongoing sensitization could be very great, potentially persisting indefinitely.

Our claim is that this is just what happens in cases of addiction. Since the addictive drugs artificially stimulate the dopamine system so powerfully, they give rise to long-lasting dispositional desires. The dispositional desires are triggered by cues surrounding the consumption of the drugs: the drugs themselves, but also, given the associative nature of the process, the places in which they are consumed, the paraphernalia surrounding their consumption, and so on. Since these are intrinsic and not instrumental desires, they are not undermined by the belief that consumption of the drugs will not be pleasurable, or that it will be harmful in some other way. These dispositional desires may persist long after the subject has stopped taking the drugs and has gone through any associated withdrawal. A cue provided by seeing the drug, or the environment in which it was once taken, or even by imagining it, may provoke a powerful occurrent desire for it; and if this results in further consumption, the whole pattern will be repeated.

This seems to fit the facts very well. Or at least, it fits some of the facts very well, the pathological facts, those concerning the way that addiction differs from ordinary behavior. But it might seem that this has taken us too far, for what are we to make of those aspects of addiction that make it seem very much like ordinary behavior? Can we preserve the idea that addicts are nonetheless sensitive to standard incentives?

The crucial point here is that, in human beings, the incentive salience process that we have sketched does not necessarily lead directly to

44. (Rosse et al., 1993); (Rosse et al., 1994); (Rose et al., 2010).

behavior.[45] It typically leads instead to cravings: to powerful desires that tend to crowd out other considerations.[46] Many philosophers make a sharp contrast between desires and intentions. Desires are the inputs to deliberation; it is quite rational to have many that conflict. Intentions are the outputs of deliberation; they are insulated from reconsideration and lead directly to action, and so they need to be consistent. Cravings seem to come somewhere between the two. While they have many of the features of standard desires, they are not easily thought of as inputs to deliberation. Rather, they lead directly to action unless something stops them. Stopping them requires self-control; to this we now turn.

SELF-CONTROL

Both philosophers and psychologists tend to view desires as a fundamentally uniform class. Roughly, they are the states that move an agent to action. In contrast, we think that they are heterogeneous. So far we have focused just on one kind, the desires, or cravings, that result from the process of incentive salience. As we mentioned at the beginning, we also have other, more rationally tractable desires: a desire to take a holiday in St. Petersburg, say, or to be healthy, or to treat a particular person well. And many of these are intimately connected with our beliefs. If we come to think that St. Petersburg is too Western to be worthy of a visit, and that Moscow would be a better destination, then our desire to visit will be undermined. In contrast, the cravings that result from the incentive salience process are not typically undermined by the belief that they are harmful.[47]

But if we have at least two different sorts of desires—together perhaps with other factors that also influence our behavior, like our habits—then the question arises of what it is that will determine what we will do. This is a difficult and complex question that we cannot hope to fully answer here. But one thing that we think has become clear in recent years is that it is not fully determined by the relative strength of the different sorts of desires. We also need to factor in a more active control on the part of the agent.

A wealth of psychological research supports the idea that self-control should be taken seriously. Self-control develops in children after the development of

---

45. This is not to deny that incentive salience effects can work unconsciously in a way that takes them fairly directly to behavior. See (Winkielman and Berridge, 2004). But such behavior is still susceptible to self-control; it is just that the subject doesn't see the need to exert it.

46. See (Loewenstein, 1999) for a good discussion of how cravings tend to narrow one's focus.

47. For an excellent discussion of such desires see (Railton, 2012). Many actual desires may combine an element of both types; indeed, the very case that Railton uses as illustrative of the more cognitive desire—a desire for an espresso—is very plausibly a case in point.

desires; it is effortful; it is depleted by various factors including stress, fatigue, and its prior exercise; and it can be developed and deployed more or less successfully.[48] A failure to behave a certain way might indicate a lack of desire to behave that way. Alternatively, it might indicate that a desire, even the kind of craving that results from addiction, is being held in check by self-control.

To say that self-control is real is not to deny that its exercise is sensitive to the agent's beliefs and desires. Agents can be well motivated to employ it, if they think that there is something to be gained from it, and that its employment will be successful. Alternatively, if they think that it will bring little benefit, or that the benefits can be gained more easily another way, or that it is unlikely to succeed, they will be far less likely to employ it, and even if they do initially employ it, given that it is effortful, they will be far more likely to give up.

As we have seen, the pathology of addiction means that addicts will experience strong cue-driven cravings long after withdrawal is over, especially at particular moments such as when a drug cue is encountered in a moment of stress or emotional excitement. But this is not the end of the story. While there is some evidence that addictive drugs can diminish self-control by damaging the prefrontal cortex,[49] there is no reason to think that addicts lose it altogether. Indeed, the fact that addicts can get themselves off their addictions is strong evidence that it is not lost. Controlling cravings may be tremendously hard work, but that is not to say that it is impossible. Understanding when it is that addicts will continue to consume and when they will not thus requires an understanding of how their cravings interact with their self-control. While we do not have even the beginnings of a real account here, we identify the following factors as very likely to be relevant to the pattern of activity that we remarked on at the outset, in particular the responsiveness of addicts to incentives, and their tendency to escape their addictions in their late twenties or early thirties:

    (i) *The strength of the self-control system*
       There is evidence that self-control, regulated primarily by the prefrontal cortex, continues to develop in strength into the midtwenties, typically maturing rather earlier in women than in men.[50]
    (ii) *The efficiency with which the self-control system is employed*
       A great deal of research indicates that there are techniques that enable agents to better deploy their self control. Forming prior

48. For general discussion of the evidence and of some of the mechanisms involved, see (Holton, 2009).

49. See for instance, (Volkow et al., 2004).

50. See, for instance, (Luna and Sweezy, 2004); (Goldstein et al., 2009); and, for a popular review, (Sabbagh, 2006).

intentions and then acting on them without reopening the question of what to do seems important. Similarly, mindfulness techniques can enable agents to stand back from their desires in ways that make their self-control more effective. It is still an open question how effective such techniques can be against the kinds of cravings engendered by addiction, but initial research indicates that they can make a difference.[51] Again, skill in using the self-control system is something that we might expect to increase with age.

(iii) The role of desires

Addicts who have strong motivations for giving up rather than continuing are more likely to employ their self-control to overcome cravings. And it does seem likely that the concerns about partners, families, and careers will become more pressing as people reach their late twenties and early thirties. Conversely, since dopamine levels start to fall from the teenage years onward, the power of the cravings may themselves diminish.

(iv) The role of belief

If addicts think that there is little reason to give up today, since giving up tomorrow will be just as good, there will be little motivation to employ self-control. Vague concerns about health and well-being are often of that form; there can be a sense that while giving up is something that needs to be done at some point, one more dose won't hurt. In contrast, the incentives that have been shown to work well—for instance, the knowledge that certain dismissal from a much valued job will follow a single positive drug test—guarantee a immediate cost or benefit. We suspect that much the same is true of a price rise; while it is true that paying the higher price just one more time is probably within the addict's reach, there is no escaping the fact that a higher price is being paid. The other set of relevant beliefs concern the efficacy of exerting self-control. If addicts are convinced that they will succumb despite their best efforts—if not today, then surely soon—the motivation to try will be much reduced. And here, presumably, the addict's own theory of addiction will have a part to play. If addicts think of the addiction as resulting in behavior that is quite outside their control, they will be far less motivated to try to control it.[52]

---

51. (Prestwich et al., 2006); (Kober et al., 2010).

52. A point that has been noted many times by Albert Bandura; see, for instance, (Bandura, 1999).

THE EXTENT OF ADDICTION, AND ITS RATIONALITY

We have talked about addictions that are caused by drugs—by substances that interfere directly with the dopamine system and gain their incentive salience effect from that interference. But what of the many other kinds of behavioral addictions—addictions to gambling, shopping, sex, or the Internet—that feature so prominently in current discussion? Can we give an account of them? Or is the theory we have given bound to say that they are not really addictions?[53]

Clearly our account is bound to say that there is an important difference between substance and behavioral addictions. The latter do not, so far as we know, involve mechanisms that short-circuit the dopamine system in the way the former do. Nevertheless, there is good reason to think that they, too, work through the incentive salience system and so they, too, can result in cue-driven cravings that are relatively insulated from other desires and from beliefs about what is good. Of course, if the dopamine system has not been short-circuited, then these behavioral addictions must have originated from behavior that was pleasurable, or was in some other way recognized by the agent's dopamine system as being beneficial. But the assessment of the dopamine system might be at odds with the agent's more cognitive beliefs about the value of the activity; and even if it is not, once the intrinsic desires have been established, they will tend to persist through changes in the agent's assessment at any level. Even if the agent stops liking the thing concerned, a well-established incentive salience desire will degrade very slowly. The result can be behavior that looks very like the addiction engendered by drugs.[54]

This brings us finally to an issue that we have largely skirted up till now, that of the rationality of addicts. Most ordinary choice models see addicts as quite rational, though working with unusual desires or false beliefs (perhaps there is some irrationality in how they arrived at those beliefs, but that doesn't affect the rationality of how they act upon them). Most disease models see the addict as largely arational: addictive actions hardly count as intentional actions at all, and so fall outside the scope of rationality. In contrast, the account that we

53. We have made the traditional division between substance addiction and behavioral addiction, but it could be that some substances give rise to addiction-like behavior without hijacking the dopamine system in the way we have discussed, and so should be grouped with the behavioral addictions. Sugar might be like that, and, perhaps, though here the findings are controversial, cannabis. So a more careful distinction would be between the dopamine-hijacking addictions and those that are not. But we will stick with the more traditional terminology.

54. Further evidence that drug and behavioral addictions have much in common comes from the cases of Parkinson's patients who respond to their dopamine supplement by developing addictive behavior. See (O'Sullivan et al., 2009). We leave open the question of whether other behaviors that look rather like chemical addictions—those resulting from obsessive compulsive disorder, for instance—should also be understood in the same way.

have developed here sees the addict as potentially irrational in two ways. One is familiar: if considered views about what would be best diverge from action, then both substance addicts and behavioral addicts will frequently be akratic, in ways that have at least a prima facie claim to irrationality. The second is rather less familiar. If what we have said is right, then something goes badly wrong with the process by which substance addicts (but not behavioral addicts) form their desires: substances come to be desired independently of any pleasure or other benefits that they bring. There has been much discussion in philosophy of whether intrinsic desires can be irrational. What we are suggesting is that substance addiction results from the malfunctioning of a normally rational system for creating intrinsic desires. This seems to us as clear a case of an irrational intrinsic desire as one is ever likely to find.

CONCLUSION

We started by stressing the need to find a middle path. Our attempt to find one has involved exploring the interaction between two different systems: one that regulates our desires, and one that controls which desires we act on. Addiction results from the malfunction of the first; insofar as it does not result in a complete loss of agency, that is thanks to the second. In a sense, then, both the disease model and the choice model are describing something real; but each gives a picture that is partial. We hope that we have gone some way to putting them together.

ACKNOWLEDGMENT

This paper derives from two independent papers presented at the Oxford conference. Versions have since been presented by RH at MIT, Yale, Reading, Bristol, Oslo, Cambridge, and NYU. Thanks to all the audiences at these places for their comments; and to Anna Alexandrova, Tony Dickinson, Olav Gjelsvik, Rae Langton, Neil Levy, Hanna Pickard, Drazen Prelec, Tim Schroeder, Gabriel Segal, and Nick Shea.

REFERENCES

Allan, R.W., and H.P. Zeigler 1994: "Autoshaping the pigeon's gape response: acquisition and topography as a function of reinforcer type and magnitude." *Journal of the Experimental Analysis of Behavior*, 62, 201–223.

Bandura, A. 1999: "A sociocognitive analysis of substance abuse." *Psychological Science*, 10, 214–217.

Berridge, K. 2000: "Taste reactivity: measuring hedonic impact in infants and animals." *Neuroscience and Biobehavioral Reviews*, 24, 173–198.

———— 2007: "The debate over dopamine's role in reward: the case for incentive salience." *Psychopharmacology*, 191, 391–431.

—— 2012: "From prediction error to incentive salience: mesolimbic computation of reward motivation." *European Journal of Neuroscience*, 35, 1124–1143.

——, and Morten Kringelbach 2008: "Affective neuroscience of pleasure: reward in humans and animals." *Psychopharmacology*, 199, 457–480.

——, and E. Valenstein 1991: "What psychological process mediates feeding evoked by electrical stimulation of the lateral hypothalamus?" *Behavior Neuroscience*, 105, 3–14.

Cornell, C.E., J. Rodin, and H. Weingarten 1989: "Stimulus-induced eating when satiated." *Physiology and Behavior*, 45, 695–704.

de Wit, H., and M. Chutuape 1993: "Increased ethanol choice in social drinkers following ethanol preload." *Behavioral Pharmacology*, 4, 29–36.

Dickinson, A., and B. Balleine 2010: "Hedonics: The Cognitive-Motivational Interface" in M. Kringelbach and K. Berridge (eds.), Pleasures of the Brain (Oxford: Oxford University Press) pp. 74–84.

Everitt, B., D. Belin, D. Economidou, Y. Pelloux, J. Dalley, and T. Robbins 2008: "Neural mechanisms underlying the vulnerability to develop compulsive drug-seeking habits and addiction." *Philosophical Transactions of the Royal Society of London B Biological Science*, 363, 3125–3135.

Faure, A., J. Richard, and K. Berridge 2010: "Desire and dread from the nucleus accumbens: cortical glutamate and subcortical GABA differentially generate motivation and hedonic impact in the rat." *PLoS One*, 5, e11223.

Flagel, S., J. Clark, T. Robinson, L. Mayo, A. Czuj, I. Willuhn, C. Akers, S. Clinton, P. Phillips, and H. Akil 2011: "A selective role for dopamine in stimulus-reward learning." *Nature*, 469, 53–57.

Goldstein, R., A. Craig, A. Bechara, H. Garavan, A. Childress, M. Paulus, and N. Volkow 2009: "The neurocircuitry of impaired insight in drug addiction." *Trends in Cognitive Science*, 13, 372–380.

Herrnstein, R., and D. Prelec 1992: "A theory of addiction" in G. Loewenstein and J. Elster (eds.), Choice Over Time (New York: Russell Sage Press) pp. 331–360.

Heyman, G. 2009: Addiction: A Disorder of Choice (Cambridge, MA: Harvard University Press).

Hoffman, J., and S. Froeke (eds.) 2007: Addiction: Why Can't They Just Stop? (Emmaus, PA: Rodale Press).

Holton, R. 2009: Willing, Wanting, Waiting (Oxford: Clarendon Press).

Jaffe, J., N. Cascella, K. Kumor, and M. Sherer 1989: "Cocaine-induced cocaine craving." *Psychopharmacology*, 97, 59–64.

James, W. 1890: Principles of Psychology (New York: Henry Holt).

Jenkins, H., and B. Moore 1973: "The form of the auto-shaped response with food or water reinforcers." *Journal of the Experimental Analysis of Behavior*, 20, 163–181.

Kalivas, P.W., R.T. Lalumiere, L. Knackstedt, and H. Shen 2009: "Glutamate transmission in addiction." *Neuropharmacology*, 56 Supplement 1, 169–173.

Kober, H., E. Kross, W. Mischel, C. Hart, and K. Ochsner 2010: "Regulation of craving by cognitive strategies in cigarette smokers." *Drug and Alcohol Dependence*, 106, 52–55.

Lawrence, A.D., A.H. Evans, and A.J. Lees 2003: "Compulsive use of dopamine replacement therapy in Parkinson's disease: reward systems gone awry?" *Lancet Neurology*, 2, 595–604.

Leyton, M. 2010: "The neurobiology of desire: dopamine and the regulation of mood and motivational states in humans," in M. Kringelbach and K. Berridge (eds.), Pleasures of the Brain (Oxford: Oxford University Press) pp. 222–243.

Linden, D. 2011: The Compass of Pleasure (New York: Viking).

Loewenstein, G. 1999: "A visceral account of addiction," in J. Elster and O-J. Skog (eds.), Getting Hooked (Cambridge: Cambridge University Press) pp. 235–264.

Luna, B., and J. Sweezy 2004: "The emergence of collaborative brain function: fMRI studies of the development of response inhibition." Annals of the New York Academy of Science, 1021, 296–309.

McClure, S.M., N.D. Daw, and P. Read Montague 2003: "A computational substrate for incentive salience." Trends in Neuroscience, 26, 423–428.

Moore, G.E. 1905: Principia Ethica (Cambridge: Cambridge University Press).

O'Sullivan, S., A. Evans, and A. Lees 2009: "Dopamine dysregulation syndrome: an over-view of its epidemiology, mechanisms and management." CNS Drugs, 23, 157–170.

Peciña, S., B. Cagniard, K. Berridge, J. Aldridge, and X. Zhuang 2003: "Hyperdopaminergic mutant mice have higher 'wanting' but not 'liking' for sweet rewards." Journal of Neuroscience, 23, 9395–9402.

Prestwich, A., M. Conner, and R. Lawton 2006: "Implementation intentions: can they be used to prevent and treat addiction?" in R.W. Wiers and A.W. Stacy (eds.), Handbook of Implicit Cognition and Addiction (Thousand Oaks, CA: Sage) pp. 455–469.

Railton, P. 2012: "That obscure object, desire." Proceedings of the American Philosophical Association, 86. 22–46

Redish, A.D. 2004: "Addiction as a computational process gone awry." Science, 306, 1944–1947.

Robinson, M., and K. Berridge 2010: "Instant incentive salience: dynamic transforma-tion of an aversive salt cue into a 'wanted' motivational magnet." Abstract, Society for Neuroscience, San Diego.

Robinson, T., and K. Berridge 2003: "Addiction." Annual Review of Psychology, 54, 25–53.

Rose, J., A. Salley, F. Behm, J. Bates, and E. Westman 2010: "Reinforcing effects of nicotine and non-nicotine components of cigarette smoke." Psychopharmacology, 210, 1–12.

Rosse, R., M. Fay-McCarthy, J. Collins, T. Alim, and S. Deutsch 1994: "The relationship between cocaine-induced paranoia and compulsive foraging: a preliminary report." Addiction, 89, 1097–1104.

———, M. Fay-McCarthy, J. Collins, D. Risher-Flowers, T. Alim, and S. Deutsch 1993: "Transient compulsive foraging behavior associated with crack cocaine use." American Journal of Psychiatry, 150, 155–156.

Sabbagh, L. 2006: "The teen brain, hard at work." Scientific American Mind, August/September, 20–25.

Saunders, B., and T. Robinson 2012: "The role of dopamine in the accumbens core in the expression of Pavlovian-conditioned responses." European Journal of Neuroscience, online first.

Schultz, W. 1998: "Predictive reward signal of dopamine neurons." Journal of Neurophysiology, 80, 1–27.

——— 2002: "Getting formal with dopamine and reward." Neuron, 36, 241–263.

———, Peter Dayan, and Reid Montague 1997: "A neural substrate of prediction and reward." Science, 275, 1593–1599.

Skog, O-J. 1999: "Rationality, irrationality and addiction—notes on Becker's and Murphy's Theory of Addiction" in Jon Elster and Ole-Jørgen Skog (eds.), Getting Hooked (Cambridge: Cambridge University Press) pp. 173–207.

Smith, K., K. Berridge, and J.W. Aldridge 2011: "Disentangling pleasure from incentive salience and learning signals in brain reward circuitry." Proceedings of the National Academy of Science, 108, E255–E264.

Sournia, J.C. 1990: A History of Alcoholism (Oxford: Blackwell).

Sutton, R., and A. Barto 1998: Reinforcement Learning (Cambridge, MA: MIT Press).

Tindell, A., K. Smith, K. Berridge, and J.W. Aldridge 2009: "Dynamic computation of incentive salience: 'wanting' what was never 'liked.'" Journal of Neuroscience, 29(39), 12220–12228.

———, K. Berridge, J. Zhang, S. Peciña, and J. Aldridge 2005: "Ventral pallidal neurons code incentive motivation: amplification by mesolimbic sensitization and amphetamine." European Journal of Neuroscience, 22, 2617–2134.

Volkow, N., J. Fowler, and G-J. Wang 2004: "The addicted human brain viewed in the light of imaging studies." Neuropharmacology, 47, 3–13.

Wilde, O. 1891: The Picture of Dorian Gray (London: Ward Locke and Co.).

Winkielman, P., and K. Berridge 2004: "Unconscious emotion." Current Directions in Psychology, 13, 120–123.

Wise, R. 1980: "The dopamine synapse and the notion of 'pleasure centers' in the brain." Trends in Neuroscience, 3, 91–95.

——— 1985: "The anhedonia hypothesis: Mark III." Behaviour and Brain Science, 8, 178–186.

——— 2004: "Dopamine, learning and motivation." National Review of Neuroscience, 5, 483–494.

Wood, W., and D. Neal 2007: "A new look at habits and the habit-goal interface." Psychological Review, 114, 843–863.

Wyvell, C., and K. Berridge 2000: "Intra-accumbens amphetamine increases the conditioned incentive salience of sucrose reward." Journal of Neuroscience, 20, 8122–8130.

——— 2001: "Incentive sensitization by previous amphetamine exposure: increased cue-triggered 'wanting' for sucrose reward." Journal of Neuroscience, 21, 7831–7840.

INDEX

Page numbers in italics indicate figures.

A.A., *See* Alcoholics Anonymous
abstinent addicts, 219, 227–30
ACC, *See* anterior cingulate cortex
accelerator effects, 257, 258–9
actor-critic models, 255–6
addiction
  behavioral addictions, 124, 264, 264n54, 265
  blameworthiness and, 234–6
  case study, 122–4
  compulsion thesis of, 2, 170, 171–5
  consequences of, 1, 42, 122
  defining, 16–17
  genetic risk for, 45
  integrative approaches to understanding, 2, 14, 219–20
  as malfunction of wanting system, 260–1
  neural mechanisms of, 6, 43–5, 101, 102, 241
  philosophy of, 230–4
  picoeconomics and, 43, 45
  prevalence of, 16
  process addictions, 1, 5
  rationality of, 264–5
  relapse, risk factors for, 170, 171
  science of, 219–30
  self-control, importance in overcoming, 70, 175

  sex addiction, 45–6, 46n7
  See also gambling addiction; substance dependence
Addiction: A Disorder of Choice (Heyman), 76
agency
  degrees of, 167, 180–1
  transformations, 53
  See also team agency
agoraphobia, 173n8
Ainslie, George, 3–5, 16, 38–9, 40, 41, 42, 44–5, 46
akratic conduct
  Ancient Greeks on, 48
  blameworthiness and, 192–3, 197, 211, 212
  as mismatch between values and intentional actions, 191–2
  reasoning process of, 49
  team agency and, 59
alcohol and alcoholism
  as defined by A.A., 73–5
  disease model of, 71, 72–7
  dry drunks, 86, 86n16
  myths of, 71, 72–4
  personality disorders and, 167
  as spectrum disorder, 75, 81–2
  withdrawal from, 72, 124–5, 171
  See also substance dependence